WHAT HAPPENS IN COUPLE THERAPY

Also Available

FOR PROFESSIONALS

Clinical Handbook of Couple Therapy, Sixth Edition
   Edited by Jay L. Lebow and Douglas K. Snyder

*Common Factors in Couple and Family Therapy:
The Overlooked Foundation for Effective Practice*
   Douglas H. Sprenkle, Sean D. Davis, and Jay L. Lebow

*Couple-Based Interventions for Military and Veteran Families:
A Practitioner's Guide*
   Edited by Douglas K. Snyder and Candice M. Monson

Helping Couples Get Past the Affair: A Clinician's Guide
   Donald H. Baucom, Douglas K. Snyder, and Kristina Coop Gordon

*Treating Difficult Couples: Helping Clients with Coexisting Mental
and Relationship Disorders*
   Edited by Douglas K. Snyder and Mark A. Whisman

FOR GENERAL READERS

*Getting Past the Affair, Second Edition: A Program to Help You Cope,
Heal, and Move On—Together or Apart*
   Douglas K. Snyder, Kristina Coop Gordon, and Donald H. Baucom

What Happens in Couple Therapy

A Casebook on Effective Practice

edited by
Douglas K. Snyder
Jay L. Lebow

THE GUILFORD PRESS
New York   London

Copyright © 2024 The Guilford Press
A Division of Guilford Publications, Inc.
370 Seventh Avenue, Suite 1200, New York, NY 10001
www.guilford.com

All rights reserved

No part of this book may be reproduced, translated, stored in a
retrieval system, or transmitted, in any form or by any means,
electronic, mechanical, photocopying, microfilming, recording,
or otherwise, without written permission from the publisher.

Printed in the United States of America

This book is printed on acid-free paper.

Last digit is print number: 9 8 7 6 5 4 3 2 1

The authors have checked with sources believed to be reliable in their efforts to provide
information that is complete and generally in accord with the standards of practice that are
accepted at the time of publication. However, in view of the possibility of human error or
changes in behavioral, mental health, or medical sciences, neither the authors, nor the editors
and publisher, nor any other party who has been involved in the preparation or publication
of this work warrants that the information contained herein is in every respect accurate or
complete, and they are not responsible for any errors or omissions or the results obtained from
the use of such information. Readers are encouraged to confirm the information contained in
this book with other sources.

Library of Congress Cataloging-in-Publication Data

Names: Snyder, Douglas K., editor. | Lebow, Jay, editor.
Title: What happens in couple therapy : a casebook on effective practice /
   edited by Douglas K. Snyder, Jay L. Lebow.
Description: New York : The Guilford Press, [2024] | Includes
   bibliographical references and index.
Identifiers: LCCN 2024019694 | ISBN 9781462554744 (paperback ; alk. paper)
   | ISBN 9781462554751 (hardcover ; alk. paper)
Subjects: MESH: Couples Therapy--methods | Professional-Patient Relations |
   Case Reports | BISAC: PSYCHOLOGY / Psychotherapy / Couples & Family |
   RELIGION / Counseling
Classification: LCC RC488.5 | NLM WM 430.5.M3 | DDC
   616.89/1562—dc23/eng/20240529
LC record available at https://lccn.loc.gov/2024019694

Editors' note. The case illustrations in this book are based on the authors' clinical practices. In all
instances, names and identifying information have been changed.

To our friends and colleagues—from those just beginning their careers to those with decades of experience. Our journeys together have brought much joy and inspiration.
—D. K. S.
—J. L. L.

About the Editors

Douglas K. Snyder, PhD, LMFT, is Professor of Psychological and Brain Sciences at Texas A&M University, where he also served as Director of Clinical Training for 20 years. Dr. Snyder has engaged in clinical practice and training of couple therapists since the 1970s, and is a clinical member of the American Association for Marriage and Family Therapy (AAMFT). He is coauthor or coeditor of several books, including the *Clinical Handbook of Couple Therapy, Helping Couples Get Past the Affair,* and *Couple-Based Interventions for Military and Veteran Families.* Dr. Snyder has served as editor of the *Clinician's Research Digest* and as associate editor of the *Journal of Consulting and Clinical Psychology* and the *Journal of Family Psychology.* He is a recipient of the Distinguished Contribution to Research in Family Therapy Award from AAMFT, the Distinguished Contribution to Family Psychology Award from the American Psychological Association (APA) Division 43 (Society for Couple and Family Psychology), and the Distinguished Psychologist Award from APA Division 29 (Society for the Advancement of Psychotherapy).

Jay L. Lebow, PhD, ABPP, LMFT, is Clinical Professor of Psychology at Northwestern University and Senior Scholar at The Family Institute at Northwestern University. He is coeditor of the *Clinical Handbook of Couple Therapy* and a past editor-in-chief of the journal *Family Process.* Dr. Lebow has engaged in clinical practice, supervision, and research on couple and family therapy since the 1970s, and is board certified in family psychology and an approved supervisor and clinical member of AAMFT. His numerous publications focus on the practice of couple and family therapy, the relationship of research and practice, integrative practice, and intervention strategies with divorcing families. Dr. Lebow served as president of the Society for Couple and Family Psychology of the American Psychological Association (APA Division 43) and on the board of directors of the American Family Therapy Academy (AFTA). He is a recipient of the Lifetime Achievement Award from AFTA and the Family Psychologist of the Year Award from APA Division 43.

Contributors

Donald H. Baucom, PhD, Department of Psychology and Neuroscience, University of North Carolina at Chapel Hill, Chapel Hill, North Carolina

Adrian Blow, PhD, Department of Human Development and Family Studies, Michigan State University, East Lansing, Michigan

Anthony L. Chambers, PhD, The Family Institute at Northwestern University, Evanston, Illinois

Andrew Christensen, PhD, Department of Psychology, University of California, Los Angeles, Los Angeles, California

Carrie U. Cole, PhD, The Gottman Institute, Seattle, Washington

Donald L. Cole, DMin, The Gottman Institute, Seattle, Washington

Barbara M. Dausch, PhD, Veterans Affairs Eastern Colorado Healthcare System, Aurora, Colorado

William J. Doherty, PhD, Department of Family Social Science, University of Minnesota, St. Paul, Minnesota

Celia Jaes Falicov, PhD, Department of Family Medicine, University of California, San Diego, San Diego, California

Mona DeKoven Fishbane, PhD, Chicago Center for Family Health, Chicago, Illinois

James L. Furrow, PhD, Couples and Family Therapy Program, Seattle University, Seattle, Washington

Shirley M. Glynn, PhD, Veterans Affairs Greater Los Angeles Healthcare System, Los Angeles, California

Rhonda N. Goldman, PhD, The Chicago School, Chicago, Illinois

Sarah E. Griffes, MS, Department of Human Development and Family Studies, Michigan State University, East Lansing, Michigan

Steven M. Harris, PhD, Department of Family Social Science, University of Minnesota, St. Paul, Minnesota

Rebecca Harvey, PhD, Department of Marriage and Family Therapy, Southern Connecticut State University, New Haven, Connecticut

Jay L. Lebow, PhD, The Family Institute at Northwestern University, Evanston, Illinois

Erica A. Mitchell, PhD, Department of Human Development and Family Studies, Michigan State University, East Lansing, Michigan

Tammy Nelson, PhD, Integrative Sex Therapy Institute, Los Angeles, California

Arthur C. Nielsen, MD, Department of Psychiatry and Behavioral Sciences, Feinberg School of Medicine, Northwestern University, Chicago, Illinois

Reenee Singh, DSysPsych, The London Intercultural Couples Centre, London, United Kingdom

Douglas K. Snyder, PhD, Department of Psychological and Brain Sciences, Texas A&M University, College Station, Texas

Ellen F. Wachtel, PhD, private practice, New York, New York

Serine Warwar, PhD, Centre for Psychology and Emotional Health, Toronto, Ontario, Canada

Danielle M. Weber, PhD, Department of Psychology, University of Georgia, Athens, Georgia

Contents

CHAPTER 1   Voices in Couple Therapy: Journeys with Master Clinicians   1
Jay L. Lebow and Douglas K. Snyder

CHAPTER 2   Emotion-Focused Therapy for Couples   8
Serine Warwar and Rhonda N. Goldman

CHAPTER 3   Integrative Couple Therapy with a Surprising Twist   26
Ellen F. Wachtel

CHAPTER 4   Integrative Psychodynamic Couple Therapy in the Presence of Enduring Personality Dysfunctions   43
Arthur C. Nielsen

CHAPTER 5   Gottman Method Couple Therapy and Healing from Betrayal   62
Carrie U. Cole and Donald L. Cole

CHAPTER 6   An Integrative Relational–Neurobiological Approach to Transforming Couple Vulnerability Cycles   79
Mona DeKoven Fishbane

CHAPTER 7   Integrating Common Factors in Couple Therapy   99
Sarah E. Griffes and Adrian Blow

CHAPTER 8   Discernment Counseling with a Couple on the Brink   119
William J. Doherty and Steven M. Harris

CHAPTER 9	Therapy with Black Couples: The Intersection of Race and Class *Anthony L. Chambers*	139
CHAPTER 10	Addressing Gender, Class, and Racism in a Mexican Transnational Couple *Celia Jaes Falicov*	157
CHAPTER 11	Therapy with Intercultural and Interfaith Couples *Reenee Singh*	176
CHAPTER 12	Affirmative Therapy for Queer Relationships *Rebecca Harvey*	196
CHAPTER 13	Couple Therapy with Older Adults: Navigating Challenges and Building on Opportunities *Douglas K. Snyder*	216
CHAPTER 14	Couple Therapy with Young Adults: Navigating the Transition to Parenthood *Erica A. Mitchell*	234
CHAPTER 15	Integrative Behavioral Couple Therapy with Military and Veteran Couples *Barbara M. Dausch, Shirley M. Glynn, and Andrew Christensen*	252
CHAPTER 16	Couple Therapy and Sexuality: Promoting Intimacy and Connection *Tammy Nelson*	271
CHAPTER 17	Couple Therapy and Spirituality: Finding Faith in Love *James L. Furrow*	287
CHAPTER 18	Working with Couples Encountering Serious Illness: It's More Than Medical *Donald H. Baucom and Danielle M. Weber*	305
	Index	323

CHAPTER 1

Voices in Couple Therapy
Journeys with Master Clinicians

JAY L. LEBOW
DOUGLAS K. SNYDER

"I wish I could be in the room with them—not just to see and hear—but somehow to be inside their head to know what they're thinking and feeling, how they're deciding to do this instead of that, whether they ever struggle along the way like I do."

So many times we've heard similar sentiments expressed by our supervisees and junior colleagues. They've read about the theories and models of couple therapy—for example, in the *Clinical Handbook of Couple Therapy* (sixth edition; Lebow & Snyder, 2023) or one of its earlier iterations. They've studied the case vignettes that expositions of these approaches often include. Some have gone online or pursued other venues for accessing videos of developers of these models or other senior clinicians demonstrating the therapeutic process. Each additional mode of learning and experiential engagement promotes a deeper understanding of the underlying principles and techniques, and some of their nuances. But nearly always, something is missing—a sense of the therapist's decision process, a feel for the flow of real therapy and, most of all, access to the moment-by-moment subjective experiences of the master clinician—those internal thoughts, feelings, and even somatic experiences of the therapist that contribute to the therapeutic process, whether implicitly or explicitly. It's through such intimate descriptions of what actually evolves in the course of working with couples that the flow of therapy and the factors most crucial to positive outcomes most distinctly emerge.

This is the reason for this casebook—why we approached master clinicians across a broad spectrum of approaches to couple therapy, distinct populations, or specific issues and encouraged them to describe their work in a unique way—one that invites you, the reader, into their own internal experiences, their inner dialogues, in a far more transparent and at times even vulnerable way. The enthusiastic responses from these couple therapists we invited to join in this collective effort were remarkable. Each of our contributors to this casebook embraced the opportunity to engage with you in conversation about not only *what* they do, but just as importantly *what it's like* for them to share in the intimate and intricate process of couple therapy. The complex decisions and relational challenges leap out in each narrative, as do the rich algorithms in the maps of our expert therapists. Each speaks to you in the first person: "What did I witness? What was I thinking and feeling as I tried to make sense of my experience and deliberated our next steps together?" Each of them invites you to join in the journey with them along the way.

WHOM WILL YOU ENCOUNTER?

These are master clinicians, each and every one. The best couple therapy involves a great deal of highly specialized skillfulness. There is such wisdom in the practice of the therapists in this casebook. Although the couples in focus vary in their problems and these therapists enter with different theories to guide them, always present is a keen ability to assess and understand, to ally, to adapt to the case, and a parsimony of action that characterizes those who have mostly done the proverbial 10,000 hours of deliberate practice sessions previously (Gladwell, 2008).

That said, you'll encounter them at different points in their career trajectory—some earlier, and others later. Some developed the particular therapeutic model or approach reflected in their case narrative. Others draw upon well-established therapeutic approaches but speak to the nuances of adapting these to specific populations or to particular issues frequently described by couples in therapy. Still others have created their own integrative methods of practice. Collectively, these master clinicians reflect varied theoretical orientations, areas of expertise, and backgrounds. But their skillfulness and wisdom are evident throughout—in the depth and complexities in how they think, their attunement to self as well as the couple, the nuances of selecting and pacing specific interventions, their subtleties of language in the therapeutic process, and their skill in bringing you—the reader—into the entire experience.

You'll also encounter couples contending with a broad spectrum of issues across the lifespan. They diverge in nationality, culture, race and ethnicity, sexual and gender identities, and aspects of both individual and couple functioning. These couples are drawn from our authors' clinical practices; in all instances, names and identifying information have been changed.

WHAT PATHS WILL THE JOURNEYS FOLLOW?

Each chapter adheres to a prescribed structure with four common elements:

1. A brief introduction to the theoretical approach, specific population, or particular issue illuminated through the case narrative
2. Methods of engaging in initial assessment and case formulation
3. The evolution of the therapeutic process across beginning, intermediate, and concluding phases—however these are conceptualized (as explicit or indeterminate as they may be)
4. Further reflections and implications from both personal and clinical perspectives.

Within this structure, each of our master clinicians shares a narrative of multiple journeys. The first is a journey of self—how they came to be the person and therapist they are, oftentimes reflecting a unique fusion of personal and professional heritage. In this introduction to the case narrative, they share how they came to adopt the particular approach to couple therapy they're about to describe, or how they were drawn to work with a particular population or couples confronting a specific relationship challenge. Distinguishing features of the therapeutic approach, clinical population, or specific issue are then illuminated to provide the context for the case narrative that follows.

Two additional journeys are then interwoven as each clinical narrative unfolds. One is the journey of the two partners and their relationship. How did they come to be who and where they are? What steps do they take over the course of the therapy—whether venturing forward or retreating back, moving toward or away from one another, in concert or out of sync? The second journey is that of the therapeutic relationship. How do the couple and therapist work toward safety and trust? How do they co-design the journey? How does the therapist translate a complex therapeutic framework into a language and map that make sense to the couple? Which steps necessarily precede others? When, if ever, does the therapeutic journey end? What pauses occur along the way, and for what purpose?

The final journey our master clinicians invite us to join is one that continues after the therapy journey itself has ended. What have we learned? When and how was the therapy helpful, and when and how perhaps not? How have we grown along the way? What can we take from this journey to inform the next?

WHAT SHOULD I LOOK FOR ALONG THE WAY?

Every case narrative illuminates the therapist's skillfulness in harnessing common factors essential to effective therapy and integrating these with specific interventions tailored to unique aspects of the couple (Sprenkle, Davis, & Lebow, 2009). Primary is their ability to form strong therapeutic alliances in ways that go well beyond simply joining in a positive way with partners. Notice how our therapists find ways to develop alliances with both partners as individuals and with the couple as an entity, and help to restore or create an alliance between the partners. Observe how they navigate the perilous space of keeping alliances with partners in balance and how they avoid or repair split alliances in which one partner feels more allied to the therapist than the other. And look for how they do this even around specific issues or at times when one partner may well need much more attention than the other. Our therapists use different terms to describe their connections to couples (e.g., therapeutic or multipartial alliance, joining, attunement), but all reflect a caring and empathy for each partner while also addressing their contribution to the problems for which they're seeking therapy—accentuating the shared mission toward reducing partners' distress and increasing intimate and joyful connection.

Notice also how our expert clinicians all speak to the importance of fostering hope. Couples who enter therapy are often demoralized about their relationship—mired in conflict or in strategic retreat. Partners understandably become disheartened when ensnared in anticipation that any efforts of their own will be met with the other one's dismissal or turning away. Yet each of our contributors conveys their own hopefulness and abiding belief in the potential for change. The resilience of these master clinicians' positive expectancies likely emerges from considerable experience in working with distressed couples who are demoralized and can't see a path forward, only to witness couples adapt and transform. Fostering hope isn't about promoting some idealized fantasy but, instead, is about offering a path toward some better possibility and pledging to travel that path with the couple even if they falter along the way.

And what might that better possibility be—where might the journey lead? For some, the path forward lies in disrupting dysfunctional patterns of behavior (e.g., the demand–withdraw cycle or other forms of spiraling negativity) and promoting more functional patterns (whether communication skills, emotional support, or other forms of positive exchange). For others, the better possibility comes about by changing how partners think about themselves and each other—for example, reframing negative reactivities as residual coping strategies from painful developmental experiences in family-of-origin or other prior relationship—and harnessing this new understanding toward more compassionate responding. For yet others, it evolves from deepening emotion in pursuit of more intimate connection. And for still other couples, the path forward comes about by facilitating partners' acceptance of inevitable differences or failings and moving past resentments to reach greater reconciliation to these limitations. As you join our therapists and couples along these various passages, notice how movements in each of these domains—behaviors, thoughts, or emotions—mutually influence one another and at times interact in synergistic ways.

All of our master clinicians articulate their theories of how couples change and their preferred methods of intervention. The narratives they share illuminate numerous specific techniques—some of which typify various schools of therapy, while others are simply favored ways of speaking or framing problems that are idiosyncratic. However, even here, you'll discover how much these therapists share in common with one another. All of them translate their formulations and methods to their couples in transparent ways using straightforward language to promote their shared mission. Notice how so many of these expert therapists, regardless of theoretical orientation, are pluralistic or integrative in what they do. The cognitive-behavioral therapists work with emotion, and those centered on emotion create time-outs. All offer education or advice when warranted. And each adapts their interventions in the wake of the partners' responses and the couple's progress along the way.

Closely related here are underlying frameworks to couple therapy that transcend practitioner and orientation. Almost all of these therapists seem keenly attuned to the foundational role of attachment and adopt various strategies to restore or create partners' attachment when it is compromised. They attend to individual differences in identity and social location—for example, gender and sexual identity, race, class, or culture—and incorporate an intersectional viewpoint in considering their relevance to partners' lives and specific implications for the couple therapy. These therapists draw on experience and relevant literature to anticipate challenges that accompany various stages of life—for example, transitions to parenthood or retirement—as well as unexpected events that provoke predictable challenges such as infidelity or serious emotional or physical illness. And most all personify multifocal lenses for understanding and intervening in their couples' journeys as they move back and forth from the couple dyad to the individual partners; from the partners' and couple's histories back to the present and future; from the couple relationship to considerations of broader systemic influences—their extended families, their community and significant others—and how these either support or undermine the couple's well-being. From a systemic perspective, individual partner dysfunctions may sometimes contribute to relationship dysfunction, but relationship difficulties can similarly arise in well-functioning individuals for myriad other factors. Yet, although highly systemic in their practices, these also are not therapists who shy away from exploring individual contributions to relationship problems.

Our expert therapists also demonstrate considerable flexibility both in the structure of the couple therapy and how they think about the outcomes. Most of the case narratives involve a single therapist meeting with both partners conjointly, typically in a therapy occurring over an extended period with a reasonably clear beginning and end. But there are exceptions—including a cotherapy by two therapists meeting conjointly with the couple (a fairly rare form of practice today given cost considerations despite its illustrious history and obvious utility), a "marathon" therapy conducted over a 3-day period (a newer emerging format of couple therapy), and several courses of therapy with "soft" beginnings or endings in which the couple returns periodically to work on either recurring or emergent issues (now a frequent pattern in couple therapy). Even the treatment system may vary or expand over time—transitioning between individual and couple sessions (always with explicit understandings regarding the goals and boundaries of confidentiality in either format), or including family members outside the dyad in brief consultative liaisons.

Observe also how flexible and nonjudgmental these expert clinicians are in conceptualizing goals and outcomes. Couple therapy is a far more complex journey than simply leading to success or failure. More typically, the therapy aims to facilitate informed decisions about how to move forward along paths more likely to end painful ways of interacting and promote healthy and joyful lives—whether partners stay together or move on separately. Couple therapists can help identify processes needing attention and can intervene to gauge the potential of altering those processes, favoring "couple" solutions over individual ones. However, ultimately the partners choose whether to stay with one another. Having someone present who doesn't want to work on the relationship almost inevitably vitiates the chances of therapeutic progress, whether the couple decides to separate or not.

Note as well how frequently couple therapy centers not on profound relationship dysfunction but rather on how to remain connected and build on relational strength in encountering life transitions and common problems. Couples go through transitions; encounter illness, age, and deal with extended family; live in the vicissitudes of a racist heteronormative society; and struggle with myriad other factors. We can see that some of the best couple therapy begins with partners fairly well anchored to one another, who draw on the therapy to be more resilient and overcome adversity. Notably, "we" solutions often work better than individual ones when encountering life's challenges.

Finally, take advantage of this unique opportunity to experience the introspective humility that each of our master clinicians embodies. Notice how they acknowledge uncertainty at various points along the therapeutic journey and ask themselves questions with which any of us may wrestle. Are they understanding the couple's struggles and contributing factors in all their complexity? Can they confront this or that dysfunction without jeopardizing the therapeutic alliance? Should they disclose to the couple about themselves—and if so, when, how, and to what purpose? When is the "good" good enough? When does a decision to end the relationship reflect therapeutic success or failure? What does the therapist wish they had done differently? Even these expert therapists show themselves not to be afraid of describing their errors. Some tell us about moments when it becomes clear they've missed an essential aspect of a case. Others report engaging in good work with a couple only to have the couple decide to part. In considering such disclosures, we can appreciate that even the best therapists make mistakes, struggle with clients who report on their lives selectively, and have to contend with how powerful some factors beyond the therapist's control may be for a couple's outcomes. Consider the valuable lesson illuminated through such reflections—that the best journey may be realized by pausing along the way to contemplate the ambiguity of various signposts and then ponder potential gains or setbacks along any particular path.

WHAT'S NEXT?

We've sequenced the case studies by three broad groupings:

- The first seven narratives describe specific models or approaches to couple therapy. Two of these reflect more narrowband methods—emotion-focused therapy for couples and discernment counseling with couples on the brink of divorce. The remaining five all speak to more integrative approaches, sometimes highlighting a specific feature such as substance abuse, personality dysfunction, or infidelity.

- The next set of seven narratives describes couple therapy with specific populations diverging along various markers of social location (e.g., race, class, culture, and gender or sexual identity), age (young or older adults), or other context (military and veteran couples). As in the first set, each of the narratives in this second set also highlights a specific feature such as discrimination and marginalization, transition to parenthood or challenges of aging, conflicts involving jealousy or money, or struggles regarding children or extended family.

- The final three narratives describe critical ways of conceptualizing and approaching therapy with couples around three common challenges—physical and sexual intimacy, matters of faith and spirituality, or encounters with serious physical illness. The perspectives shared in these narratives transcend any specific therapeutic approach (although each draws on an explicit model of therapy) to enhance the reader's understanding of the core dynamics distinguishing partners' struggles and principles of effective therapy in each of these domains.

These case narratives in couple therapy can be read in any order—each stands alone, and each is incremental to the others. Depending on where you are in your own professional journey, you might want to view these therapists as models (they do such a wonderful job of demonstrating how to think as a couple therapist, how to track feelings, and how to intervene—offering language so easily applied to other couples) or consider how they work compared to how you do. You can choose to engage with one of your favorite clinicians or a familiar therapeutic approach. Or perhaps you're hoping to delve deeper into working with a particular population or specific issue you've already encountered. We hope you'll also seek out the unfamiliar—those approaches, populations, or issues you have yet to encounter or aren't certain you would even want to encounter. None of us knows our future. More importantly, we all have opportunities to shape and expand our futures by venturing into the unknown. These master clinicians encourage you to join them, and they offer to guide you through less familiar territory.

As editors, we offer brief introductions to each of the case narratives—perhaps similar to trail guides preparing you for new expeditions—pointing out highlights to anticipate, and offering a sampling of prominent features and subtle nuances. Go slowly as you engage with each narrative, pausing along the way to reflect on the moment. What are you experiencing—and how does that compare with the internal dialogue and feelings shared by the therapist? What do you wonder about? What can you take away not only about this particular approach to therapy, or this population or specific issues, but also about yourself as therapist? About the phrasing and pacing of specific interventions? Or about openness to emotions, to internal debates, to sharing aspects of yourself with the couple? Embrace the journey and discoveries along the way!

REFERENCES

Gladwell, M. (2008). *Outliers: The story of success.* New York: Little, Brown.
Lebow, J. L., & Snyder, D. K. (Eds.). (2023). *Clinical handbook of couple therapy* (6th ed.). New York: Guilford Press.
Sprenkle, D. H., Davis, S. D., & Lebow, J. L. (2009). *Common factors in couple and family therapy: The overlooked foundation for effective practice.* New York: Guilford Press.

CHAPTER 2

Emotion-Focused Therapy for Couples

SERINE WARWAR
RHONDA N. GOLDMAN

> *Editors' Comments*
>
> In this illuminating exemplar of emotion-focused therapy for couples (EFT-C), Serine Warwar and Rhonda Goldman explicate both the underlying principles and clinical processes of this evidence-based treatment with a gay interracial couple. They describe how EFT-C has evolved from its original experiential–systemic formulation—incorporating more recent developments from contemporary emotion theory and expanding its emphasis beyond attachment to address core issues of identity and attraction. The structure of EFT-C has a linear yet flexible, five-stage sequence, but note how the therapy is guided by multiple in-session process diagnostic "compasses" that inform decision making throughout the process regarding when and how to intervene around any specific issue.
>
> Observe also the relative balance of teaching communication skills versus creating opportunities for deep emotional connection—and how promoting the former is always in service of the latter. From an EFT-C perspective, developing and maintaining deeply intimate relationships require a safe context for partners to express and respond empathically to vulnerable, soft emotions. When couples are unable to do this on their own, the therapist creates that safe milieu and then helps partners identify the recurring negative interaction cycles that interfere with those more intimate exchanges, as well as enduring sensitivities that either partner brings into the relationship that trigger disruptive reactivities.
>
> Warwar, the therapist for this couple, illuminates this couple's recurring negative cycle and sensitively helps the partners recognize how each of their individual histories renders them less secure and more reactive with each other. And Warwar's interventions are tailored through awareness of the various marginalization and discrimination experiences that both partners have sustained as members of sexual or racial minorities. Though not the central focus of the couple therapy, these influences and their intersection contribute importantly to the context in which interventions are crafted.

> This chapter also effectively speaks to the challenges of conducting EFT-C for any therapist with any couple. Note how a highly attuned therapist attends to not only the partners' emotional processes but also their own emotional experiencing throughout the therapy both as a "compass" and as a mechanism for modeling vulnerability and empathic joining.

For me, Serine, I find it deeply fulfilling to be present when partners disclose their underlying pain and vulnerability, and soften toward each other; I experience great joy and beauty in witnessing the bravery clients demonstrate in being vulnerable, and being a facilitator of their emotional transformation. Additionally, in codeveloping the emotion-focused therapy (EFT) model for resolving emotional injury in couples (Greenberg, Warwar, & Malcolm, 2010), I was amazed and inspired when I realized that even couples who had long-standing issues that seemed unresolvable could not only heal but also breathe new life into their relationships if I could guide them in a process to connect with and reveal their underlying heartfelt emotions and needs; many of these couples had tried many therapies before resolving their issues using this approach.

And for me, Rhonda, working with couples was a natural fit, as I have always taken great pleasure in helping people resolve conflict. I love the dynamic and lively atmosphere that happens in the couple therapy room. Working in depth with people's emotional pain allows for rapid and meaningful change. I never quite know what's going to unfold within sessions, and I love the challenge that it brings. I find myself in awe everytime I see people dig deep into internal emotional resources that perhaps they did not know they had. As the codeveloper of the EFT-C model, I continuously witness the power of the model to help people find courage to authentically connect from within their vulnerable selves.

EFT-C (Goldman & Greenberg, 2013; Greenberg & Goldman, 2008) comes from the humanistic–experiential tradition that sees emotion as both fundamental in guiding experience and functioning and as a primary source for change in therapy. This model integrates systemic interactional theory and thought, updating it with modern emotion theory. Emotion regulation in couples is viewed as a core process that organizes motivational systems of attachment, identity, and attraction. Attachment systems are related to our needs for security and closeness, as well as our concerns regarding the availability and responsiveness of our partners. In contrast, identity systems are related to our needs for self-coherence, self-esteem, and mastery, and are maintained by the recognition and validation that we seek and are provided to us in our relationships. Additionally, being seen, heard, valued, and understood by our partner leads to strong bonding. Our relationships are considered most functional when governed by positive emotions, and the attraction system involves positive emotions of interest, liking, and attraction. We couple because we like our partner's way of being, spending time with them, how they make us feel, and seeing the world through their eyes.

EFT-C focuses on promoting authentic relating between partners. The sharing of genuinely felt, vulnerable emotion is seen as creating an important path toward healing and is considered the glue that helps create and maintain secure bonding. A strong emotional bond allows partners to connect and together tackle the challenges and complexities of modern living. The aim of treatment is the transformation of negative cycles into more virtuous cycles governed by positive emotions. These negative cycles are typically driven by protective emotions that are secondary and extremely damaging to the relationship. The current five-stage, 14-step treatment process is described in detail by Greenberg and Goldman (2008) and updates an earlier nine-step model proposed by Greenberg and Johnson (1988). The current model further elaborates working the two major dimensions of attachment and identity and distinguishes a third dimension, the attraction and liking system. Based in part on our development of EFT for individuals, this approach to couples further specifies how to work with individual processes within a couple's context such as the historical origins of primary painful sensitivities and vulnerabilities, blocks to accessing core vulnerabilities, and self-soothing.

EFT-C COMPASSES FOR ASSESSMENT AND INTERVENTION

To guide moment-by-moment assessment of processes and interventions throughout therapy, there are important EFT-C compasses that we use. First, the therapeutic relationship compass is important because it's necessary that each partner feels safe to reveal vulnerability throughout the treatment process. Thus, a strong alliance with the therapist is monitored ongoing as the therapist takes a read of the degree of safety that each partner feels toward revealing vulnerability throughout the treatment process.

In addition, the compasses we use to inform interventions include the cycle, emotion, task, and stage of treatment; they are all important orientation systems and can be considered together as they intersect with and inform each other. The cycle compass is initially used at the beginning of treatment to determine what the couple's particular cycle is; that is, who is the pursuer and who is the distancer? Or who is the coercive, dominant partner and who is the submitter? As therapy progresses, therapists continue to refer to the cycle as a guide to determine what each partner in the ongoing cycle is doing. Are they in the secondary cycle—locked into angry, blaming pursuit, knocking against passive, resentful withdrawal—or have they moved toward the primary cycle, attempting to access, allow, or reveal more vulnerable emotions such as fearful insecurity or enveloping shame? The assessment compass is used throughout as we continually assess and intervene in reference to the cycle as we focus on restructuring the negative cycle into a more positive cycle and reframe couples' ongoing conflicts in relation to their cycles. Later, as things improve, we help couples understand how they've transformed their negative cycles and how they're now cocreating their positive cycles. The emotion compass operates on a moment-by-moment basis and guides therapists to focus on which emotion a person might be feeling at a given moment (sadness, anger, shame, fear, or joy) and what type of emotion it might be (primary, secondary, or instrumental) to direct interventions; therapists provide holding responses that help clients share vulnerabilities, or deepening responses that help clients undo blocked emotion and work toward transformation of stuck or problematic emotions. The task compass helps therapists engage in marker-guided tasks across the therapy; these are in-session indicators of which interventions would be helpful moment by moment. For example, as markers arise, a therapist might systematically and evocatively explore a recent or past interaction, internally focus on one partner's subjective experience, focus on an emotional injury, focus on an intra- or interpersonal block, suggest an enactment, consider homework, or recommend a specific course of action.

The stage-of-treatment compass takes a read of where in the process the couple might be. Are they in the early stage of treatment or still forming and solidifying the bond? Has the cycle been understood and reframed including secondary and primary emotions, and have the historical origins of primary emotions in each partner been identified? Have primary emotions and needs been accessed, deepened, elaborated, and revealed to partners? Have emotional blocks and protective walls been explored? Have emotional vulnerabilities been received by partners and interactions been restructured? Have interactional shifts been attained, consolidated, and integrated—including an exploration of old, negative cycles versus new positive cycles? Such considerations are important when selecting specific interventions depending on the stage of treatment, as illustrated in the couple therapy with Jake and Hiro.

INITIAL ASSESSMENT AND CASE FORMULATION

The referral came by email addressed to me (SW), written by Jake and including his fiancé Hiro:

"Dear Dr. Warwar,
I'm seeing Dr. Rhonda Goldman for individual therapy, and she referred me and my fiancé Hiro to you. We're having difficulty with our communication and it's very stressful. I hope you can see us. We'd like to start therapy as soon as possible! We can make ourselves available to you at any time next week.
Thank you kindly, Jake and Hiro"

I find that I can learn a great deal about a couple from the initial contact, even before meeting with them. First, it stood out that the email was from Jake, writing to me directly, with his partner included on the email. In couple therapy, there is often one person leading the initiative to seek therapy, and I wondered if this was Jake. Second, I noted the urgency of wanting to start therapy immediately. In terms of the presenting issue, couples frequently present with "communication issues" and it's a very general and nonspecific way of describing the problem, which is usually symptomatic of deeper issues; this always makes me curious about what the source of these underlying communication issues is. From my first contact with a couple, I'm curious about and try to understand each partner's pain and how they may be protecting it. I strive to understand the core needs each partner is trying to meet, how those relate to their earlier relational experiences, and how they contribute to the difficulties between them.

After welcoming a couple into the office and introducing myself, I usually start the session by asking how each partner is feeling about being there. Couples are usually nervous about coming to therapy and I strive to put them at ease, offer a sense of what to expect in the overall therapy process, and try to address any immediate concerns or questions. To this end, I said the following to the couple:

> ME (SW): Let me tell you a little bit about what to expect. Today, I want to hear about your relationship concerns and what brings you to couple therapy at this time, and also more generally about the two of you as a couple. My goal is to understand what you need help with and to make sure that I can help you with your

relationship concerns, and to see if it feels like a good fit for us to work together. I also want to make sure that this is a safe space for you to open up about your issues.

I find it helpful to inquire whether the couple has been in therapy before and what their experiences have been, as I want to consider their past experiences, negative or positive, in providing an explanation of what to expect of our work together. Experiential teaching is an important part of therapy that involves providing psychoeducation and rationales that are tailored to each partner's current process and needs. The relationship compass is particularly important in the early sessions and an important task in building safety and trust is to provide experiential teaching as needed. Neither Jake nor Hiro had been in couple therapy previously, and only Jake had been in individual therapy, which was with his current therapist (RG). In providing psychoeducation about the therapy process, I explain to couples that EFT-C is an approach that has some structure to it and that there's a different focus in the beginning, middle, and later phases of therapy, and that the first few sessions of therapy involve learning more about their relationship, as well as getting a history of their sensitivities and vulnerabilities that may affect their relationship. In addition, I describe how the next phase involves focusing on identifying and deescalating their painful negative cycles. My experience is that couples are relieved to hear that there's some structure, because it's common that couples come to therapy when they're experiencing chaos and distress in their relationship.

Jake and Hiro were an interracial, gay couple who had been in a relationship for 4 years, living together for 2 years, and were engaged to be married. Jake was a White, 41-year-old male, originally from Canada, and Hiro was a 39-year-old Asian male, originally from Japan, and had immigrated to Canada with his sister and his parents when he was 12. To provide therapy that can promote the best outcomes, I emphasize an intersectional lens in understanding each partner. Sometimes partners' intersections are obvious, and other times they only become known when we're exploring each partner's individual history. I observed that Jake spoke with a mainstream Canadian accent and Hiro spoke with a mild, Japanese accent. My clinical practice is in downtown Toronto, which is often touted as being one of the most culturally diverse cities in the world. Given that Hiro and Jake were an interracial, gay couple, with Hiro being a person of color, I noted that race, ethnicity, gender, and sexual orientation would be relevant to explore with them as I learned more about their personal histories. People who are minorities have often had negative discriminatory experiences that can leave them feeling generally more unsafe and self-protective. Consequently, building trust and safety in the therapeutic relationship can understandably present more of a challenge, especially in an EFT-C approach, which requires partners to express their deepest emotional pain and vulnerabilities.

The first stage of EFT-C—validation and alliance formation—begins with establishing a safe and collaborative therapeutic relationship by empathizing with each partner and validating each partner's pain. The experiential teaching and psychoeducation I provide in the early sessions helps to create a safe therapeutic space to do the deeper work. In addition, when I provide empathy and validation of each partner's core painful feelings, it helps to calm each partner's anxiety and soothes the hurt of not being heard by their partner. However, it can be challenging at times to validate each partner's pain without alienating the other person. With Jake and Hiro, I noticed that neither partner was reactive to what I was saying to the other, so I felt that I could validate each of them without concern that the other would feel invalidated.

I observed that Hiro appeared to be the less talkative partner of the two, as he was quiet and often looked down at the floor, not making eye contact. Jake took the lead in initiating the conversation and answering my questions and seemed more active. In general, what I see in front of me in session is usually the same negative cycle that plays out in the couple's relationship. Assessment is process diagnostic, conducted throughout the course of therapy to guide my interventions, requiring a close attunement to the couple's moment-by-moment process, and includes assessing types of emotions expressed, partners' responses to my interventions, negative and positive cycles, and stages of treatment. From an EFT-C perspective, within the negative cycle there's often a more passive partner and a more active partner. I noted that Hiro's nonverbal behavior of looking down at the floor and being more withdrawn might indicate either underlying shame or fear, so I was curious to know which one of the two it was.

In this first session, I learned that Jake was frustrated with Hiro, because he felt that Hiro wasn't following through with various promises—for example, not communicating with Jake when his work schedule changed and then coming home late without letting Jake know in advance. What was even more upsetting to Jake was that Hiro was unreachable if he tried to call him. Jake described a situation in which he needed Hiro's help with something and said angrily, "I can't trust that he'll be there when I need him!" Furthermore, Jake reported that when he tried to speak with Hiro about any of these issues, Hiro would get upset and "shut down," and the conversation would be unproductive. In response to Jake's comment, Hiro responded in a defeated tone, "He's right, it's my fault; he deserves a better partner than me. I can't do anything right." I empathized with and validated each partner's experience:

> ME (SW): Jake, it sounds like you get upset because you feel that Hiro isn't following through on what he says, and you feel that you can't rely on Hiro to be there for you when you need him. You get worried when you can't reach him, and you don't know how to have a helpful conversation about it with him, and it sounds like this is very painful for you, yes? And for you, Hiro, it sounds like you feel that you're disappointing Jake, and you feel very badly about this and you blame yourself?

Part of building an alliance in the first stage is to pay attention to the partners' presenting narratives to identify how their issues and concerns indicate core problems in areas of attachment and identity, and to be able to reflect this to them. This builds the alliance as partners feel relieved when they have their vulnerable identity- and attachment-related concerns named. I keep in mind that attachment sensitivities are related to concerns about safe connection and feelings of security, and identity sensitivities are related to feelings of shame or invalidation. With Jake, I observed that he seemed to be feeling insecure and anxious, as he was worried about Hiro not being responsive and dependable. Hiro seemed concerned about issues related to identity, as feelings of shame were implied in both what he expressed and in his body language. I checked my tentative understanding of this with both partners; they resonated with it and were able to elaborate on more specific examples. In EFT-C, partners are viewed as the experts of their own experience. I try to help each partner find their own voice, emphasizing the importance of the back-and-forth dialogue, and privileging each partner's understanding. To do this, I use what we call "empathic conjecture"—that is, empathic guesses offered tentatively in an exploratory and inquisitive manner with an intonation of a question to invite the person to experientially collaborate on the response. In the intermediate stage of therapy, empathic conjectures are particularly important, as they help partners to access core vulnerabilities.

It's important to foster a sense of hope in the first session. Although this occurs in part by validating each partner's expressed concerns, instilling hope can also be facilitated by highlighting any strengths or positive qualities that you see in the couple. For example, it was apparent to me that Hiro and Jake really loved each other and cared about their relationship, and I shared this with them:

> ME (SW): I hear that these issues are very painful, but I can also see how much you love each other and care about the relationship, which is a strength of your relationship. It's why you're both so upset about what's going on; if you didn't care, you wouldn't be so troubled by it. Every relationship goes through ups and downs, and every couple can benefit from having some help at times. I'd really like to help you with your relationship concerns if you feel comfortable working with me.

Hiro and Jake expressed a sense of relief that I wanted to work with them and indicated that they felt comfortable with me. There was already inherent trust, as Jake's therapist had recommended me. I also felt relieved to hear this, as when I meet any couple for the first time, I hope they like me personally and that our initial interactions allow them to feel safe with me and that I understand each of their concerns well enough that they want to continue their work with me.

In the first session, I offer a map of treatment, which involves having a sense of what to expect regarding the overall therapy. I told Jake and Hiro that it's important to attend therapy weekly, at least for the first four or five sessions to build our alliance and allow us to work on deescalating their negative cycle. I also explained that the first few sessions would be spent getting an in-depth relationship history, as well as a personal history from each of them to help me understand them better. As many couples do, they asked me how long the therapy takes. I find this difficult to determine until I get to know the couple better and understand the complexity of their issues. I explained that long-standing issues can take more time to resolve, but that on average a short-term course of therapy can be anywhere from 16 to 20 sessions.

BEGINNING PHASE OF THERAPY

Stage 2 of EFT-C involves negative cycle deescalation. Identifying the negative interactional cycle as the relational problem that needs to be changed, and each partner's position in the cycle, is important in reducing partner blame and conveys the central message that "It's not your relationship that's the problem, it's the problematic cycle that you keep getting stuck in!" I strive to understand each partner's observable behavior in the cycle and not let partners impose intention onto each other's actions. An example of this is when Jake says about Hiro, "He ignores my calls and doesn't care that I'm waiting for him." I reflect to Jake, "So it sounds like what happens is that you call Hiro when he's late and he doesn't answer, and then you keep calling him without a response from him? Jake, I can imagine that this is painful and that you feel ignored, but let's try and stay with Hiro's words and actions, not what you *think* he feels or means." Although I want to validate Jake's feelings, it's important for me not to agree with Jake's assumptions about what Hiro is intending or feeling when he doesn't answer Jake and comes home late.

When I'm identifying the negative cycle, I focus on what I see in front of me or, if the couple is recounting what happened during a past conflict, what I would observe if I were watching a video of the couple's interactions. A question I find helpful to ask is "What would I see if I were a fly on the wall if I was observing a specific fight you had? Tell me about what happens." This brings the cycle to life in the session, so that I can understand how these observable problematic protective emotions and behaviors are expressed for each partner. To get at each partner's role in the negative cycle, I explore with that partner, "What do you say and do in this fight?"—and when I understand this, I turn to the other partner to find out "When your partner says and does that, what do you say and do in response?" and so on, to see how the cycle intensifies and evolves from interaction to interaction. I want the couple to tell me about a *specific* conflict they remember, not just generally how they fight, and it doesn't matter what conflict they choose, because couples tend to have the same cycles in their conflicts.

In getting Jake and Hiro to tell me about what happens during a specific conflict, they tell me about an argument they have when Hiro comes home late from work. I learn that the negative interaction begins after Jake confronts Hiro when he comes home and criticizes and blames him, and in turn Hiro withdraws and shuts down. Their cycle is a pursue–withdraw cycle or, more specifically, a criticize–shut down pattern. Specifically, Jake would criticize Hiro for not being responsive to his requests and needs, and question him angrily, "Why didn't you tell me that you would be home late? You're always late! You could have called or at least answered me when I called you! That's so rude!" In response, Hiro typically gets quiet and doesn't say anything, and appears shut down and sometimes starts to cry and says something to Jake like, "I'll do better." In turn, Jake replies angrily, "You're not responding to me!" Furthermore, when Hiro gets tearful and quiet, Jake reports that he gets angrier, because he feels that his concern is being dismissed by Hiro, and he says something to Hiro like, "Now you're being selfish and making it about you!" Jake's response results in Hiro becoming even more shut down. I describe the cycle as I understand it to them:

ME (SW): (*to the couple*) You're stuck in this negative cycle that seems painful for both of you and difficult to get out of. Jake, when you're upset with Hiro, you say things to him that sound critical and accusing, like "Why were you late, or why didn't you answer my call?" And Hiro, in response you shut down and withdraw, put your head down and get quiet, sometimes you cry, but ultimately you're not responding to Jake's questions. (*turning to Jake*) That gets you more upset with Hiro, and then (*turning to Hiro*) you shut down even more, and you (*turning to Jake again*) get even angrier and say critical things. Does that fit?

JAKE: Yes, that's it exactly!

HIRO: Yes, that's what happens, and I get so upset that I've let him down, I can't face him. [They're both relieved and have notably relaxed in having their negative cycle named. I see this as a positive sign that I've named the cycle accurately, and this is a relief to me, because it means that I can help the couple deescalate their conflict and get into the deeper emotional work of identifying their primary vulnerable emotions that their cycle is protecting.]

ME (SW): I can see how difficult this cycle is and that it's painful for both of you, but what you say and do in this negative cycle isn't really what's going on inside. I get the sense that for you, Jake, although you get very upset and angry with Hiro, you instead may be feeling insecure or worried about your connection with him? And for you, Hiro, I get the sense that when you cry and withdraw, you actually feel very badly that you're disappointing Jake and that it's difficult for you to face him when you feel like you've let him down, maybe you're even feeling some shame? (*Hiro nods.*) Your negative cycle is what's hurting your relationship and I'd really love to help you with this.

It's not typically relevant or helpful to indicate who starts the negative cycle. For example, even in Jake's and Hiro's relationship, it's difficult to know whether it's Jake who starts the cycle by criticizing or Hiro who starts the cycle by being late and not responding to Jake, or something else. What's important in negative cycle deescalation is to clearly identify what each partner says and does, and to emphasize that the cycle intensifies with each interaction—using the language of "the more and the more" which captures its cyclical nature; for example, "The more you do this, the more he does that and, in turn, the more you do this."

To help with cycle deescalation, EFT therapists assess identity- and attachment-related emotions to identify the historical origins of what each partner is sensitive and vulnerable to and to make sense of how this may get activated in their relationship. This helps to reduce partner blame and helps each person feel compassionate and understanding of their partner's sensitivities. Sensitivities can be thought of as lenses through which a person views their world and relates to situations in which threat to attachment or identity is experienced. An attachment sensitivity/vulnerability involves concerns about security and safety relating to closeness in the relationship, "Are you going to leave me, or are you going to be there when I need you?" Attachment concerns can be indicated by fears of abandonment or feeling suffocated in a relationship. In contrast, an identity sensitivity/vulnerability involves concerns about shame or invalidation (e.g., "Am I good enough?"; "Am I going to be invalidated?"; or "Do my emotional needs matter to you?").

I assess sensitivities by empathically exploring each partner's experiences in forming relationships, with special attention to family-of-origin and previous relationships in relation to connection, comfort, validation, past traumas, and how they adapted. I find it helpful to explore what feels problematic in relation to unmet childhood needs. Questions I may ask include "Did you feel loved and why?"; "Did you feel safe and why?"; "Did you feel like you were good enough and why?"; "In your family, who would you have turned to when you had a bad day and what did they say and do?" Furthermore, when determining who's sensitive to attachment issues and who's sensitive to identity issues in the couple's relationship, I find the following questions helpful: "Who typically wants the most emotional closeness in your relationship?"; "Who's the most sensitive to criticism?"; "Can you turn to your partner when you're feeling hurt or scared? What happens when you do? Do you feel understood and validated by your partner?"

I spent the rest of the session getting a history of Jake's and Hiro's sensitivities and vulnerabilities, encouraging them to speak about their personal histories from a vulnerable place. In inviting one partner to open up about their history, I work to create a safe space by encouraging the other partner to be a receptive listener by providing information about what to expect. I find it helpful to say something like "You may or may not know what your partner is sharing about their history, but I ask you to listen with care and compassion, and I may turn to you at times and ask you what you know about this and how you feel. This will feel more one-sided than what we will usually do in therapy, but I'll also take time later to learn about your history, too."

I learned that Jake and Hiro each had difficult childhoods. Jake was the oldest of three children, and his father abandoned the family when he was 10 years old; consequently, his mother was coping with financial stress and raising three children on her own. She relied heavily on Jake to take care of his younger siblings. Jake felt abandoned by his father and was anxious growing up, and his mother was always working and unavailable. He felt that there was no one there to turn to and felt confused about why his father left. As the oldest, he felt that he was responsible to hold things together and take care of his two younger sisters, who were 5 and 7 years old when his father left the family. Jake had a previous 5-year relationship in which he was engaged, and his fiancé cheated on him and broke up with him shortly after Jake found out about the affair. This was a few years before he met Hiro. Given his childhood and previous relationship history, it made sense that Jake's sensitivity was about security, as he felt unexpectedly abandoned by both his father and his fiancé. And in relation to his family, he felt overburdened, unsupported, alone, and anxious in both his childhood and adolescence. During our session, Jake was emotional at times, especially when he talked about his family. Hiro was quiet but appeared to be listening attentively. When I asked him if he knew about what Jake shared, he replied, "Jake did tell me most of this, but to hear him talking about it with you, it helps me understand more about how it affected him." I observed that Jake smiled at Hiro in response, and I had a sense that he felt acknowledged and perhaps even understood by Hiro.

In turning to Hiro, I learned that his father was very critical and shaming, and placed high expectations of success on him. Hiro didn't feel like he could be himself and felt that he had to adhere to his father's standards. Hiro was born and raised in Japan until his family immigrated to Canada when he was 12 years old. Recognizing that culture is an important intersection, I asked whether there was anything about growing up in Japan or the Japanese culture that would be helpful for me to understand. Hiro expressed that in his family, being raised Japanese meant that his identity, reputation, and responsibilities were deeply connected to his family, and that his own emotional needs were not considered. Hiro didn't come out as being gay to his family until he was in his mid-30s, because he felt that this would not be accepted. As an adult, when he did finally disclose to his parents that he was gay, they were quite upset and distanced themselves from him. Although they had met Jake, they were not supportive of the relationship, and Hiro currently had a very strained relationship with them.

I explored with Hiro what it was like for him to immigrate to Canada, acknowledging that it could be difficult to move here when English wasn't his first language and that, although Toronto is a diverse city, unfortunately, racial discrimination still exists. He appreciated my directness about recognizing that these intersections might be difficult, and he seemed much more vulnerable with me as he opened up about having a difficult time in school as he was bullied and experienced racial discrimination. Another relevant issue for him was that because he recognized that he was gay early on and didn't feel comfortable to come out to others publicly, he had felt very uncomfortable in social situations throughout his life. I learned that he currently struggles with feeling like he's never good enough and has always felt that he's had to work extra hard to succeed. When his family came to Canada, his parents told Hiro that people would judge him for being Japanese and that he had to be perfect so he wouldn't give people a reason to find fault with him. This explained why he currently had difficulty setting boundaries at work when his boss asked him to stay late or when his work wasn't finished. Jake's and Hiro's heartfelt disclosures of suffering and emotional pain deepened my feelings of compassion and emotional connection with them—and this increased my optimism that I could be helpful to them.

Hiro's emotional disclosure about feeling like he had to be perfect was very beneficial for Jake to hear, as much of this was a surprise to him. It was moving for me to experience Jake tenderly putting his arm on Hiro's shoulder to soothe him, and for me to see that Hiro was able to find comfort in his touch as he leaned toward him. I felt hopeful and saw this as a positive sign that Jake could comfort Hiro's pain, but at the same time I wondered if this was something that Hiro could do for Jake in their relationship, since Jake's core complaint seemed to be that he couldn't rely on Hiro to be there for him. In asking about this, I learned that Hiro was able to comfort and soothe Jake when his discontent or distress wasn't about Hiro or their relationship. This made sense to me given that Hiro's difficulty in being responsive to Jake was related to feeling shame about disappointing Jake. I also reflected to them that it was a strength of their relationship that they could both comfort each other at times. In couple therapy, to offset a tendency to focus solely on problems, it's therapeutic to notice and highlight positive behaviors and strengths.

I also asked what their experiences were like regarding being a gay couple given that they are part of a marginalized minority. They described very different experiences growing up. Jake's mother, siblings, and friends were very accepting of him being gay; he came out to family and friends in his early teens and they warmly welcomed Jake's past partners, as well as Hiro. In contrast, growing up, Hiro felt that he wouldn't have been accepted by his family or friends if he revealed he was gay and, as a result, he was selective about who he came out to socially. Furthermore, given his experience of racial discrimination, he felt less comfortable and free to be himself in his daily interactions in the world. Jake and Hiro both acknowledged that the reality of being a gay couple meant that they had to be more mindful of their surroundings when they were in the general public and not in the safety of friends. When asking about partners' intersections, our approach is to be curious, accepting, and validating of each partner's experiences and not to make any assumptions about how these may impact them.

Highlighting the origins of each partner's sensitivities is fundamental to cycle deescalation, because it decreases partner blame as each partner develops a greater understanding of why the other is sensitive and reactive to certain things. To Jake, I validated that it seemed that he was sensitive to feeling abandoned and alone, and that this made a lot of sense given his past childhood experiences; and to Hiro, I validated that his feeling of not being good enough was something that made a lot of sense given his past childhood experiences in addition to the racial discrimination he continues to experience. Hiro's difficulties in setting boundaries at work and communicating his needs were related to feeling that he had to be perfect and to overcompensate for being Japanese. Each partner agreed that their emotional needs weren't attended to in their families of origin and that this was something that they had in common. I helped them reframe their problem as being related to these underlying vulnerable sensitivities that fueled, but were obscured by, their negative cycle.

INTERMEDIATE PHASE OF THERAPY

After I deescalated Jake's and Hiro's negative cycle and acquired an understanding of their sensitivities and vulnerabilities, I shifted my focus to helping each partner access and express their primary vulnerable emotions underlying their negative cycle to reveal their heartfelt feelings and needs. We label this work in Stage 3 as accessing underlying feelings. In this stage, we encourage partners to express vulnerabilities and self-doubts to prepare them to ask for what they need and receive comfort and validation. These disclosures change partners' interactional stances and allow them to become more approachable, emotionally expressive, and communicative. It is this display of vulnerable emotions that's so important in changing interactions in relationships. We facilitate enactments, having partners face one another and share vulnerable feelings to create a new experience and a softened response from each other. This is the heart of EFT-C—the core mechanism that transforms the couple relationship.

To facilitate Hiro and Jake expressing their underlying feelings to each other, I drew once again on empathic conjecture (Goldman, Vaz, & Rousmaniere, 2021), in which I try to reach behind each partner's wall of self-protection and help them put words to their underlying vulnerable emotions and needs, some of which are implicit but may not be attended to or expressed. In this context, empathic explorations are intended to help partners explore the emerging edge of their experiences, where implicit emotion or bodily felt sensations can be turned into conscious experiences of specific emotions by offering language to something that hasn't been clearly defined previously. I offer these therapist responses tentatively to invite partners to elaborate on and differentiate their emotional experiences; that is, I always offer empathic conjectures in collaborative coexploration and communicate a respect for each partner's inner experience. Empathic conjecture is especially helpful when partners aren't sure of what they feel, as it allows them to turn their attention inward and see whether what's offered resonates with their internal experience. Empathic conjectures are often more helpful than asking questions about how one feels, because they help partners stay connected to an internal experiential process and out of their heads. I used empathic conjecture to identify the underlying feelings in Jake's and Hiro's negative cycle:

ME (SW): (*turning to Jake*) When you come to Hiro and you appear upset and angry with him, questioning him, "Why didn't you let me know that you would be late," he thinks that you're angry with him, but I wonder if you check inside, if you're actually feeling worried about your connection with him?

JAKE: Yes, I'm very worried, because I don't know if he's going to be there when I need him!

ME (SW): So, really, underneath your anger is this feeling of "I'm scared that you won't be there for me when I need you?"

JAKE: Yes, exactly! He just ignores me and doesn't care that I need him!

ME (SW): (*validating the feeling underneath*) So you're saying, "Yes, I'm scared," but even now, instead of telling him that you're feeling afraid, what you *actually* say and do are different. You say things like "He's ignoring me and doesn't care," and you appear angry rather than afraid. Jake, I think it may be hard for Hiro to see that you're afraid.

JAKE: (*after a long pause*) Hmmm . . . well, I guess I never looked at it like that. At that point I'm so upset because I haven't been able to reach him.

ME (SW): (*turning to Hiro*) Did you know he was afraid?

HIRO: No, I'm surprised to hear that, he always seems so mad at me.

ME (SW): (*turning to Jake, and drawing on empathic conjecture to deepen his feelings of fear and insecurity*) So, it's like you're really scared, and instead what he sees is that you're angry with him. If you could really speak from the fear instead, it sounds like what you would say is something like "I just feel so scared and shaky when you're late and I can't reach you?"

JAKE: (*tearfully*) Yes, that's exactly it! I'm very scared than he won't be there when I need him.

ME (SW): (*to Jake*) Jake, can you tell us more about the fear? I can imagine that it's similar to this feeling you had growing up?

JAKE: (*still tearful*) Yes, I'm alone, and no one is there, just like when I was a kid.

ME (SW): (*to Hiro*) Did you know he was feeling scared? [At this point, I notice that Hiro has his head down and seems withdrawn, and I'm surprised, because I was expecting a more relational response to Jake following Jake's vulnerable disclosure.]

ME (SW): What's happening inside as you hear Jake talking about this scared, alone feeling that reminds him of his childhood?"

HIRO: (*his voice trailing off*) I'm such a bad partner.

At this point in the process, I would typically encourage Jake to turn to Hiro directly to express his painful feelings of loneliness and fear, but Hiro's self-focused response about being a bad partner (as opposed to responding more specifically to what Jake disclosed) signals to me that he may be experiencing a shame spiral, which is a nonrelational response. In this moment, I'm aware that it can be damaging to the work I'm doing with them to have Jake open up to Hiro while Hiro is in a shame spiral. I'm also thinking that this response I'm witnessing is similar to what the couple has already described that happens in their cycle—that Hiro withdraws when he feels that he's the source of Jake's discontent and this further angers Jake, and so on. If I were to encourage Jake to be vulnerable to Hiro at this time, my fear is that Hiro wouldn't be able to respond to Jake's vulnerability, which would then reactivate their negative cycle. As a result, I decide to work with Hiro's nonrelational response, which in my moment-by-moment case formulation I'm conceptualizing as a *block to responding*.

In both Stages 3 and 4 partners can experience blocks to revealing underlying emotions to the other, or to accepting and responding to their partner's expressed vulnerability. At this point I'm concerned about leaving Jake without emotional support and validation following his vulnerable disclosure and Hiro's nonrelational response, but I'm also aware that I need to work with Hiro directly to help him out of his shame spiral. When I'm working with blocks in EFT-C when one partner has disclosed vulnerability and the other partner is having difficulty responding in an empathic manner, I first validate the partner who is expressing vulnerability and then let them know that I'm now going to work with their partner, who's having trouble responding to them. My approach to this enactment with Jake can be outlined as follows:

Step 1: Validate vulnerable expressed feeling: "I can see that this alone, scared feeling that gets activated is very painful."
Step 2: Validate that it's painful not to have partner respond empathically: "I'd imagine that it's painful to reveal this in here and not have Hiro respond to you."
Step 3: Instill hope by reframing it as an opportunity to help them work with this in session: "This is the exact difficulty that you've been having in your relationship, and it's helpful that this issue is happening in here, as it's an opportunity for us to be able to work on it together. I am going to help you with this."
Step 4: Seek permission to shift from the vulnerable, disclosing partner and work with the blocked partner: "Is it okay with you if I turn to Hiro now to try and understand what's going on with him, and I'll come back to you?"

In working with shame, I always validate the shame but then also encourage and teach partners how to have a more relational response, even though they're feeling shame. Expressing relational shame can be helpful at times, because it conveys a partner is feeling badly for hurting the other. However if one partner's shame and self-loathing block an empathic and relational response, the impact of this is that the other partner feels alone and unattended to in their vulnerability. Hence, at this point, I turn to Hiro to work with his nonresponsive shame state.

ME (SW): What stops you from being able to respond to Jake's pain?

HIRO: I feel like I'm constantly disappointing him.

ME (SW): So, if you could put words to that feeling, it's like "I feel that I've let you down and I can't face you because I'm so ashamed?" [empathic conjecture]

HIRO: Yes, I feel like I'm not a good partner. I'm failing him, and I can't bear to see the pain I've caused.

ME (SW): But rather than being able to talk to Jake about his concerns and tell him about your shame, it sounds like you feel so much shame that what you do is you shut down and get quiet and withdrawn rather than communicating this to him? (*Hiro nods.*) I know it's not your intention, but I don't think you realize that Jake ends up feeling more alone when he tries to talk to you about this.

HIRO: (*looking up*) I don't want him to feel alone. It's just that when I see how upset he is, I feel so ashamed that I can't face him.

ME (SW): So, what you're saying is that when you appear withdrawn or shut down, you're actually feeling ashamed. It's like, "I feel like I've failed Jake and disappointed him, and I'm too ashamed to face it?"

HIRO: Yes, that's right, the shame is very deep! It's not my intention to make things worse. I can now see that it doesn't help. (*Hiro turns to Jake and looks at him tearfully, not withdrawn anymore.*) I'm sorry. I do want to be there for you.

ME (SW): (*turning to Hiro*) I can see that you're sorry for turning away from him in those moments when he needs you. (*Then, turning to Jake*) Jake, did you know that this is what was going on when Hiro withdraws?

JAKE: No, I really didn't, I was feeling very rejected, but I feel badly for him now. (*turns to Hiro*) I wish you had told me.

It's common that the pursuing partner in a relationship (in this case, Jake) pursues in a critical, blaming way and that their vulnerability isn't seen by their partner. Equally common is that the withdrawing partner (in this case, Hiro) is perceived by the pursuing partner as rejecting or unavailable, when in fact they're experiencing a shame spiral that results in not being responsive to their partner. In Stage 4, it's a partner's acceptance of the expressed vulnerable feelings that is paramount, and it's this acceptance that restructures the negative cycle into a new interaction. Building on the earlier exchange, I now turn to Hiro to help coach him to provide a more affiliative response to Jake:

ME (SW): I can see that you do care that Jake is hurting, so I want you to try something for me. I can see that you feel this deep shame, this sensitivity that you carry around from all of your earlier experiences we've talked about. Even though you're feeling shame, and I can imagine it's very painful, you said that you want to be there for Jake and I want to help you with that.

HIRO: Yes! I want to.

ME (SW): I know you do. Can you turn to Jake and tell him in your own words how it hurts you to see him suffering and that you want to be there for him? [promoting enactment of Hiro's accepting response to Jake]

HIRO: (*slowly turning to Jake*) It's true, I'm sad to hear how alone you felt in your childhood and I want to be there for you to lean on. (*then, tearfully*) I love you.

ME (SW): Hiro, can you tell him about your tears?

HIRO: I really love you and I'm sad that you doubt that. I just worry that I'll disappoint you and that I'm not good enough for you.

Now that I've been able to help Hiro provide a more relational response, I feel that it's safe to have Jake open up to Hiro. I first want to help Jake take in Hiro's accepting response—to help him allow and accept this new emotional response from Hiro. I do this by highlighting Hiro's expression of love and support.

ME (SW): (*to Jake*) Can you see the love in his face and the way he looks at you and can you take in what he's saying? What it's like inside?

JAKE: (*smiling at Hiro, who's looking at him with love and care*) Yes, I feel warm and safe and I feel so much closer to you now that you've shared how you feel. . . . I love you, too! Of course, you're good enough for me, I'm lucky to have you!

ME (SW): Hiro, can you take this in? What's it like to hear this?

HIRO: (*tearfully, with a smile*) Good!

ME (SW): (*to both of them*) Right, so it sounds like it was so important and different that, Hiro, you expressed your feelings to Jake rather than withdrawing and, as a result, Jake, you feel closer to Hiro?

JAKE: Yes, I do.

ME (SW): *(to Jake)*: Can you now turn to Hiro and tell him about feeling afraid and alone at times? *(turning to Hiro)* And Hiro, you've shown us that you're very capable of being there for Jake. Can you listen and try to understand what it's like for him?

HIRO: Yes!

JAKE: I've never had anyone I could rely on growing up and I always felt shaky, like I didn't have a safety net, and when you don't do what you say you're going to do or I can't find you, I start to panic.

ME (SW): It sound like in those moments you feel like that scared little boy who was abandoned?

JAKE: Yes, exactly.

ME (SW): Can you turn to Hiro and tell him this?

JAKE: *(tearfully)* I feel like I'm 10 years old and I'm alone, and no one will be there if I need them.

ME (SW): It sounds like you feel very scared and alone. *(Jake nods, in tears.)*

HIRO: *(putting his arm on Jake's shoulder)* I'll be here for you always. I'm sorry that I haven't been . . .

I spend some more time deepening these new responses and helping each partner reflect on what's different and new and what it feels like. For me, this is a very rewarding part of working with this couple when I can witness these meaningful changes. For Hiro, being able to be present for Jake when he's vulnerable and express that he wants to be there for him is a new, positive emotional experience that helps him feel competent in meeting Jake's emotional needs and feel that he's a better partner to Jake. And Hiro's expression of relational shame is new and helps Jake feel more compassion for Hiro and more connected to him, which helps Jake feel more secure and less alone. For Jake, expressing his vulnerability about feeling scared and alone helps him to be more vulnerable with Hiro rather than critical and blaming, and allows Hiro to see the vulnerable part of Jake underneath his protective anger.

Once partners are more accessible and responsive, to ensure enduring change in their interactions, each partner may also need to develop the capacity to self-soothe and transform their maladaptive emotional responses; these maladaptive responses usually reflect underlying unmet childhood needs or past trauma. The ability to self-soothe is also important for times when a partner isn't emotionally available or responsive. With less distressed couples, restructuring the interaction involves first developing more responsiveness to each other, as seen with Hiro and Jake; by comparison, with more dysregulated couples, the work of restructuring often first requires helping partners learn to self-soothe when the partner isn't responsive or available.

CONCLUDING PHASE OF THERAPY

Stage 5 of EFT-C, consolidation and integration, involves strengthening and supporting new interactional positions and promoting positive, nurturing, and validating cycles of interaction. In addition, this stage focuses on relapse prevention of negative cycles. I find this to be a very rewarding stage, as usually much work has transpired to get to this point.

In Stage 5, couples look and feel transformed, as partners have softened toward each other and are experiencing more positive emotions in their relationship. When couples start reporting positive experiences in sessions and changes outside the sessions, it's vital to discuss how these changes are perceived and understood. This, in turn, helps to empower partners to take ownership for contributing to the change.

It was heartwarming for me to see Jake and Hiro laughing with each other and appearing more connected and loving toward each other. In our last few sessions, I reflect on the individual and relationship changes that transformed their cycle from a negative to a positive one. I encourage each of them to articulate the changes they've made by asking them for examples of their personal and relationship growth: "Can you describe what you're doing that's contributed to your interaction being more positive?" Jake is able to recognize that if Hiro withdraws, he's not rejecting or abandoning him, as he sees that Hiro may be feeling triggered and vulnerable himself. "I feel a lot more secure with Hiro, even if he does withdraw a bit, because I now understand that it's not because he doesn't love me or want to be there for me but that he's likely feeling ashamed. So I don't get angry with him; instead, I feel sad because I know he's hurting and I ask him if he's okay." Hiro also reveals that he's now able to recognize that when Jake is upset with him, he's really feeling scared and, although Hiro may be feeling some shame, he's been able to approach Jake with a more connected relational response. "I know if Jake is upset or angry it's really that scared boy protecting himself and it's easier for me to be there for him, even if I feel like I've disappointed him, so I'm not withdrawing anymore." I'm delighted to hear about these changes and now it's important for me to spend time reflecting on, validating, and deepening these positive changes with them. Asking partners, "what's that like inside?" in relation to the positive interactions is a great way to consolidate and deepen emotional changes.

Another important component of Stage 5 is relapse prevention. It's expected that partners will get back into their negative cycle at some point and important that they remember they can also deescalate their cycle once they understand how they get themselves into it. To strengthen this awareness, I ask partners to identify what they'd do to trigger the negative cycle. This gives them the sense of their own responsibility and control of their interactions. Although maladaptive states may not be fully transformed by the end of therapy, partners are now better able to understand their own and their partner's deep vulnerabilities; they work on how to soothe and transform their own states, how not to trigger these states in their partner, and how to respond to them if they do. When I ask Jake and Hiro how they would unintentionally restart their negative cycle, Jake says, "I'd get angry and critical rather than express that I'm scared or alone." And Hiro recognizes "I'd lose myself in my shame rather than reaching out to Jake." In addition, Hiro reflects that he's working on being more honest with Jake about what his needs are, so he doesn't put himself in a position of committing to something that he can't do.

In Stage 5, we give special attention to recognizing, supporting, and nurturing newly emerging and positive emotions. Positive emotional experiences such as love, joy, and interest are independent sources of affiliative motivation that help relationships flourish. The importance of love is obvious; it involves openness to, and concern for the other. The experience of positive emotions builds a reservoir of good feelings that helps people deal with their negative feelings, and this storehouse of positive feelings helps override and transform negative feelings when they do arise. Building positive emotional experiences between partners is one of the best forms of insurance against negative feelings escalating into conflict. This is done both in the session and by assigning homework that emerges out of the aliveness of the in-session work. Given that positive emotions are often partners' goals of therapy, when couples come to sessions experiencing and expressing positive interactions and emotions on a more consistent basis, this is usually a sign that the therapy is drawing to an end.

FURTHER REFLECTIONS AND IMPLICATIONS

When we work with any couple, we find it helpful to ask the question, "What's the corrective emotional experience that we want to facilitate in session between partners to help them restructure their negative emotional interactions?" We find it especially beneficial to consider this when we're feeling at an impasse in helping a couple with their issues. It's easy when working with couples to get caught up in simply *instructing* partners on how they "should" interact and communicate with each other—for example, by focusing solely on communication skills and healthy ways of responding. Instructing Hiro and Jake would have meant instructing Jake to be more vulnerable and less critical and similarly teaching Hiro to be more responsive to Jake. However, it was significantly more beneficial to have them *experience* one another differently—that is, to have Jake be vulnerable in session and reveal his feelings of aloneness and insecurity, and for Hiro to validate him unconditionally. This was a transformative experience for this couple. Furthermore, having Hiro express his shame in a more relational way and be responsive to Jake in session provided Jake with a sense of security, and in turn provided Hiro with a feeling of adequacy in being a worthy partner to Jake. This type of transformation in EFT-C facilitates new in-session positive experiences between partners that restructure their negative cycle and helps rebuild their emotional connection.

In working with couples, we're continuously struck by the observation that no matter where people come from, what type of relationship they're in, or even what topics or issues they fight over, people bring their core pain in relation to not feeling lovable or good enough, feeling insecure, or longing for greater connection. The key and challenge to doing this therapy is to "hear through" the content, and to listen *into* the core pain. From there, the process involves validating that both partners are in pain and helping them find ways to soothe each other's pain, or meet their needs, without losing themselves in the relationship. It's an act of courage to come to couple therapy, and an act of bravery to actually take the risk and be vulnerable, and it's truly a privilege for us to be part of each couple's journey.

REFERENCES

Goldman, R. N., & Greenberg, L. S. (2013). Working with identity and self-soothing in emotion-focused therapy for couples. *Family Process, 52,* 62–82.

Goldman, R. N., Vaz, A., & Rousmaniere, T. (2021). *Deliberate practice in emotion-focused therapy.* Washington, DC: American Psychological Association.

Greenberg, L. S., & Goldman, R. N. (2008). *Emotion-focused couples therapy: The dynamics of emotion, love, and power.* Washington, DC: American Psychological Association.

Greenberg, L. S., & Johnson, S. M. (1988). *Emotionally focused therapy for couples.* New York: Guilford Press.

Greenberg, L. S., Warwar, S., & Malcolm, W. (2010). Emotion-focused couples therapy and the facilitation of forgiveness. *Journal of Marital and Family Therapy, 36,* 28–42.

CHAPTER 3

Integrative Couple Therapy with a Surprising Twist

ELLEN F. WACHTEL

> ### Editors' Comments
>
> Ellen Wachtel's case study calls our attention to the wisdom developed over the career of an experienced integrative couple therapist. She offers us access to not only what she does in therapy but also her inner dialogue about the therapy process. As you read this case study, consider how specific therapeutic strategies are used while Wachtel retains a focus on the flow of connection between partners and a few overriding messages. Note as well that while the couple sets the specific agenda for the therapy and for the sessions, Wachtel is very much in charge of the frame of the therapy. Wachtel brings a positive nonpathologizing frame to this therapy and attention to the larger issues in the couple relationship. She also emphasizes and helps the partners assume a systemic perspective in which specific behaviors and problems are viewed in the framework of recurring feedback loops within the couple, while also attending to the influence of partners' individual processes.
>
> Wachtel's case study also offers almost a manual of practical wisdom. How do you begin therapy? How does one work with couples in a telehealth environment? What do you do if the couple chooses to have the virtual session from their bedroom? Wachtel offers numerous concrete suggestions.
>
> Certainly, most striking in this case presentation is the surprise that emerges halfway through the case study (which we won't disclose here!). Wachtel models how a therapist might best deal with such a surprise (and with similar problematic processes and outcomes), giving the reader access to her inner dialogue about this aspect of the case. She reminds us that there will always be limits to what we know and what we can achieve. In this way, being a couple therapist is also a humbling experience, even if it also is one that can provide great satisfaction.

Doing couple therapy is often exceptionally gratifying. But it can also be extremely stressful, for both the therapist and the couple. Anger, defensiveness, loss of focus and the repetition of patterns that have been so clearly explicated can leave both the therapist and the couple feeling frustrated and hopeless. I vividly remember the feelings I had as a young therapist after a day of seeing couples. I was excited by the way the couple "got" the mutuality of their difficulties and were no longer blaming one another for problematic interactions to which they each contributed. But just as often, I recall my head spinning as some sessions seemed to go from bad to worse. Not infrequently, I'd wonder if I were really cut out for this. It seemed so much harder than individual therapy, and I'd feel terrible when the tensions in the session hadn't been resolved and people left as upset or angrier than when they came in. Although I had gotten my PhD in a psychodynamically oriented program, my postdoctoral training in couple and family therapy was at the Ackerman Institute for the Family, and it was thoroughly systemic. Slowly but surely (when I was no longer supervised!), I began to integrate into my work with families and couples, ideas and methods from a variety of orientations. Though my original integration was of systemic and psychodynamic understandings, it soon expanded to include cognitive, experiential, and narrative components as well. Although the particular integration I use varies from couple to couple, there are some basic principles and methods that underlie all my work. In the case I describe here, you will see these principles in action. And, "spoiler alert," you will see, too, that my methods by no means ensure straightforward success!

Let me start by saying that I see each session as an opportunity to promote healing. Though I don't always achieve this, my aim is for the couple to leave the session feeling better than when they walked in. This may seem obvious. But many couples tell me that in their previous experience with couple therapy, they would often leave sessions feeling angry and upset, but accepted the therapist's reassurance that "things need to feel worse before they can get better." Without minimizing the seriousness of a couple's distress, I nonetheless vigilantly look for any nugget of something positive on which they might build. Research has shown that feeling hopeful is a crucial ingredient for therapeutic success in both individual and couple therapy. Combating demoralization and feelings of shame is particularly important in the beginning stages of the work, but building on what is going *right* with a couple is something I do from the first session to the very last.

Additionally, in the forefront of my mind with couples, is the aim of fostering self-reflection instead of blame, and increasing each person's motivation to change and expand their sense of self. These are not "pie in the sky" goals. Rather, they are readily achievable by specific interventions and careful attention to the myriad choice points therapists face in almost every statement uttered in the session. Being more positive in sessions is not just an attitude, it is a *skill* that with practice becomes natural and habitual. Each choice point is an opportunity to positively reinforce self-reflection instead of blame, empathy, emotional generosity, and collaboration. Often, the positive underlining is given in the form of an aside from the main point. These positive "asides" are quite powerful and can significantly change the tone of the session. So, for instance, if a husband was elaborating on how his wife is oversensitive to criticism, but then adds "She says I'm too critical and perfectionistic—I think that's just an excuse—but maybe she's right, my parents *were* perfectionists," I would first make an aside that underlines the husband's openness. For example, I might say, "I just want to say that I'm struck by how, even though you are frustrated with and even angry at your wife, you are still able to acknowledge that something she said might be a little bit right about you—not so easy to do particularly when you're upset." Then I would switch back to the content but, again, looking for something I could respond to that might further the goals of self-reflection, converting complaints to longings, and mutual problem solving.

Additionally, I use choice points and selective attention to steps in the right direction to further various aspects of my integrative orientation. Thus, if I think more focus on feelings rather than cognition would be useful for a particular couple, I'll look for moments when that is happening and build on those instances. Or if a couple is too emotionally reactive and would benefit from some soothing self-talk to calm themselves down, I'll look for the very occasional instance of soothing self-talk to underline and acknowledge.

Central to my particular integrative approach with couples is my effort to get an in-depth understanding of each person as an individual. One of the ways I do this is by using the genogram as a way not only to understand family patterns but also, and perhaps even more importantly, as a window through which I can glimpse each person's psychic reality—their values, world view, longings, vulnerabilities, strengths, anxieties and assumptions about love, trust, and committed relationships—aspects of their assumptive world about which they might not be fully aware (Wachtel, 2018b). I use this in-depth understanding of each person in two ways: first, to help the couple collaboratively brainstorm ways to prevent the vicious circles that result from the ways each partner's "legacy issues" intersect with the other's; and second, to find ways that they can work as a team to help each other with whatever individual issues each might be struggling (Wachtel, 2018a).

INITIAL ASSESSMENT AND CASE FORMULATION

When I'd scheduled Matt and Lara for a virtual first session in June 2020, I was more than a little anxious. I'd been working virtually for a few months, but they were the first couple I'd be seeing whom I had never met in person. Added to this was the fact that to escape the confinement of a New York City apartment during the prevaccine COVID lockdown, I was in a rental house that had a not-so-reliable internet connection and I was still experimenting with different chairs and pillows to see if I could make myself as comfortable as I had been in my beloved office chair.

Prior to the session I had sent them this instruction: "I'd like to replicate as much as possible the experience you would have if I were seeing you in my office. So please sit together somewhere where I can see more of you than just your face. And make yourself as comfortable as possible. If you were in my office, I'd ask you to sit together on the couch and I would be offering you some coffee or tea before we got started."

At the appointed time, I admitted them into my virtual office and was taken aback to find them stretched out on their bed! "Oh my," I thought to myself. They took my instructions more literally than I had imagined or intended. They soon explained, however, that their kids were home because their schools had instituted remote learning during the lockdown and there was no place for privacy in their apartment except in their bedroom. I've always tried to be flexible, and seeing people virtually has certainly accelerated my learning curve on that!

We were meeting at 9:15 in the morning. In answer to my "Hello, nice to meet you" greeting, Lara responded by saying "Yes, I'm glad we're meeting. I barely made it on time." She went on to explain that since she'd been up, she had walked their dog, given the kids breakfast, broken up an argument between their two boys and checked that they each were properly enrolled on their iPads for school that day. Five or six minutes before our session was to begin, Lara had come into their bedroom with a cup of coffee for herself and for Matt, whom she had woken up in time for our meeting. She sounded tired and worn out. "I let him sleep because he's had terrible insomnia and was up all night with stomach problems."

I started the session by explaining how I generally do a first meeting. "We'll spend a little bit of time with each of you telling me why you're seeking couple therapy, but today we won't go into detail about the issues or start working on them. If it's all right with you, I'd like to spend most of the session getting a sense of what drew you to each other, what made you commit to one another, what were the good things in the relationship in the beginning, and what if any of those things are still present despite the problems you are having. I do this because it's an occupational hazard of couple therapists to forget about the good stuff. After all, you're coming with problems and, understandably, that's what sessions focus on. So, it's important for me to have deeply ingrained in my psyche the good things that were and might still be there in your relationship, so I don't lose sight of the big picture."

Matt was 46 and Lara was 47; they'd been married for 15 years and had known each other for 2 years before getting married. They had two boys, ages 13 and 9. Matt worked in a small public relations firm owned by Lara's mother, and Lara was a self-employed speech therapist specializing in work with severely physically disabled children. Here's how they each described why they were seeking couple therapy.

LARA: I've been superfrustrated for a while. When we have an argument, Matt withdraws. He doesn't talk to me for days at a time. We have a little office in the back of the apartment—one of the kids uses it now during the day for school—but as soon as it's free, Matt basically hangs out in there. And it seems like we're getting into arguments a lot. I know being cooped up together in the apartment doesn't help, but it's been this way for a long time—way before COVID. I know he works very hard and he's working nonstop trying to save the business during this crisis—but still, everything about the house and kids and everything else is something I take care of. And when I ask him to do something, he says he'll do it but then forgets or does it way after it needed to be done. I get annoyed and then he's mad at me for criticizing him, and we don't talk for days at a time. I guess I just reached my limit. I don't want to live like this.

MATT: To be honest, I didn't want to do this. We did couple therapy once before, about 6 or 7 years ago, and we both found that we'd argue even more when we left the session. We learned some things about our patterns and what the therapist called the "dance we do," but we'd leave the session angry and we both thought, "This isn't going anywhere." But you came highly recommended and Lara was so insistent that I finally agreed to do it. (*He paused briefly, then went on.*) Lara's description was right: We've become distant from one another and we're arguing a lot. But Lara doesn't get how critical she is—she's constantly telling me to do this and that and that I messed up by not doing it on her time frame. She doesn't seem to understand or care about the stress I'm under in the business right now. I can't talk to her about it, because I work in her mother's firm, and she always takes her mother's side when I try to tell her what's going on in the office. I get it. It's hard to be in the middle like that. But sometimes I think she's more loyal to her mother than to me. But it's true, Lara does have a lot on her plate. I do, too. But maybe I don't express enough appreciation for everything she does."

At this point I told them that they had each given me exactly what I'd wanted—just a little bit of an understanding of what was going on. "I know you both have a lot to say about your perspective on what the other said, but, as I described earlier, if you can hold off on that, I'd like to get a clear understanding what brought you together and made you feel you could make a life with one another, before getting more detail about the issues that have brought you here."

Lara had tremendous admiration for Matt's intelligence. But most importantly, she felt that he was a generous and deeply good person. I asked her to elaborate on that and she gave several examples of how touched she was by Matt's kindness to friends and strangers alike. "And we had a lot of fun. Of course, we were young and partying a lot, and probably drinking too much, but we laughed so much. It was great."

Matt in turn described Lara "as the kindest, most loving person I'd ever met. And I loved her family. They were so warm and accepting." In answer to my question about what, if any, of the things they'd felt in the beginning were still there, despite the difficulties they were having, Matt exclaimed, "It's *all* still there," sounding shocked by the question. "Everything. I still think she's the kindest, most loving person in the world."

Lara was a little more subdued in her answer. "I still feel he's a deeply good and incredibly intelligent person. But maybe it's me, I'm not finding him so much fun anymore. His withdrawal and anger, and my resentment of it all, is really getting in the way. We seem so separate—not soul mates anymore."

The session ended with my giving them feedback. I started by summarizing my understanding of what they each felt concerned about in the relationship. I told them that they were in "agreement"—using this word emphasizes a commonality between them— that the relationship had become tense and that they were both unhappy with the distance that had developed between them. Though there were immediate stresses (e.g., COVID isolation, business worries, children at home doing remote learning) these stresses seemed to have exacerbated some long-standing issues that had not been resolved.

If at all possible, and sometimes it just isn't, I include in the feedback some of the positives that I've trained myself to observe. With Lara and Matt this was easy to do. For instance, even though Matt had not wanted to do couple therapy, he was fully present and participatory. Additionally, Matt ended his defense of himself in response to Lara's complaints, by extending an olive branch, saying, "Maybe I don't express enough appreciation." Lara had laughed in acknowledgment of Matt's comment about how they had learned about the "dance they were doing with each other." They had shared a joke about this, and it was clear that Lara could still find Matt amusing.

The reasons they each had given for why they fell in love and decided to make a life with one another were deep ones, involving admiration and respect for the other's values and way of being in the world. Additionally, they were not harsh, or out for the jugular as so many couples are when they've reached the point that they're seeking couple therapy. They seemed to be able to be disappointed, frustrated, and angry without losing touch with the love they have for one another. They corrected me on this one. "We're on good behavior here," said Lara. "It gets pretty bad—we say things to each other that are really, *really* bad."

"I'm a fighter," added Matt. "I'm not proud of it, but I know how to hurt someone if I'm mad. But, you're right, I don't think it ever gets to feeling we don't love each other anymore."

Although it is usually possible to find something affirming to say, feedback must be authentic. Few couples interact as lovingly in a first session as did Matt and Lara. Not infrequently, couples treat each other disrespectfully and make toxic and hurtful comments. When that's the case, I might say something like this:

> "You each are so hurt and angry that it was difficult for you to listen to the other without mobilizing a counterattack and striking back in a way that would wound the other. Of course, this may feel good in the moment but it gets you nowhere in terms of having a happy and satisfying relationship. One of the first things we'll need to work on is staying calm and having a mind-set of really wanting to understand what your partner is feeling. This should be possible, because there still seems to be some affection between you—I noticed you laughed together for a moment—and you each claim to still love one another. But you've gotten into a habit of communicating in a way that's hurtful and unproductive."

BEGINNING PHASE OF THERAPY

At the beginning of our second session, Matt and Lara each said that it had been a long time since they had thought about the positive things they once had, and to some extent *still* had, with each other. My pointing out some strengths they had as a *couple* had been particularly meaningful to them, and I knew that I had begun to form a therapeutic alliance with them as a *team*. The alliance with a couple is separate and distinct from the alliance with each of them as individuals.

I then asked them to tell me anything about themselves that they thought was important for me to know. I explained that I would eventually want to go into a good deal of detail about their family history, but for now, I just wanted to be sure that I knew some basics that could be important in helping me understand some things that might have had an impact on who they are and what each of them brings to the relationship. "It could be anything—not only from your childhood but also from when you were an adult—anything that is important in your life, even something that may have happened to a friend or a family member. Anything at all that's important for me know in terms of giving me some background about where you are coming from. And it could be good things, too—adventures, big successes in business, sports, winning the lottery!" In recent years, I've begun to ask this question, because I realized that the couple's urgency to start working on their difficulties often meant delaying getting family history and other information that would provide context and texture to them as individuals. Originally a stopgap measure on my part, I came to see it as not only a valuable source of factual information but also a way of learning about the personal narrative that each person told about themselves.

Matt started by saying that he has a brother just 11 months older than himself (as well as an older sister) and that they have very different personalities and are not particularly close. "I could go on and on about my family. My mother has a big problem with gambling. She once stole a lot of money from me to pay a gambling debt but eventually gave it back. They're self-involved. Almost never make time to see our kids."

Lara joined in. "Matt's family is very different from mine. My family is crazy about Matt, and they pretty much have adopted him!"

Lara's parents had emigrated to the United States and "they both worked incredibly hard to make ends meet. I was a latchkey child but I understood, and it was okay. I felt for them. They'd been through so much. They lost a 6-month-old child to sudden infant death syndrome before I was born."

I then followed up on the question I had asked them to think about at the end of our first meeting: "What do you know about yourself that makes you not always the easiest person in the world to be married to?" This question sets an important tone—our work together won't be about blame and fault. Rather, we'll look at what each person contributes to the difficulties and what they can do differently to make things better.

Matt started by saying he knows he is very competitive. Once he's arguing, he holds his ground and must win. It takes him a long time to cool off. "Lara can just let it go—she wants to pretend that it never happened—but I can't. I guess I hold grudges, though I try not to."

Lara said that she becomes very anxious when they argue. "I hate confrontations. I'm a peacemaker." She also said that she likes to do things quickly and is impatient with delay. This comes up with the children, as well as Matt. "I'd like to be more mellow and relaxed—not as compulsive about getting chores done right away."

We started by exploring how these characteristics entered into the difficulties they were having. In the first few sessions of my work with couples, I ask them to recount in detail a recent instance of an argument or the kind of tension or bad feeling that led them to seek couple therapy. My aim is to get a handle on both the type of content that triggers them and the reciprocal patterns of interaction that are leading to problems. I state from the outset, however, that once I've heard a few of the arguments, we will not be using the sessions to unpack the upsets of the prior week. Rather, we'll focus on more big picture issues such as how to maintain closeness, how to get back to the positives they had in the beginning of their relationship, how to quickly resolve conflicts when they occur, and how to keep their relationship lively and sexually intimate. I gave them this preview to whet their appetite. The sooner we resolve the immediate tensions, the sooner we can get to things that would enhance their relationship, not just restore peace. Couples are heartened by this, and it lays the groundwork for my later interruption of their rehashing of arguments to focus instead on wishes and ways to enliven their relationships and grow closer.

Initially we worked on what happened after they had an argument. I asked Lara to describe how she feels when Matt is cold to her and days would go by without any friendly contact. I encouraged her to bring the feeling back and to see where she feels it in her body. She answered, "I feel a sense of emptiness. I'm so lonely. So alone. I don't know what to do. I don't know how to bring him back. I don't think he understands how awful it feels."

As Lara spoke, Matt began to get annoyed—disputing that he'd been so distant and going back to the *reason* for his anger in the first place. It was helpful to me to see his "hot under the collar" agitation and the defensiveness that followed. We worked on what he could do to stay calm in the session. Heightened physiological arousal can be addressed in a variety of ways. I often find it useful to suggest some deep breathing and suggested that

Matt try that. I also asked him to center himself in the here and now by paying attention to the weight of his body against the surface of the bed on which he was sitting. We explored, too, what kind of self-talk he thought might be calming to him, for instance, saying to himself, "Lara is the woman I love" or reminding himself that staying calm is a "win–win strategy" (a term he often used).

In the early stages of a disagreement, Matt would try to stop the conversation, but Lara would persist. She found it very difficult to leave things unresolved and would follow Matt into another room so they could keep talking about an issue. Matt would feel trapped and get angrier, eventually exploding and withdrawing.

In future sessions, I would choose the choice point that highlighted the steps—even if small ones—that each was taking to translate this understanding of their pattern into action. So, for instance, if they had a disagreement that had not escalated nearly as badly, we would look at what enabled them to prevent escalation. Success and progress are big motivators, and the more we could find some signs of change, the harder they worked at doing even better.

Pursuing an angry partner who wants to withdraw is a common problem that not only leads to verbal escalation but not infrequently can result in verbal and physical abuse. With many couples, it is important to brainstorm with them specific strategies they can use to disengage when either of them is having the "here we go again feeling" and wants to stop in what the other regards as midstream. It is often helpful to set a time to talk again, so the person who urgently feels like they still want to make their point, does not feel they are being permanently shut down, or that their concerns are being swept under the rug. Carefully spelling out what each could do to use the time apart to really cool off, and not just to better prepare their argument, is an important part of the work.

As the work proceeded, both Matt and Lara felt that they were making some progress. Promoting memories of their deep connection, and focusing in the session on the positive nuggets that were embedded in their upset, had led to less conflict at home. Matt worked on staying calm and being less defensive. When they did argue, Matt, understanding how hard it was for Lara, would make an effort to stay connected even when he was taking the space he needed to cool off. Lara, in turn, was trying hard to let Matt retreat from an unresolved conflict, understanding that he needed time to calm down.

But the work was only beginning, and much of what they were each bothered about had not been resolved. Lara was still quite upset with Matt's preoccupation with his own stresses and physical ailments: "He's checked out. I can't count on him to take care of things—and he's much less involved with the kids than he used to be." And Matt was angry that Lara was allied with her mother and that "she doesn't understand the unfairness of what's going on at work." At this point, I saw them as having made some progress. They were arguing less, and when they did argue, it didn't escalate. They seemed more in touch with love and tender feelings for one another. But clearly, we had only just begun.

INTERMEDIATE PHASE OF THERAPY

Now that things had calmed down between them, it was time to get to the substantive issues that each had raised in the first session. It's important to deescalate arguments and help the couple recover positive feelings before trying to tackle the knottier problems on which their arguments are based. With the goodwill and calm that they have built, daunting differences are more manageable, and they can be a team in finding solutions to problems that seemed unsolvable.

As mentioned earlier, Matt worked with Lara's mother (to whom he referred by her first name "Sally") in a small public relations firm that she had built up over the past 30 years. About 10 years ago, she had invited Matt to work with her. Over the years, he functioned more and more as a partner. Lara's mother, who at the time of our work was in her early 80s, left much of the day-to-day work and decision making to Matt. The business was structured so that Matt was officially an employee, not a partner. Two years previously, Lara's mom felt they needed more executive-level help and she talked to Matt about inviting her nephew Erik to work with them. Matt liked Erik very much but resented that Erik was getting paid almost as much as himself, even though he was completely inexperienced: "I know it takes time to get up to speed, but he's been there long enough that he shouldn't be messing up as much as he does. I have to double-check everything and undo his mistakes. But I'm really stuck here. If I try to talk to Sally about it, she shuts down the conversation. She just doesn't want to hear about it. I back off then—I don't want to cause some family rift."

Lara felt stuck in the middle between her loyalty to her mother and that to Matt. "My mother loves Matt like a son, but she's frustrated with how he works, and she complains about that to me. She complains about how many days he comes in late because of stomach problems or migraines. It's very upsetting to me. I want to be supportive of Matt, but my mother is in her 80s and I'm worried about how stressed she is."

At this point Matt interjected, "Sally has no idea how much work I do at home at night—it's really frustrating. And she has no idea how much of Erik's work I end up doing."

At this point Matt, Lara, and I had a decision to make. Clearly, there were larger family issues here, and we could convert the work to family therapy. Sessions would include Lara's mother and perhaps her nephew, too. When I raised this possibility, Lara and Matt both strongly objected to that. They felt they needed to work on their relationship and didn't want Lara's family to know that they had sought couple therapy.

Lara felt that in order for her to better set boundaries with her mother, Matt had to have a conversation with Sally, so that they could straighten out the tension between them. He agreed that was the right thing to do, but several weeks went by without Matt initiating what he knew would be a difficult discussion: "I'm afraid I'll say things that I'll regret and don't want to blow up in anger."

I then strongly suggested that he, Erik, and Lara's mother see a therapist I know who specializes in working with small family businesses. Matt agreed that was a good idea, but again, using Lara's words, "dragged his feet" on talking to his mother-in-law about this possibility. Lara became increasingly upset by the delay. Like Lara, I am someone who takes care of things quickly, and I found myself strongly identifying with Lara. This is one of the hardest parts of being a couple therapist. We often have strong reactions to couples' issues that parallel our own. Much more than with individual therapy, couple work stirs what psychodynamic therapists call countertransference. To counteract my bias, I worked hard at framing this as their having different styles and rhythms. Matt needed to let ideas percolate before he acted on them. Lara, on the other hand, took action very quickly. Weeks went by, with Lara becoming increasingly upset. "It's not just this. I can't get him to see a GI specialist either. He's not following through on anything. He's got bad stomach problems, insomnia, migraines, and he's not taking care of any of it. He's completely let himself go. You don't know what he usually looks like—20 pounds lighter, fit, well-groomed—not at all the person you're seeing now." I was struck by Lara's introjection and began to wonder if Matt was clinically depressed. But rather than divert the conversation to that topic, I made a note to myself to revisit this comment as soon as I saw an appropriate opening.

Matt finally did speak to Lara's mother about seeing a family business consultant, who met with Matt, Sally, and Erik in various combinations, and some progress was made. Within that structure, Matt was able to discuss that he felt he was not being adequately respected or compensated for the very significant contribution he had made to the growth of the business ever since he had come on board. Lara's mother had understood, and they were making some structural changes that would address a number of Matt's concerns.

Lara also worked on setting boundaries with her mother, and we discussed how to lovingly remind her mother that she didn't want to hear complaints about Matt. We then also talked about how Matt and Lara wanted to handle Matt's talking with Lara about work stresses. "I know it's tough on Lara, and I guess I just have to respect that. She's very close to her mom, and I love Sally, too, and I understand why I shouldn't really complain to Lara about her."

At this point in the work, it seemed that *some* progress was being made. But at the same time, Matt was not functioning well at all. He was exhibiting many symptoms of depression. He agreed with what Lara had said in an earlier session, that he had let himself go, gained a lot of weight, didn't shower regularly, and was irritable with the kids. But Matt attributed this to the changes in his life due to the pandemic and stated that he didn't *feel* depressed. Nonetheless, he was willing to see a psychiatrist for an evaluation. Once more, it was several weeks until he actually followed through on the referral, and Lara became increasingly frustrated and despairing.

Matt liked the psychiatrist and in addition to being prescribed medication for depression, he had regular Zoom meetings with her. We all breathed a sigh of relief as a result of Matt's willingness to talk with a therapist and that he seemed to accept that the diagnosis of depression was correct. Lara understood that it would take a few weeks for the medication to take effect, and she tried to be patient. But she was concerned that not only wasn't she seeing some gradual improvement but also she felt that Matt wasn't making any effort and was just relying on the pill to kick in. "He's still staying up very late and not even trying to get on a normal sleep schedule." The psychiatrist he was working with referred him to a sleep specialist for a one- or two-session consultation to learn better sleep habits. Sensing that Lara was at her wit's end, Matt followed through on the psychiatrist's suggestion. Still, nothing changed. By now Lara was both fuming and despairing. "What's the point? He went to the sleep specialist, but I don't see him trying to do one thing that the doctor suggested."

Once, in the middle of the night, Matt wrote Lara a letter about how much he loved her and how he wanted to be a better husband. They had a very emotional session about that letter, and Lara felt relieved that Matt was finally understanding what she had been going through. But 1 week went by and nothing changed. Then another week went by, and still Lara didn't see any effort on Matt's part. And then another week with no change. One night Lara wrote Matt a letter about how she loved him but didn't see how they could keep living together in this situation. I worked with them on how Lara could handle Matt's depression in a way that would be more helpful to him and more comforting to herself.

Then one day, before our next session, I got a call from Lara. Matt was in a residential rehabilitation facility. He had confessed to her that for the past 2 years he had been addicted to cocaine!

Readers who have experience with addiction must be scratching their heads at this point. How could I have missed something so obvious? Of course, I asked myself that repeatedly, often in the middle of the night! I have very limited experience with cocaine addiction, and I took solace from the fact that the psychiatrist, sleep expert, and family business consultant were as clueless as I had been.

Matt had been home from rehab for several weeks when he called to say that they had a lot to discuss and wanted to see me as soon as possible. I barely recognized Matt. His unruly hair had been tamed, he was freshly shaven, and he had lost a lot of weight. Most strikingly, there was an alertness to his manner that I had never seen.

The session started with Matt apologizing to me, as he had to all the other therapists who had tried to help him. This was not a pro forma apology. It was clear that he felt sincere remorse. It was important that he did this because, despite my understanding that what had happened was part and parcel of addiction, I felt I'd been made a fool of and felt irritated. I wasn't proud of feeling this way and was relieved that my too personal sense of betrayal all but vanished once I started working with them again.

Matt went on to tell me about the full extent of the addiction. It had started about 6 months before the outbreak of COVID. He'd been at a 50th birthday party for a client. "I guess I wanted to show him that I was young and cool." Matt described it as feeling great, and he realized that he'd been "in a rut." In the beginning, he used it only once or twice a week, and only when out with buddies from work. Soon he craved it more and more. "Someone at work knew a dealer, and he got it for me. I wanted to protect my family, and I never dealt with the dealer directly, so he didn't know who I was. After a while, I wasn't enjoying it at all. I felt sick without it and I needed more and more of it just to feel okay. I'd get up the middle of the night to use it—I hid it in the back of the bathroom cabinet. I tried to stop a few times but just couldn't. It's hard to explain what it's like, but I thought I'd die without it."

Lara, according to Matt, had been "incredibly supportive." "Coming home to so much support is amazing. I know I won't relapse because of that support." Hearing this, a red flag went up for me. I wondered if Matt was putting too much of the responsibility for his recovery on Lara. And I was also concerned that so much appreciation of her supportiveness didn't allow Lara to express the full range of her feelings.

I decided to be very explicit about my concerns and said, "Lara, how is that for you? Matt is so appreciative of your support and it's a big part of why he feels he won't relapse. But that's a lot of responsibility on your shoulders."

Before Lara could answer, Matt corrected his statement. "No, no. Of course, I have to stay clean on my own and it can't depend on whether Lara is being supportive. I know that a lot of people relapse—and some of the people in my group already have. But I'm sure I won't. Drugs, drinking . . . they don't interest me at all anymore."

"I'm relieved you raised this," said Lara. "I've been so scared of him relapsing. I feel I have to be very careful about what I say to him. I really don't think he'll relapse, but if he did, I don't know if I could go through it again."

With this go-ahead, Lara began to talk about how deeply shaken she was about all the lies Matt had told. "I was so worried about his stomach problems—he was always running to the bathroom, and I was so frustrated that he wouldn't go to a doctor and check out what was going on." She understood that it was an addiction that "had hijacked his brain," but she had always assumed that they were so close that there would never be secrets between them. The deception he'd engaged in was "like a stab in my heart. I had trusted him 100%." She felt terrible that the deep and profound trust she had once had was gone forever. Matt understood this and vowed to do anything to regain her trust. This sounded good, but we soon hit some pretty significant bumps in the road.

In order to finance his drug addiction, Matt had been retained by a few private clients and did not disclose this work to his mother-in-law. He justified this to himself by saying that these were old high school friends for whom he was informally doing some public relations work and they paid him what they wanted—well below what his firm would charge. Lara was again pulled into a loyalty conflict. Matt had been very appreciative of how supportive his mother-in-law had been when she realized that so much of what she had been concerned about was due to addiction. Matt teared up when he described it. "She gave me a big hug. So loving. So supportive." Lara felt strongly that Matt needed to tell her mother about his side business. Matt disagreed. At this point I asked them to look at each other instead of at me, and asked them each to talk from their hearts about what they felt in regard to this issue. But each also needed to listen to the other with a mind-set of "what makes sense to me, what can I understand, what can I agree with" rather than listening with the mental set of waiting to rebut and advocate for their own position. At first, Matt had trouble with this. He felt it was important to correct what he regarded as Lara's exaggerations and inaccuracies. I reassured him that there would be time later for that, but asked for now that he try listening for what he could agree with and what was right. "I get why this is difficult. It takes some practice because it's not the way most people listen. But I think if you have a joining mind-set, it might be easier than you think." When they each had finished explaining what they felt, I underlined how well they had done in actually listening to the other's point of view. As I do with many couples, I suggested that they let what the other said percolate for a while rather than coming to some agreement there and then. Often people soften their position a bit when they don't feel boxed in and pushed to resolve something immediately. They left that session feeling heard, and feeling good about how they had interacted with one another around a difficult topic.

The following week, Matt said that he had discussed the issue with his rehab group and decided that Lara was right and he needed to talk with his mother-in-law about what he had done. There was some give on Lara's part, too. She felt that as long as she knew he would tell her mother the truth, she could live with his timetable, which was to tell her after they had all been together on Thanksgiving, just a few weeks away.

As I said earlier, I have very little experience working with drug addiction. But I was struck by how much the work with Matt and Lara resembled my work with couples who are trying to recover from an affair. So, for instance, Lara was heartbroken that some basic faith she had that they were a "we" and had no secrets from one another had been shattered. I explained that, in my experience, scars can heal and deep trust can be restored, but it requires a *daily* experience of the other being up front, transparent, and open. Lara disliked how suspicious she had become, but when Matt didn't tell her small things that she knew weren't important, she felt depressed and worried about their relationship. "I know it's stupid, but really, if he would tell me everything—like letting the kids stay up later than we agreed—I think it would help."

Matt had trouble with this. "I don't want to be judged constantly. I don't want to feel like I have to report to you about everything I do."

In rehab, Matt realized that he had a lifelong habit of preferring to finesse a situation rather than have conflict. He was committed to tackling this head on and knew that at the core of his drug use was a massive avoidance of difficult feelings. I encouraged him to include noticing times that he might be *omitting* something in his communication in his efforts to overcome avoidance, when he just didn't mention some small thing to which Lara might have a negative reaction. Lara thanked me for mentioning that. Important omissions can be as hurtful as outright lies. It helped Matt to think about the effort he would make to be honest with Lara not as *reporting* to her but as working on an issue central to his recovery.

We went on to discuss one of the reasons that Matt avoided conflict. Matt described being overwhelmed by the anger he felt once an argument began. "I love my brother and we mostly get along, but boy, when we were kids, the fighting was bad." Though his brother was the bigger and stronger of the two, Matt was skilled at knowing the "cruelest" (his word) and most shaming things to say. When Lara and Matt did argue, that side of Matt was activated, and to avoid being "mean" (again, his word) he skirted around issues so there would not be an argument.

Lara chimed in, "Well I'm no saint either when we argue. I say things that hurt you, too, but that doesn't make me avoid telling you the truth."

Here was an important choice point. I could focus on the anger in what Lara said, or I could say something that joined them in problem solving. I choose the latter because it both reinforced self-disclosure and helped them join together in healing. Here's what I said: "Lara, I know you are angry with Matt about this, but I'm also so impressed with how open you are being about how hostile you, too, can be in an argument. I think we need to talk more about how you both can tone down conflicts when they arise."

At first, this all seemed quite hypothetical. In the months since Matt had returned home from rehab, they had not had *any* arguments of the type they had had before. But finally an old-style fight had erupted. It involved Matt not telling Lara that he had gotten a speeding ticket. They had both said things that were so hurtful and mean that they didn't want to repeat them in the session.

I have found it useful to explain to couples that when they are mean in an argument, it's because they are dissociating or cutting off an awareness that this is a person they love and who loves them. They've lost a sense of the whole person, and in those moments they are fighting with an *enemy*, not their loved one. I revisited with them what we had talked about early in our work—finding ways to calm themselves down physiologically (e.g., pausing and taking some deep breaths), as well as talking themselves down emotionally by using self-talk that would help deescalate their emotions. I recommended that they get a book called *Instant Calm* (Wilson, 1995) that describes 100 different methods to calm down very quickly, so that each could experiment with some techniques they thought might work for them.

In order to stay emotionally in touch with the fact that the person one is angry with is *also* the person they love, I suggest that it might be helpful for couples to create a "Reminder" photo album in which they put particularly endearing photos of their partner that trigger the memory of the love and warmth that they have felt in the past. They could also print out one or two of those photos and put them in a very prominent place—the refrigerator door or a bathroom mirror, so that they have easy access to images that stir the positive memories of the other. It is, of course, difficult to do this when agitated. But some couples calm themselves down by taking a bathroom break and this would be a good time to try to reconnect emotionally by looking at these images.

Photos can be particularly useful for addressing the upset that often follows an argument. Matt took a long time to calm down. And though he had shortened the period he needed to withdraw, it was still difficult for him to let go of the fight. Intrigued by the photo idea, Matt reported that he had printed out a photo but hoped that they wouldn't have that kind of argument again, so the photo wouldn't be needed.

For Lara, the issue wasn't so much what she said when angry, but rather the intense loneliness she felt when Matt was withdrawn. Lara didn't think looking at photos would help at all, and I agreed that she shouldn't bother with that if she sensed it wouldn't work for her. It was clear to Lara that the intense discomfort she felt until she and Matt were "good" with each other was related to how alone she felt while waiting after school for her mother to return home. Matt said, "But I'm home," and joked that he should send Lara a text saying "home soon." Lara, laughed and said that yes, that would help. I laughed with them and commented that though they were joking around, underneath the lightheartedness there was deep caring and a wish to help each other feel better.

Another similarity to working with affairs is the issue of how much the injured party has a right to ask of the other. Lara wanted Matt to stop being friends with Charlie, someone Matt had been close to for several years. Charlie had told Lara that he had known about Matt's addiction but never confronted him or thought that it was his obligation to tell Lara. "He said that he thought you needed to hit bottom before you'd be open to help. That's fine for him to say, but you were drinking, too, and could have OD'd. Didn't he worry when you had a fender bender with the kids in the car?" Furthermore, Lara felt that Charlie was someone who had often encouraged Matt to drink too much and to buy luxury items they could not afford. Matt believed that Lara was unfairly scapegoating Charlie and that she had misunderstood him when he told her that he knew Matt was addicted. "I think he didn't literally know—maybe just suspected it." In one of their heated discussions about this, Matt mentioned that Lara had a friend whom he disliked, and he didn't ask her to stop seeing that person. This comparison incensed Lara, and she felt that by equating the two situations, he was minimizing the seriousness and unique stress on the marriage that had resulted from his behavior while addicted.

Matt experienced this request as punishment and was angry about that. "How long am I going to have to pay for this?! Am I always going to be the bad guy—one down in every disagreement we have because of what I put you through?" It took several weeks to work this out, but eventually they arrived at a compromise with which they both could live. Matt agreed not to meet or talk to Charlie for 6 months, at which point they would revisit the decision. They both agreed that their feelings could evolve in that time.

I commented and underlined how positive it was that they each could envision a change in their position. "Neither of you is digging in and agreeing to the compromise with a mind-set that in 6 months, you'll have to battle it out again because what you think and feel now is set in stone. That's really terrific."

In the next session, Lara said something that, again, was very familiar to me from my work with couples trying to recover from an affair. "One of the worst things for me about what happened is that I don't like who I've become. I hate setting rules and telling you what to do. I hate being suspicious and worried all the time."

Touched by what Lara said, Matt reassured her that though he initially resisted what felt like a demand to stop seeing his friend, he really did understand. "I get it, I really do, and I'm sorry about it."

I underlined what Matt said—it was not about Matt complying with rules, but rather acting in a way that would ease Lara's pain. Matt agreed. "Yes, that's right. Sometimes I get a little annoyed, but really, I do understand and want Lara to trust me again."

CONCLUDING PHASE OF THERAPY

As the months went by, Matt's and Lara's confidence that Matt would not relapse increased. Commenting on how much Matt had changed, Lara said, "He's up front. Doesn't harbor resentments. Deals with things right away instead of procrastinating or avoiding difficult situations."

Matt added, "I think we're closer than ever. I tell her everything. We laugh, we touch a lot, we're having sex again—honestly, I think it's the best it's ever been with us."

Sometimes I felt concerned that Lara felt pressure to agree with Matt that everything was wonderful. I also wanted to counteract any pressure she might be feeling by my emphasis on the gains that they had made. With this in mind, I asked Lara if there was anything that she had been hesitant to raise. Two issues came up. Lara was concerned that Matt had an addictive personality and that his new interest in collecting guitars felt too intense. Matt countered that except for one or two of them, he was not "attached" to these guitars and considered them an investment. He had studied the guitar market and believed that he would sell the guitars at a profit. Additionally, Lara was concerned that in investing in guitars, he had made a big financial decision on his own, and we revisited earlier conversations about trust and transparency. Matt agreed to show Lara a spread sheet on what had been bought and sold, and for the time being this particular issue was resolved.

"There's something I'm embarrassed to talk about," said Lara the next time we met. "I consider myself a pretty secure person, and I don't like the insecurity I'm feeling." She went on to say that she felt excluded from the close friendships Matt had formed with his rehab group. She wanted to be his confidante and felt badly in particular about Matt's conversations with a younger woman who had been in rehab with him. She did not think Matt was having a sexual affair or even an "emotional" one, but she felt that this relationship took away from the special place in Matt's life she thought she had. Matt was touched by the vulnerability Lara had shown in saying this and in response explained in detail the kinds of talks he had with this woman, which were not at all like his conversations with Lara. Additionally, he arranged for Lara to meet her, as well as all the members of his rehab group. Lara liked them and understood that there was no need to be threatened by these relationships.

At this point, I raised with them the possibility of meeting less frequently, and we started to meet every other week instead of weekly. Increasingly, the sessions felt a bit forced. We all were straining to use the time meaningfully. It was clearly time to stop. Both Matt and Lara expressed sadness about totally stopping our work. It wasn't that they felt they really needed to keep seeing me to maintain the gains they had made but rather that they would miss me and our time together. I shared with them that I felt the same way and that I, too, was finding it hard to say good-bye. We talked about how we had not only worked well together but we also just seemed to *click* with each other on a personal level.

We went back and forth with one another about what date should be our final session. Lara was apprehensive about the holidays. "I don't really think Matt will relapse, but I know that with all the parties and socializing, I'm going to be very nervous." At first, Matt took offense at this. He was confident that being around alcohol and possibly even drugs would not be a problem for him and was irritated that Lara had some doubts about it. But as happened many times before in our work, Matt very quickly challenged his own reflexive irritation and was able to respond to Lara with empathy. I took this as an opportunity to once again highlight the progress Matt had made in his ability to catch himself in what he called "the old habit" of responding defensively.

My work with Lara and Matt never came to a hard stop. I invited them to contact me whenever they felt like a session or two would be useful. I explained to them, as I do to all couples with whom I work, that they should not regard contacting me as a sign of failure or a need to start all over again. Couples often take me up on this invitation. Sometimes they ask *me* to contact *them* in a few months to see if they want to come in, and I'm okay with doing that. I send myself a reminder on my Google calendar to be sure to follow through on that request. These tune-up sessions are often one-time meetings just a few times a year. We start by reviewing what has been going well and then brainstorm on areas where they need a little help. I have seen Lara and Matt five or six times in the past couple of years. Matt has not relapsed, and they've maintained the gains they made during our work together.

FURTHER REFLECTIONS AND IMPLICATIONS

The first thing I'm hoping that the reader will take away from this case study is the power of finding nuggets of strength and using those observations to foster hope and motivation to change. Though the particulars of this case were far from typical, the methods I used apply to work with all couples. By noticing and underlining the moments when each person is showing empathy, being less defensive, really hearing the other, or taking in my comments and suggestions, I help build attitudes and states of mind that over time lead the couple to more easily resolve what at first may seem to be daunting differences.

The second takeaway is the importance of rooting for a couple as a "we." When I asked Matt and Lara for permission to describe the work we had done in a composite case study, I also invited them to write me a note about what they each felt had been helpful or not so helpful, both before and after Matt's addiction was disclosed. They wrote me separate notes, and it was striking that they each mentioned what we would call the "therapeutic alliance" with them as a couple. Lara said, "You raised issues and concerns, while all the while being on our team and making us see why we love each other."

And Matt said, "You never pitted us against one another. This is so important to me as I'm ultracompetitive, but this never felt like one of us was wrong or right. It always felt like we should work this out as one entity, and we succeed and fail together."

Though these are powerful methods, many other factors contributed to the successful outcome in this case. Matt's excellent rehab program had helped him gain insight into himself. In my initial formulation, I had not realized how important a role avoidance of conflict had played in Matt's life. I also had underestimated the role of drinking in the "fun" they had together prior to having children. My work with them was enhanced by the therapy Matt was getting in his rehab work.

Additionally, they had good medical insurance that paid for rehab and allowed them to work with me for as long as it seemed useful. Often couple therapists have only a limited number of sessions to accomplish something. That makes it all the more important that the focus of the work is on the way couples communicate and resolve differences rather than the resolution of a particular issue in itself.

Another factor that contributed to the success of this work is that this couple did not have years of accumulated bitterness and anger. Though they had been having some marital difficulties even prior to Matt's addiction, the love they had for one another had not eroded. Lara wrote that prior to knowing about Matt's addiction, she'd been enormously frustrated by trying to figure out "where my beautiful, fun-loving husband" had gone. Sometimes, by the time couples seek therapy, the good feelings they had for one another are very distant memories. It is the work of therapy to try resuscitate the dormant love but, of course, that is not always possible.

Last, this case was a reminder of the importance of humility. I was stunned by my failure to even think that Matt might have a problem with addiction. Later, I was surprised by some of the things Matt and Lara mentioned in their posttherapy notes. Matt felt that I had modeled being open to criticism from him, and that helped him be less defensive. "You acknowledged when what you said was off-base and tried to understand why I was annoyed at you and then apologized." And Lara mentioned that the time I used a personal anecdote to show how love is expressed in the small things of daily life (my husband puts out my vitamins) was an important moment for her.

Writing about this couple has made me a bit nostalgic. I believe that looking for the strengths and good in people rather than the pathology not only makes the work more effective, but it also fosters our attachment to them. I've never said a final good-bye to them and I'm fine with that!

REFERENCES

Wachtel, E. F. (2018a, July/August). Becoming a therapist for each other: How to deepen couples therapy. *Psychotherapy Networker*.

Wachtel, E. F. (2018b). *The heart of couple therapy: Knowing what to do and how to do it.* New York: Guilford Press.

Wilson, P. (1995). *Instant calm: Over 100 easy-to-use techniques for relaxing mind and body.* New York: Plume.

CHAPTER 4

Integrative Psychodynamic Couple Therapy in the Presence of Enduring Personality Dysfunctions

ARTHUR C. NIELSEN

> When the one you love keeps hurting you, when the one who hurts you doesn't try to make it better, when the one you need abandons or frightens you, when the one you know becomes impenetrable or unknown to you, when the one who knows you no longer recognizes you—these are the ubiquitous traumas of love lost.
> —Virginia Goldner (2014, p. 403)

Editors' Comments

Art Nielsen offers an integrative approach to tackling the unique challenges of couple therapy when one or both partners have enduring personality features that interfere with their relationship. Even at lower levels of intensity, underlying issues stemming from individual personality can play a crucial role in relationship difficulties. These disruptive patterns can also be explicated and addressed in couple therapy—reducing their negative impact on the couple relationship. At higher levels of intensity, personality disorders may sabotage not only the partners' relationship but also the couple therapy.

    Nielsen clearly explicates the foundational psychoanalytic lens he adopts to understand the repetitive, exaggerated, and disruptive emotional and behavioral responses each partner brings to their relationship. Grounded in this approach, he methodically but sensitively explores both partners' developmental histories through an extended assessment process before beginning "formal" therapy sessions. Nielsen then expands that process to promote partners' enhanced understandings of themselves and each other. Harnessing the opportunities for corrective emotional experiences in the couple therapy, he models empathic responsiveness and then creates enactments of caring and emotional connection between partners within—and subsequently outside of—the couple therapy. Into this core framework, Nielsen skillfully and systematically integrates the tools and benefits of family systems, emotionally focused, cognitive-behavioral, and psychoeducational models.

> There is much to be learned from this chapter—ranging from explicit lists of principles of therapy with personality disordered clients or goals of a first session to gold nuggets interspersed throughout (e.g., the naming of relational "allergies" and the "Three C's" for handling escalating conflicts). Importantly, Nielsen notes that the goal of couple therapy is not the elimination of emotional sensitivities or behavioral reactivities left over from early experiences, but rather promoting their recognition and improved management to reduce their negative impact. Speaking to his internal experiences throughout the therapy, Nielsen shares how such work can be both humbling and deeply satisfying.

Intimate relationships are challenging for most people. They're even more challenging for individuals with significant personality dysfunctions, character pathology, or personality disorders, who often progress to the relationship hell described by Goldner above. Integrative couple therapy for such problems is something I've written about extensively (Nielsen, 2016, 2022) and illustrate in this chapter, while highlighting the utility of psychodynamic concepts.

I was a psychiatric resident at Yale in the 1970s when I saw my first couple in therapy. As someone who had taken many lessons growing up (in music, sports, dance), it made sense to me that I would meet with a couple and coach them on how to improve their communication (the almost universal couples' complaint). I wouldn't just hear them tell me what was wrong; I would witness it live and offer advice like a coach. Later, I dubbed this the *Talk-to-Each-Other Model*, or *Couple Therapy 1.0*, and it still serves as the scaffold for my work, as I usually focus early in therapy on the vicious cycles that interfere with the couple's communication and erode friendship, intimacy, and trust.

After Yale, I studied structural family therapy at the Philadelphia Child Guidance Clinic, psychoanalysis at the Chicago Psychoanalytic Institute, and behavioral interventions while teaching an undergraduate course on marriage. Each of these overarching approaches to couple therapy—systemic, psychodynamic, and behavioral/psychoeducational—improved my results. I call these "upgrades" to Couple Therapy 1.0 and have attempted to work out how to integrate and sequence them.

DYSFUNCTIONS OF PERSONALITY

Everyone has a "personality"—the internal psychology that makes us behave relatively consistently in different contexts—but enduring *maladaptive patterns of personality* compromise both individual and interpersonal well-being. Categorical varieties of personality disorders or dysfunctions—antisocial, borderline, histrionic, narcissistic, avoidant, and obsessive–compulsive—are useful ideal types, but current research favors a dimensional approach (American Psychiatric Association, 2022). Certain dimensions of personality merit therapeutic attention, including attachment security, self-esteem, emotion regulation, mentalization (psychological mindedness), empathic capacity, and maturity of ego defenses. Less healthy functioning in any of these areas leads to problems in intimate relationships, including excesses of dependency, anger, blame, distrust, grandiosity, entitlement, vengefulness, violence, shame, guilt, depression, distancing, addictions, affairs, and pretty much all the other problems we see in clinical couples.

From a psychodynamic perspective (Leone, 2008; Nielsen, 2017; Solomon, 1998), individuals challenged by personality dysfunctions present with exaggerated fears (negative transferences), unmet desires and needs (positive transferences), and maladaptive defenses (security operations, survival strategies). They fear and expect that others will reject, control, abuse, or criticize them. These expectations lead to anxiety (that needs won't be met), to depression (when needs are not met, including due to anxious avoidance), and to intensified security operations (like blaming and distancing) that make matters worse and confirm negative expectancies. Partners' negative reactions (both understandable and those resulting from their own personality issues) tend to confirm negative expectancies and maintain maladaptive relating. By contrast, secure persons enhance relationship success by self-disclosing when in need, listening when a partner is upset or critical, forgiving when a partner is unavailable or frustrating, and providing affirmation and pleasurable experiences that boost their partner's spirits.

Psychotherapy with individuals challenged by personality dysfunctions attempts to reduce these maladaptive expectations and behaviors while increasing the desirable attributes and skills of more mature people. To accomplish this, we employ the tools common to all psychotherapies as we attempt to illuminate what is going on (to add insight), facilitate corrective experiences, and teach and encourage better ways to meet fundamental human needs.

Facilitating Insight

To increase insight, we must look for the upstream sources of distress—the hidden issues that evoke shame, guilt, anxiety, and attachment insecurity—that power downstream secondary emotions (like anger and hopelessness) and maladaptive coping (like fight or flight). Doing so often uncovers prior traumatic experiences in our clients' lives. When it does, this not only helps explain maladaptive behaviors but can also render them less off-putting to partners, who can now see them as "psychological allergies" or adaptations to past stressors. Better than individual therapy, couple therapy can provide partners with metaphorical owner's manuals of each other that can make them more comprehensible and easier to live with.

Corrective Experiences, Facilitating Listening, Improving Attachment Security

Another advantage of couple therapy is the opportunity to disconfirm negative expectancies of partners in real time. Since, arguably, the greatest traumas inflicted by intimate partners on each other (per the opening quote) are combinations of neglect and negation, the core corrective experience in much couple therapy is helping partners to be heard, usually first by the therapist, then by their partner. This improves internal working models that usually include varieties of attachment insecurity.

Facilitating Emotion Regulation

The ability to regulate one's emotions when upset, and especially to calm oneself when under fire, is a vast topic containing much practical advice relevant to couple therapy (Fruzzetti, 2006; Nielsen, 2016, Chap. 12). Distinct from teaching specific skills (time-outs, deep breathing), a more general target and outcome of successful couple therapy is self-soothing accomplished by improved self-talk, what psychoanalysts refer to as "the self-analytic function." Ideally, a person whose emotions are boiling over can "stop and think," become curious about themselves and their partner, and consider ways to make things better.

Countertransference

Especially in couple therapy involving partners with personality dysfunctions, therapists must monitor their own emotional reactions. To do this, I imagine what frustrations and disappointments I might have if I were married to either partner, and I pay particular attention to negative feelings I have during sessions. Noticing a reflexive inclination to side against an obviously offensive partner is particularly important. If I can reframe, uncover, or give coherent voice to that partner's concerns, this often improves the repellent behavior, the couple's relationship, and the therapeutic alliance.

Non-Personality Variables and Coping Ability

While personality dysfunction is both common and routinely leads couples to seek therapy, other problems also cause conflict and distress and require our help. Taking a biopsychosocial approach to diagnosis, we should also assess biological issues (like depression, substance misuse, or physical illness), external stressors (like those from work, family, or prejudice), and the conflicts these and other life choices can elicit (like whether to relocate to a different city or to have another child). While the following case foregrounds personality problems, much couple therapy (as illustrated by other chapters in this book) is complicated by such matters that stretch our clients' personal capacities to cope.

INITIAL ASSESSMENT AND CASE FORMULATION

My 18-month therapy with Dan and Akira began with an email request via my website. Dan wrote that he had heard positive things about me from colleagues and wondered if I had time to see him and his longtime girlfriend, as they were considering moving in together. I phoned Dan, and we talked briefly. I try to keep such calls short so as not to jeopardize therapeutic neutrality, since the person calling is almost invariably more committed to therapy, whereas their partner may be more skeptical and require more work to convince them to trust me and give therapy a try. In this brief call, I learned that the couple, both divorced and in their early 50s, lived separately and were planning to buy a place together, with an eye toward getting married.

The opening phase of treatment is never easy for clients or therapists. We are all anxious and trying to make sense of what's going on. As I begin initial couple meetings, I remind myself of the following overlapping goals that I try to meet before time runs out:

- Develop an alliance with both partners while maintaining neutrality.
- Understand the couple's reasons for coming, including why they've come now.
- Place the current problem in its developmental context.
- Observe the couple "doing their problem" in their characteristic interaction cycle.
- Provide some therapeutic help and hope.

- Summarize my view of their primary problems.
- Obtain feedback.

Session 1

Dan canceled our first appointment, explaining that something had come up at work. This made me wonder about his or their ambivalence, and about how his prioritizing work might cause problems as, indeed, turned out to be the case. At the rescheduled first session, both Dan and Akira arrived on time. After we were seated, I began, as I usually do, by speaking to both of them: "I understand from Dan that you're having some trouble prior to moving in together and possibly getting married. How would you each describe what's been going on, and how do you think I can help?" I tailor this opening to reflect what I've already learned. If couples seem particularly anxious or slow to begin, I add: "It's hard to come to talk about your troubles with a stranger and to summarize what's upsetting you." As I listen to their responses, I'm curious about who will speak first, how each will react to the story the other tells, and how their stories match up.

Dan was eager to talk, though his voice trembled, revealing his anxiety. He shared his fears of saying anything that might upset Akira. His mood shifted up and down in the session, and he often seemed uncertain of himself. Akira was more reserved, though full of pep once she got going. She was more stylishly dressed, in keeping with her career (see below). She listened attentively, her face showing an effort to control her reactions, but not really disagreeing with Dan's account of their problems. Akira's attempts to control herself and Dan's anxiety about upsetting her made me think that I might be witnessing, out of the gate and in a more muted form, the key personality issues that caused problems, ones that would interfere with discussion of whatever other problems they might have.

Here's what I learned as they took turns telling me their story: Dan was a 55-year-old, Jewish physical therapist, divorced 7 years previously, with three children (one in college and two in high school, living with their mother). Akira was a 52-year-old Japanese American graphic designer, divorced long ago after a brief, unhappy marriage, with no children. I imagined that both would be fearful of repeating past marital mistakes including, of course, marrying "the wrong person." I also wondered whether cross-cultural differences, his ex-wife, or his children might be causing problems.

This was their first couple therapy, though Dan had undergone considerable psychoanalytically oriented individual therapy, which he believed had helped him. They had been together for 5 years. "Okay," I thought, "they've had considerable experience with each other. This isn't an impulsive decision to move forward. Had they gradually overcome doubts about marriage but were now getting cold feet? Why?"

They agreed that they had very much liked each other at first, though Akira had been quite wary. She had been "burnt" many times while dating and feared being overwhelmed or controlled by a man. Dan had seemed different to her. She really appreciated that he had liked her intensely, though the way he expressed this could "feel a bit creepy." Above all, Akira liked that he didn't say, "My way or the highway!" as she had been taught that all men do. Dan liked that they could talk about so many diverse topics and that Akira appreciated what he had to say.

I always ask what drew partners to each other because of its almost unsurpassed value in flagging issues of importance, unmet needs, and fears of potential disappointments. In this case, Akira's fears of being controlled and her desire to be given an equal say sounded important. Though commonplace, it was noteworthy that they each emphasized how they were drawn to a person who admired them. Both wanted to know that they mattered and made a difference to each other. However, the way they stressed this suggested uncertainty about whether these qualities could be taken for granted or sustained.

They came to therapy now because of frequent, painful relationship ruptures that occurred without much warning and could last for days. These usually began when Dan was upset or irritable—most often after a stressful day at work. Akira would become distressed and, if her distress exceeded her capacity to manage it, she would stop talking and leave the room, leaving Dan alone with his initial distress and panicked that she might leave him for good. He would then blame himself for "being too needy."

This pattern was worse when Akira was trying to help Dan with a specific task, like moving furniture. At such times, she would also start to blame herself, believing that it was her responsibility to fix the situation. She noted—insightfully, I thought—that this was how she had often felt with her mother and siblings as the oldest child in her family. As it did with Dan, excessive self-criticism added to Akira's distress and her tendency to flee.

These blowups were the main reason their relationship had been slow to move ahead. Indeed, when I asked them, they weren't quite sure whether they were engaged, though they blamed this on their difficulty finding a ring that Akira, as an artist, would appreciate. Here, I thought that this lack of formal commitment must make their ruptures more frightening and their commitment even more uncertain.

Much of the anxiety Dan brought home related to work, which was stressful and mattered deeply to him. More than that, to my mind and to Akira's, he simply worked too much. Many dual-career couples get into trouble simply because they have too little time together (Nielsen, 2022, Chap. 11). This was true of these two, as Dan worked 6 days a week and came home late most nights. I recalled my suspicions about his canceling our first session due to work, and I now had a taste of what being married to him might be like.

Things had recently become worse, as Akira's work had fallen off. She had more free time, and she wanted to spend it with Dan. Dan admitted that his focus on work was partly driven by overly intense, irrational financial fears. He worried that if he wasn't sufficiently attentive, his patients would go elsewhere. Because their combined income seemed realistically sufficient, I wondered what else might be fueling Dan's financial worries. I also noted the reemergence of Dan's abandonment fears, this time evoked by his patients.

The couple then told me how they can both be critical and perfectionistic, something they worried about as they spent more time together. They mostly share values and agree on things, but when they don't, each can feel stung by the lack of agreement, which they take as personal criticism.

Their accounts of their problems showed strengths, as well as vulnerabilities. Both partners seemed intelligent, motivated to do better, willing to consider their own roles in their problems, and had better-than-average insight into what was going on. Compared to many couples with more severe personality dysfunctions, their ability to not locate all blame in their partners was a big plus and made me hopeful. The issues they described—fears of subjugation, abandonment, and criticism—revealed insight, as they all felt accurate to me, but I worried that these (most likely) lifelong fears might not be easy to alter. Their survival strategies of hard work, perfectionism, and self-criticism also cut both ways and might not be easy to modify.

As the session ended, I said to them:

"I'm glad you've come, and I think you're in the right place. I think I can help you. Although I'm just getting to know you, here's briefly what seem to be your problems: First, approaching greater commitment to each other stirs up some fears, fears that may be lifelong and have roots in both childhood and previous relationships. It also seems that when Dan is anxious and upset and wants to talk about it, you two have trouble doing that. Akira then feels overwhelmed, burdened, and self-critical, so that sometimes she flees the scene. This makes matters worse, as Dan feels even more upset. There is also disagreement and concern about how much time Dan spends at work and whether you have enough good times together. Does that sound about right?"

The couple agreed. I then asked, as I always do, "How was this session? Was it what you expected? Was there anything I said that rubbed you the wrong way or that you disagree with?" and later, "Do you think you can work with me?" Both said that it was pretty much what they'd expected, that there wasn't anything objectionable, and that they thought they could work with me. These questions encourage feedback from clients who might otherwise be afraid to express doubts or disagreement. Research shows that this is especially important with couples like Dan and Akira who aim to please and are slow to voice dissatisfaction.

I then handed them my basic intake questionnaire, explained my plan for our next diagnostic sessions, and worked out times for those meetings. All of this went uneventfully.

This was a typical first session for me, as it focused on the presenting problems and did not attempt to get much history other than what the couple brought up spontaneously. I thought we did pretty well in meeting my priorities, including focusing on the current problem and its dynamics while beginning to form an alliance with both partners. I didn't ask them to "talk to each other" to show me their problematic interpersonal process because I got a taste of it at the beginning, and because they did a credible job of describing it as I later summarized to them. I assumed (correctly) that we would witness it later as therapy progressed.

As for my countertransference feelings, I mostly enjoyed being with them due to the strengths I've noted. But as I tried to imagine myself married to each of them, I was able to access some negative feelings, feelings I term "usable countertransferences," which would inform my work going forward. I felt a bit annoyed by Dan's canceling the first session, something that fit with Akira's experience. It also wasn't hard to imagine that I would feel frustrated and annoyed if he was always ruminating on his anxieties, if she fled conversations when I was upset, or if I had to tiptoe around all the time because each was so highly sensitive to criticism. I left the session feeling optimistic and curious about what would come next. As I always do, I wrote down topics that I thought would be good to cover soon: sex, his kids, her career, friends and family, and shared pleasurable activities.

Session 2

This time Akira was late, and I got to witness Dan's anxiety about her commitment (to him, not just to the therapy) and her perfectionism, as she got quite flustered after keeping us waiting only 4 minutes. I always begin the second session by asking how the couple reacted to our first session. There was good news and bad news. They both had liked the first session, had told each other so, and—heeding my implied suggestion that they might benefit from more good times together—they had enjoyed a nice brunch afterward. But they had trouble when Dan wanted to have sex later "to celebrate."

This led us to discuss their sex life a bit, an item already on my agenda. Akira's libido was lower than it had been, but mostly their sex was still satisfying. What had made her balk was something different: Not feeling in the mood, she experienced Dan's suggestion as "phony," "tying a bow around our problems" (minimizing them) and "forcing me to take care of his feelings." After I encouraged him to talk to her directly, Dan said that, on the contrary, he didn't want to sweep things under the rug, but that her rejection had hurt his feelings, which was also how he could feel when she preferred to be alone. Here, I offered a simple suggestion (if these work, great; if they don't, we can find out why): When she wanted to decline an offer to be together, Akira could tell Dan that she loves him but needs some time alone and then provide him a specific time when she would be available.

But because Akira's complaint confirmed the pattern of her feeling burdened by Dan's feelings, as discussed in our first session, I wanted to do more than offer advice; I wanted to explore what might make my advice hard to follow, thus integrating behavioral psychoeducation with psychodynamic exploration. After I asked how it had felt when she was called upon to comfort or console him, she associated to memories of having to do just that with her emotionally overdramatic mother, who "from as early as I can remember" involved her inappropriately in problems with her father (especially their financial differences). Hearing this, I thought it might explain some of the heat behind their financial squabbles, as these replayed her parents arguing about money. Akira's mother would require that Akira TOTALLY AGREE WITH HER (all caps in my notes). Her mother would also sometimes blame her for the mother's distress. In other situations when Akira was upset (e.g., much later when Akira was getting divorced), her mother would make things worse by saying that she herself was the one who was most upset. To give Akira the sense that I understood and empathized with this parent–child role reversal, I said it would be like an emergency room doctor being more upset than a patient who had been in an auto accident. She appreciated that validation, as I next labeled (interpreted) this as a "transference allergy" she had to situations when Dan appeared in need of emotional assistance. When this happened, I said, she'd panic, become angrily conflicted about what to do, and sometimes flee the scene, just as she had learned to do as a defensive strategy with her mother.

Though I didn't say this at the time, I speculated that her avoidant attachment style, developed to cope with her engulfing mother, might partially explain why Akira had found a workaholic partner both appealing (because his time demands might be few) and distressing (because his anxiety would require responsiveness). More surprising, we could now understand why Akira could experience Dan's efforts to comfort or please *her* (as with lovemaking after their brunch) as inauthentic, selfish, and "more about him."

After what amounted to a bit of "witnessed individual therapy" with Akira, Dan recalled some of his own traumatic experiences with his father. Once, when Dan had thrown a pillow at one of his sisters, his father had overdone the punishment—telling Dan he couldn't go to a circus performance with the family and making Dan write 1,000 times, "I will not be mean to my sister." But when his father returned home that night, he had gone to Dan's room and broken down, crying while apologizing, so that, as with Akira's mother, it was now all about his father's distress, not Dan's. I thought to myself, "These are partners with similar sensitivities who've gravitated toward each other."

As this session ended, we all felt closer and hopeful, as "model scenes" (a psychodynamic term of art) from their childhoods had emerged that partially explained some of their current problematic interactions. But could their ingrained patterns be changed? Wasn't it true, I wondered, as psychoanalysts now believe, that Freud's early theory of simply remembering and "abreacting" childhood traumas wasn't enough? Indeed, what seemed helpful here (and would continue to be mutative over the course of this therapy) was not simply the remembering of painful childhood scenes but receiving empathic responses from a partner who "softened" as they gained understanding of the experiences that had shaped their lover.

Questionnaires

After the session, I reviewed their responses to my questionnaire, which covers the bases of most couple issues and assesses levels of distress, commitment, respect, insightfulness, "love languages," and goals for therapy. Besides standard questions, it has room for free-form elaboration to encourage self-examination.

Dan's responses confirmed what he had shared as a major problem: They have trouble when he talks about his stress, during which Akira is "too dismissive of things that bother me." He added that during their fights, "My partner seems to view my words or actions more negatively than I mean them," and he "has trouble viewing himself as good or valuable." He would like more sex and more time together "just talking." But compared to most couples I see, Dan had few complaints, said many positive things about the relationship, and rated himself and Akira as strongly committed to each other. I noted that Dan's ratings of their mutual commitment reflected a divergence between his conscious beliefs written here and his emotional reactions in moments of conflict.

In her questionnaire, Akira was also mostly positive about their relationship and saw them both as strongly committed. She also wanted more positive time together but confessed that "Dan doesn't always 'know' me because I don't tell him about myself." Like Dan, she saw their biggest problem occurring when he was upset and expected her to help him feel better. She often felt overly responsible, while he felt rejected. Although she knew he wanted "more empathy," she would like him to say, "Don't worry; I'll take care of it." She knew he wanted more sex, but she wasn't always in the mood.

Individual Sessions

As part of my standard diagnostic phase, I meet once alone with each person. My goals are to improve the therapeutic alliance, to hear "whatever would be hard to say with your partner present," and to learn more about the person's history. In her individual session, Akira again focused on their problem of her becoming overwhelmed when Dan was distraught and wanting to talk about it. My understanding of this deepened as she told me more about her childhood, the subject of most of this meeting.

Akira's psychological problems began early, even before the stress of immigration. As a little girl growing up in a nice suburb outside Tokyo, she was already unhappy as a shy but "adventurous" tomboy who received much criticism for not wanting to dress or act like a traditional girl. She preferred keeping to herself, often going alone to explore the woods, where she would sometimes experiment with bugs, taking one wing off dragonflies to watch them fly in circles. Here I thought I was hearing about the beginning of her proclivity to go off by herself when upset.

Akira's mother felt superior to others and believed she had come down in the world after marrying Akira's father. She forbade Akira from playing with neighborhood children, whom she looked down on as coming from lower social classes. Her mother could be charming and full of energy (like Akira), but she had strong ideas about how Akira should behave. One younger sister had rebelled openly, and her youngest sister had coped by remaining dependently incompetent. As the oldest, Akira was tasked with being the strong, healthy one, expected to supervise and care for her younger sisters (a role she continued to fill years later).

Things got still worse when her family moved to the United States when Akira was 12. Not knowing English, for her first 2 years, she hardly spoke at all and again felt isolated from peers. Her father had hoped for a better job but ended up downwardly mobile, depressed, and strapped for money. Again, Akira mentioned her parents' loud, angry fights over money. Later, when they achieved financial stability, her parents guilt-tripped their girls for "the sacrifices we made to give you a better life."

Nonetheless, Akira gradually did well in school, discovering her love of painting and graphic design around which she built a successful career. She met her first husband in college. He was "a very nice man" who supported her and calmed her. However, she wasn't attracted to him, sex petered out, and there was "no chemistry," so she broke it off after about 3 years. Since then, she had "gone solo."

After hearing this painful story, I not only felt I understood where Akira's marital troubles came from, but I also really admired her liveliness, her openness with me, and that she had found a way to make her life work. I could see how her relationship with Dan might have unsettled her established, solitary routine. Specifically, Akira was thrust back into the caretaker role she had been required to fill with her mother and sisters, something that felt unfair and burdensome.

Dan's individual session was more complex. While he was open with me, he rambled (as is typical of anxiously attached adults) and he was not particularly adept at describing people (especially his parents). He emphasized that he felt angry with Akira when he wasn't allowed to be upset, something he also experienced with his ex-wife.

Dan was a middle child, with sisters older and younger, growing up in various Cleveland suburbs. Like Akira, he had suffered during several family relocations that had disturbed his friendship networks. His mother was "a worrier" and not someone he could seek out for help. His accountant father also seemed unapproachable. Like Akira's parents, Dan's parents fought a lot, which led to a distressing divorce when he was 10. His mother quickly married a family friend with whom she'd been having an affair.

Dan's earliest memory (always a good question to ask) fit with how he felt for much of his life: In it, he "was surrounded by many older/bigger men and felt small and lost." Like Akira, Dan felt alone, different, and silenced as a small child (the last due to a speech impediment). Like Akira, he later found a "home" (his term) in theater and singing groups from middle school on, including during an attempted acting career. He loved playing roles he could lose himself in, while earning audience approval. Despite some success as an actor, he reluctantly gave that up (due to low pay and anxiety during auditions) to become a physical therapist.

Prior to marriage Dan had had many unsuccessful "infatuations" that left scars. He was drawn to his ex-wife because, unlike his parents, she was low key and calm. He was still upset that his wife had left him 8 years earlier. It remained unclear why his marriage had ended.

From Dan's history, I could see the roots of his insecurity, of his desire for approval, and of his wish to finally find a home. I could see why he would be upset more than average when he and Akira fought, because this resembled his parents, whose fights had led to their divorce. And I could see how, despite what might seem to be dramatic cultural differences, this couple shared much in common. As children, both had been forced to relocate, had few friends, experienced trouble speaking, and suffered from emotionally impinging, critical, and warring parents. Later, both found happiness in hard work and in a love of the arts. While explaining their specific personality weaknesses, these shared experiences were also a source of mutual attraction and, with help from me, might help them understand each other better.

BEGINNING PHASE OF THERAPY

The first formal therapy session: I began by providing a summary of where I thought we were so far, pretty much what I'd said at the close of our first meeting, but with more detail about how the impact of Dan's and Akira's early lives might explain their reticence about marriage and troubles being close. After establishing that we were on the same page, I outlined my basic format for our meetings:

> "In most sessions, I'll leave it up to you to pick a topic to discuss. That's because you will know better what is most pressing and important. I reserve the right to bring up things I think might need attention. Most times, I'll encourage you to talk to each other, and I will listen and try to help. Like a music teacher or athletic coach, this will help me see what you do and how you interact, so that I can help you do better, including when I'm no longer present. Obviously, this plan fits with your central problem of talking to each other when Dan is upset."

And so we began. They did surprisingly well in this first formal therapy session, as they followed my direction and tried to explain to each other their distress and needs. Initially, I was more a witness, representing the task of safely opening up to each other.

His voice shaking a bit, Dan returned to how he sometimes felt rebuffed when he wanted sex. He explained that it wasn't just sex he wanted, but "closeness." Controlling her impulse to become defensive, Akira replied that Dan's recent request for sex had felt the same as when he pressed her to discuss stressful situations, like the previous night, when he wanted to talk about a patient with chronic lung disease. That had felt "simply too close and too much." His distress felt almost contagious, so that she had become short of breath, like the woman he'd been describing. Recalling this now made her feel like leaving my office.

Witnessing their problem in the session, with a comforting nod of recognition to Akira, I stepped in and spoke to Dan: "I get how you can feel alone and want to bridge the gap after a long day by having sex or by talking about distress left over from work, but anticipating that Akira won't respond as you'd like makes you anxious [as it had as this session opened]. My guess is that you convey this additional anxiety to Akira. When it comes to wanting sex, *that* must not be very sexy." They both laughed in agreement. "And when you describe a scary scene at a nursing home, Akira can feel overwhelmed and then turn away."

Both nodded, giving me permission to wonder how they might "meet in the middle," where Dan could feel close and Akira could feel less compelled to do as he wanted, with sex or by soothing his distress about work.

Akira responded, in keeping with what we'd learned about her situation with her mother. "You're right. What gets me going is feeling forced to act or feel a certain way. Like when a colleague shocked me recently by saying, 'I hate Italians!' and expected me to agree. I felt that way when my mother told me how to dress, and when kids made fun of me for being a tomboy and shamed me for not wanting to talk when I came to the United States." Here, she started to cry softly, and Dan reached over to hold and comfort her.

After that, Dan said he didn't need her to agree with him or match his feelings or desires (unlike her mother, I thought), only to recognize them as valid; otherwise, he could panic and feel alone. I said that both had felt alone, unprotected, and stressed by their parents, who "had overshared their own distress," and that this might help us understand both the desire to be close and "find a home" (voiced by Dan) and the desire to be free of impingements by fleeing to a safe distance (voiced by Akira). The session ended on this deeper, somewhat somber note.

INTERMEDIATE PHASE OF THERAPY

Despite the auspicious beginning, and as is typical with such couples, considerable work and much repetition in the here and now (not that different from our first formal therapy session) were required over the next year of weekly meetings to alter this couple's problematic, automatic personality predispositions. Some paradigmatic and revealing sessions follow.

Session 6

Akira said she was feeling more alone (Dan was still coming home late) and out of sorts now that her work, which had occupied her and boosted her self-esteem, had fallen off. To cope, she had gone for a walk but then feared that others she passed might blame or even attack her, an Asian American, after President Trump had labeled COVID the "Chinese flu." Reminded of the many times she'd been unfairly criticized as a child and thinking she might have been angry at American racism, I noted how she'd coped with her loneliness and anger as a girl by "going into the woods and torturing dragonflies." My tone aimed to make her childhood behavior sound almost sensibly cathartic. She got it and her mood lightened. She agreed that years of criticism and racism had stung, and then corrected me, explaining that she had not so much wanted to torture the dragonflies as "to see if they could fly with only one wing" (that is, despite adversity, like her). To me, this illustrated a corrective experience between us, witnessed by Dan, who'd also been a supportive listener. Akira, feeling alone and dispirited about her work, had gone for a solitary walk, her childhood survival strategy. But the walk had triggered memories of childhood bullying, racism, and exclusion, stirring more feelings of loneliness, anxiety, and anger. Now, sharing those feelings with us, Akira felt understood, validated, and accepted.

Session 7

We reviewed a big fight. Akira had made fun of Dan over how he had cut some fish she had prepared. His self-esteem had taken a hit. Now, in the session, she admitted surprise at the intensity of her criticism. Like other partners shocked by intense fights over minor events, this had stunned them. Subsequent discussion, moderated by me, revealed Dan's sensitivity to criticism (I recalled his father's severity) and Akira's anxiety over his apparently imperfect behavior ("Only a child doesn't know how to cut fish!"), which recalled her mother's incompetence and, when Dan had become upset by her criticism, her mother's inability to regulate her emotions. As the therapy went forward, Akira began to own her fears of herself or others being less than perfect. On this day, she acknowledged not showing Dan how she wanted things done and how she might be "a bit of a perfectionist."

This was another escalating dance of "interlocking negative transferences"—his to his father, hers to her mother. This fight was about sensitivities to criticism and imperfection. It was different from the one we had discussed before, which occurred when Dan was upset or wanted sex. In both situations, each partner experienced a "transference allergy"—a hot button—that rendered them unable to regulate their emotional responses or assist their partner who was growing increasingly upset. I suggested that they give this one a name to recognize it when it began. Dan suggested "Reginald." We all thought this name apt, as their mutual perfectionism was captured, lampooned, and contained by reference to a British sitcom character with that name, familiar to both, who was often "miffed."

Session 8

Despite the pandemic and being together more, they laughed over the fact that they had no big fight to review with me! The session focused on Akira's distress/anxiety/anger at her mother, whose anxiety had risen due to the pandemic. Her mother had told everyone else in the family to come down on Akira for not calling her more often. As in childhood, Akira, as the oldest, was frequently the target of her mother's anxiety and criticism. As a teen, Akira had rebelled, telling her mother she was a "bad mother." Her mother had responded by slapping and punching her. Akira then ceased rebelling, alternated between feeling angry and guilty, and thought she "had no mother." Today, she found it helpful when I suggested that her current "anxiety" might signal suppressed anger, and she confirmed this by relating recent nightmares in which she was "violent or angrily lecturing others."

Dan listened attentively and then wondered, "Is this why I can't be allowed to be anxious?" Her account also reminded him of his childhood, when no one attended to him when he was upset. What he really wanted now was not so much permission to be anxious (as he conceded that he often is), but for Akira to listen and simply hang in there with him. For Akira to do that, to remain calm and present, I suggested that it might help if she didn't feel inner pressure to "solve" the problem du jour, as her mother had pressed her to do in childhood and currently.

Session 9

Dan and Akira had had another fight, the kind that had brought them to therapy. A planned evening at home had been spoiled, as each felt unappreciated and criticized. In their usual pattern, Akira had felt that she was trying to help, but Dan had felt criticized. He had sworn at her, calling her a "micromanaging bitch." She had countered, calling him "an abuser," and had fled the scene. Both then had wondered if their relationship would make it. (Another Reginald!)

In the session, their concern for each other and wish to make up prevailed, as I helped them unpack what had happened and apologize. After they had repaired their bond and settled down, I spent the remaining time on psychoeducation, beginning with recommendations for time-outs—including that the person leaving the scene should commit to a time to resume the discussion and that, in the interim, both should try to discern what nerves had been touched.

I then shared my overarching recommendation for handling escalating fights: to follow The Three C's by attempting to remain calm, curious, and caring. I suggested some strategies to restore a degree of calm, especially deep breathing, and noted how curiosity also fosters calming. I said that fights over what seemed like nothing (like this one, again in the kitchen) were always about something significant, so that searching for "hidden issues" and core sensitivities, as we had been doing, would help. As concerns the third C of "caring," I recommended turning empathic attention to their wounded partner, something that almost always helps. Going forward, we had many opportunities to discuss their efforts "to follow those C's" and some additional rules for regaining composure. To make my points stick, I told them that these worked for me and that "When my friends ask how Dr. Couple Therapy Expert is in real life, my wife reports that my shift to active listening really works for her!"

Sessions 10–12

These were productive sessions, with Dan and Akira mostly in good humor as they "talked to each other" in sessions with progressively less help from me and attempted to follow The Three C's and be less picky with each other. They talked about buying a home and their wedding plans. Choosing a wedding ring allowed us to revisit Dan's sensitivity to criticism and Akira's to being held captive to Dan's preferences.

The legacy of living in families with parents who so frequently lost it emotionally made Dan and Akira extremely alert to each other's moods, something I compared to my hypervigilant cat. What then helped was showing them how they relied too much on their childhood strategies of guessing each other's states of mind rather than discussing them. While cats can't ask about what's going on, they could. They now cut each other more slack as they learned that their mind reading had been excessively negative.

After another round of Reginald, Akira shared her fear that to make their marriage work, she must perpetually "walk on eggshells," a situation reminiscent of how everyone had had to cater to her mother's sensitivities. We all knew that Dan could be easily hurt, and she and I felt better when Dan acknowledged that and said he didn't want Akira to always be on guard "like Nielsen's cat." But when he followed this empathic apology with an attempt to soothe her by giving her a hug, she pulled away, saying she experienced this more as "something for him, not really for me."

While one hopes—and over time usually observes—that better partner behavior will be registered as corrective emotional experiences that modify underlying pathological schemas (here, Akira's negative maternal transference), this is often not the case. One of the major advantages of couple therapy is that when this occurs, we are on the spot to focus attention on how hard it is for the partner to let down their guard and see the world differently.

With this in mind, I began with an interpretation: "Akira, your skepticism here—rejecting Dan's hug, believing him insincere and, like your mother, in need of care from you—certainly protects you from disappointment, as in the adage 'The pessimist is never disappointed,' but this also robs you of what you most desire: a loving husband who wants to comfort *you*, not just one who needs you to comfort *him*."

Akira listened but didn't jump for joy as she took in what I thought was good news. So, I followed up with a homework assignment designed to chip away at her maternal transference in an experiential way. When the time seems auspicious, I use homework to help partners test their basic assumptions about each other outside the consulting room. I said, "As a child, you had to fend for yourself, remaining ever on guard about your mother's moods and needs, unable to ask her for help. I'd like to see if you can take a risk to reverse that pattern. This week, at some point, ask Dan for some form of emotional help." Akira listened and high-energy, can-do person that she was, accepted my challenge.

Session 13

Acknowledging and experiencing how hard it was for her to ask for emotional help, Akira had, nonetheless, taken up my homework challenge, as she had told Dan of her fear that his children might come to live with them and create problems (the "burdensome mother" theme again). Dan had reassured her, telling her this was unlikely and that his kids were "mostly low maintenance." As the session closed, they mentioned that they had successfully cleaned her apartment together and enjoyed sex afterward.

Session 14

Just when I thought that their big fights might be in the rearview mirror, they had another. It began when Dan tried to explain that he was not intending to pathologize Akira for having tortured insects (I can't recall why he had brought *that* up) but understood it (as I did) as a way to cope in childhood. Nonetheless, she experienced this as needlessly critical and intrusive, and after fighting back briefly, she fled the apartment and later gave him the silent treatment for 3 days. In the tense, controlled session that followed, I suggested some images Akira might use to create more mental separation when she felt forced by Dan to see things his way. She especially liked the image of a protective windshield that controlled what she would let in.

Session 15

Dan and Akira were doing well as they discussed the joint purchase of a condo. Sad that other buyers got the one they preferred, they associated to regret about their prior marriages. Dan was palpably moved when Akira told him how much she respects how hard he works. In the ensuing months, they hardly ever mentioned anxiety about money, something I explained to myself as being due to Dan's unrealistic worry about money having concealed deeper, now much reduced, anxieties about respect and commitment. Similarly, I no longer heard complaints about too little time together (time spent together was up), which I thought was due to Dan's lessened fears of having too little money, losing patients, or losing Akira—all resulting in fewer hours at work. These positive developments show how some problems solve themselves as relationships improve.

Sessions 16–22

Akira and Dan continued to do well, openly sharing concerns and satisfactions about moving into a new home. They were less crabby and more accepting and supportive of each other. This positive behavior continued to disconfirm their transference fears; meet their needs for support, affirmation, and companionship; and, consequently, reduce their need to use their childhood survival tactics. In short, their vicious circles, including Reginald, which we sometimes joked about, were becoming benign ones. Feeling better and more confident, they reduced the frequency of sessions to once every 2 weeks.

Their move to a new home evoked memories of the stress and trauma both had experienced during childhood relocations, especially hers to America and his Hamlet-like experience of his mother moving so soon after her divorce to marry his stepfather. But now, unlike their insecure attachments of childhood, they had each other. Akira had Dan to help, and her appreciation reduced his belief that no matter what he did, it was never enough. In one important conversation, she explained how important her art had been to her as a child, something he, as a once-aspiring actor, understood. She then consoled him for having changed careers, and he comforted her for having parents who never valued the arts.

Sessions 23–26

Like others who avoid talking about sexual problems until other issues are settled and this feels safer, Dan returned to wanting more frequent sex. They agreed that sex was 90% great but felt bad about their desire discrepancy. After I helped them to make this a "joint problem like others requiring discussion," we brainstormed about what might help. While Dan's compliments didn't do much for Akira (who preferred action to words), going out to dinner or doing some of the aforementioned housework helped Akira get in the mood. They agreed that masturbation for him would also be okay when she wasn't available or in the mood. All this talk felt intimate, not just practical.

CONCLUDING PHASE OF THERAPY

Session 28

About 2 weeks before their wedding, they began the session almost speechless, still terribly upset about a fight 3 days earlier. Fueled by anxiety about a final commitment to marriage, this blowup engaged deep desires, not just familiar fears. Dan had been triggered when Akira wanted to replace the blanket on their bed. This reminded him of his childhood "blankie" and of how he had felt displaced and less loved after his sister was born. Even more than his wishes for sex, the current blanket represented "the one thing I should get to choose!" Unfortunately, Akira felt unfairly attacked by him and thought that she was the one making more accommodations in their new home. When Dan lost it and started yelling that she was just like his selfish, controlling ex-wife, she had freaked out, again reminded of scenes of her parents fighting.

But they had been this way before. We were able to slow it down and "make a short story long" as we uncovered the familiar triggering sensitivities and then attempted repair. Trying to normalize what I imagined would be fights like this in their future, I spoke of their need to accept transference allergies in themselves and each other, reminded them that time-outs can help, and noted that when a row like this happened again, they might think to themselves, "We've been here before and we know what to do," rather than, "Oh, no, this marriage is hopeless!" To end the session, I suggested that they hug. They did so for quite a long time, which seemed to help. The hug was made more authentic, corrective, and complex as Dan pointed out—with a trace of anxious, hostile humor—that he was "doing this for Akira, too, not just for himself!"

Session 29

Akira and Dan were feeling happy and close a few days after their wedding. Akira had been moved to tears as she read her vows, including when registering that she would now have someone with whom to grow old. We celebrated their happiness and then reviewed several discombobulating moments that revealed some persistent anxiety about their future together.

Sessions 30–34

In the five monthly sessions that followed, there were occasional (but now familiar) dust-ups. But, immunized by me, as in Session 28, they had hung in, turned toward each other, solved the moment, and regained their composure. While doing so, they had come to know each other's sensitivities—especially how each could feel easily criticized, how each felt they had to sacrifice too much for the other, and how Akira could feel pressured to fix Dan's behavior and feelings. This knowledge helped them not to take things quite so personally and to remain calm, curious, and caring. Each time they did so, they gained confidence that they could do it again and that they might truly "grow old together," as Akira had imagined at their wedding.

In our final session, they expressed their gratitude, mentioned Reginald and my scaredy cat, and were happy to know that my door was always open. I felt happy for this couple, even as I worried that we might not have done enough. That was 4 years ago and, so far, they have not returned.

FURTHER REFLECTIONS AND IMPLICATIONS

Can self-centered, emotionally dysregulated, insecurely attached, and painfully defensive people—people cursed with personality dysfunctions—become more mature, connected, and loving? That question is answered positively in the fanciful "psychotherapies" presented in Charles Dickens's *A Christmas Carol* and Danny Rubin's film *Groundhog Day*. In both of these stories, characters must face their pasts and learn new skills on the way to self-awareness and happier lives with others. It turns out that love is the answer, but getting there is not so easy. Can couple therapy help? What are its strengths and limitations?

My work with Akira and Dan demonstrates how couple therapy can help, as they worked on lifelong problems of insecure attachment, dysregulated emotions, sensitivity to criticism, negative expectancies concerning relationships, and inadequate interpersonal skillfulness—the personality dysfunctions identified in this chapter's introduction.

My initial formulation held up pretty well, as it explained their sensitivities, attachment styles, and the vicious cycles these could create. When Dan anxiously approached Akira for either comfort or sex, this upset her, as it repeated her experiences with her intrusive, demanding, critical mother, who had saddled her with too much responsibility. Her main defense was to flee, as she had both as a child and as she had later as a single (avoidantly attached) adult. But Akira's flight left Dan feeling alone and rejected, as he had felt in childhood and after his divorce. Their other negative cycle occurred when Akira, imagining that Dan was as incompetent as her mother, and upset that her world wasn't quite under her perfectionistic control, became inordinately critical of Dan, thus recreating his experience with his critical father and aggravating his own internalized self-criticism. He would often respond with a counterattack that touched Akira's own sensitivities to criticism and lack of control. In both cycles, the partners would feel deeply wounded and alone as they retreated to separate corners.

The couple therapy showed the value of an integrative psychodynamic approach that increased insight, provided corrective experiences, and taught some relationship skills. Akira became better at responding to Dan's (now less anxious) requests for comfort and sex, less likely to see them as burdensome and self-serving. She also became better able to ask for what *she* needed (see Nielsen, 2023). Both became less sensitive to criticism, less likely to dole it out, and more openly appreciative of each other. When conflicts surfaced, they were better able to manage, to empathize, and to repair the damage. Their shared intimacy in therapy and their ability to bounce back from conflict gave them confidence in a shared future, now that they believed they had made the right choice by daring to be close when that had seemed iffy. All this resulted in more good times together, more proof that their painful childhood experiences need not repeat, and more "love in the love bank" to buffer inevitable disappointments.

This case is typical in illustrating the value of countertransference awareness, the need for repetition, the benefits of empathic listening, humor, and an improved sex life, and the growing capacity of partners—no longer so thrown off by each other—to meet each other's basic needs for support and appreciation.

While this case ended well, others with more severe character pathology often don't. Some couples can still make it if we add more frequent meetings, more structure during sessions, separate individual meetings, psychoactive medication, drug/alcohol treatment, or intensive individual therapy. My work has benefited from all the above add-ons when appropriate. Possibly the most important modification is the need to pay still greater attention to negative countertransference feelings. In more troubled patients, one must work harder to see the vulnerability and unmet needs that are covered by distasteful behavior. But even with such additions and therapist self-examination, some couples give up and accept devitalized parallel lives, some divorce, and (my least favorite outcome) some remain stuck in co-created hellscapes maintained by a mix of external constraints and internal enacted benefits. We couple therapists must accept our limited power.

On a more positive note, working as a couple therapist for more than 40 years has been endlessly fascinating (it engages life's great issues), never boring (no two people are alike and, when fighting, they definitely keep you awake), and rewarding (as it fills a need to help others, leaving most partners happier and wiser, if not completely free of their personality limitations). In the end, many of our couples free themselves from *Groundhog Day* repetitions, and many, like Ebenezer Scrooge, find that love is the answer.

REFERENCES

American Psychiatric Association. (2022). *Diagnostic and statistical manual of mental disorders* (5th ed., text rev.). Washington, DC: Author.

Fruzzetti, A. E. (2006). *The high-conflict couple: A dialectical behavior therapy guide to finding peace, intimacy, and validation.* Oakland, CA: New Harbinger.

Goldner, V. (2014). Romantic bonds, binds, and ruptures: Couples on the brink. *Psychoanalytic Dialogues, 24*, 402–418.

Leone, C. (2008). Couple therapy from the perspective of self psychology and intersubjectivity theory. *Psychoanalytic Psychology, 25*, 79–98.

Nielsen, A. C. (2016). *A roadmap for couple therapy: Integrating systemic, psychodynamic, and behavioral approaches.* New York: Routledge.

Nielsen, A. C. (2017). Psychodynamic couple therapy: A practical synthesis. *Journal of Marital and Family Therapy, 43*, 685–699.

Nielsen, A. C. (2022). *Integrative couple therapy in action: A practical guide for handling common relationship problems and crises.* New York: Routledge.

Nielsen, A. C. (2023). Asking for things and listening to criticism: Two fundamental challenges in intimate relationships and targets for couple therapy. *Psychoanalysis, Self, and Context.* [Special Issue on Couple Therapy], *18*, 262–280.

Solomon, M. F. (1998). Treating narcissistic and borderline couples. In J. Carlson & L. Sperry (Eds.), *The disordered couple* (pp. 239–284). Bristol, PA: Brunner/Mazel.

CHAPTER 5

Gottman Method Couple Therapy and Healing from Betrayal

CARRIE U. COLE
DONALD L. COLE

> *Editors' Comments*
>
> In this exposition of Gottman method couple therapy, Carrie and Don Cole offer a marvelous introduction to this evidence-informed approach and specific interventions aimed at three distinct aspects of a couple's relationship—friendship, conflict management, and shared meaning. Respectively, and particularly in combination, these promote positive exchanges, reduced negativity, and a deeper foundation for connection around core values. Conflict and emotion are viewed not as barriers but rather as potential paths toward mutual experiencing. These Gottman method interventions now permeate most couple therapy.
>
> In the case narrative offered here, the Coles describe how these foundational elements of the Gottman method are adapted to address the impacts of one partner's emotional involvement with someone outside the couple's relationship. Note the authors' explicit model within the Gottman method for promoting healing from betrayals—their sequence of "atonement, attunement, and attachment." They deliver specific interventions within that model in a sensitive and clinically nuanced manner. The theory or prescribed interventions never supersede the constraints or opportunities defined by specific characteristics of the partners, their relationship, or the therapeutic process in that moment.
>
> Other unique aspects of the Coles' case narrative also bear noting. Their interventions with this couple are delivered in a "marathon" format—across 3 days for 6 hours each. And Carrie and Don conduct their work with this couple as cotherapists. Both are highly useful and impactful, but rare ways of offering couple therapy today given the time and expense involved. Note their discussion of specific strengths and potential limitations of this marathon format. Follow as well their internal decisional processes as they discern which of them will respond to which partners around which issues, and at which points in the therapy. As you delve into the Coles' narrative of this interesting

> work, consider how the unique aspects of marathon or cotherapy might be adapted to other therapeutic approaches or specific issues described in this *Casebook* and how this therapy might have been different if offered in a traditional once-a-week format with one therapist.

We've been fascinated by relationships for as long as we can remember. No two relationships are exactly the same. Even if one person were to leave one relationship and get into another, the new one is quite different from the prior one. What makes relationships work? How can relationships go from feeling like one is in heaven to feeling like one has fallen into hell? One of the things that drew the two of us together was our mutual interest in relationships.

Early in our careers, we would see individuals in therapy who reported that their primary struggle was their relationship with their romantic partner. It seemed that they could benefit from couple therapy. However, when that person brought their partner into therapy, it was quite another story. The partners might angrily attack one another for their misdeeds or, worse, sit in stony silence. Yet they loved each other and wanted to stay together. In the beginning of our careers, we felt woefully inadequate to help them. We weren't totally ignorant about couple relationships and the research on relationships. In fact, we had both read John Gottman's work. However, reading about the destructive behaviors that cause relationships to end didn't automatically mean that we knew how to treat the couple sitting in front of us. It was painfully clear that couple therapy was not the same as individual therapy. Fortunately, for us and for the couples we work with, we sought Gottman training for couple therapy.

One of the first tenets of Gottman therapy is to have the partners talk directly to one another about their relationship struggles within the therapy sessions. Talk directly to each other? Weren't we supposed to keep them *from* fighting with each other? The Gottman method encourages couples to directly engage in conflict discussions with each other in our office, so that we can observe those interactions. Couples need skills to have productive conversations about their disagreements and misunderstandings, and state-dependent learning is the most effective way to learn a new skill. There's no such thing as idly sitting back in couple therapy. We had to be actively engaged and involved in the process. Just like when you learn to ski or drive a car, the first thing to learn is how to stop. We had to learn how to respectfully, yet decisively, interrupt the destructive behaviors between partners as they occurred in the therapy session.

Gottman method couple therapy is based on the "sound relationship house" theory and is grounded in the research of John Gottman and Robert Levenson that led to the ability to predict with high accuracy which relationships would succeed and which would fail (for summaries of this research, see Gottman & Gottman, 2018, 2023). Gottman and Levenson examined both healthy and ailing relationships to discover differences between the two. That examination led to an awareness that there are three systems that need to be healthy in relationships—the friendship system, the conflict management system, and the shared meaning system. Interventions aimed at promoting these systems has three phases: assessment, treatment, and relapse prevention.

We worked with the couple we describe here in an intensive form of therapy that we call "marathon therapy," because it's conducted over the course of 3 days, 6 hours per day. The assessment was conducted by Carrie the day before the therapy began, and the therapy was conducted jointly by both of us (Don and Carrie), because this is what the couple requested. It's a rare opportunity that we get to work as cotherapists, perhaps once or twice a year. Gottman method couple therapy is usually conducted by a single therapist in either traditional, weekly, 90-minute sessions or this more intense format. We love the marathon therapy! There's time to talk, to repair, and to rebuild. There's time to delve deeply into the couple's struggles and gain understanding and clarity around those issues. Couples with whom we've worked have described a transformative experience and have loved this marathon format as well. That said, there are some potential drawbacks to marathon therapy. The up-front cost may be prohibitive for some couples. In addition, they don't have the time to practice new skills between sessions, so sometimes follow-up sessions are needed to help couples maintain changes. While marathon therapy can put the couple on a trajectory toward positivity, it takes time for the habit of positivity to take root in the relationship.

INITIAL ASSESSMENT AND CASE FORMULATION

Couples are thoroughly assessed before any therapy begins. The assessment process has multiple parts and we begin by asking the couple about what brings them into treatment (their narrative), followed by an oral history interview about the development of their relationship. We then videorecord the couple having two discussions in our office. One discussion is about the events of the week, and the other is about an ongoing difference between them. They each watch the videos and rate them based on how they felt about those interactions. We observe the couple's interactions, behaviors, and conflict strategies within those videorecorded discussions. We look for issues such as the use of the four negative interaction patterns that predict divorce (criticism, defensiveness, contempt, and stonewalling). We watch for signs of flooding (entering a fight-or-flight state during conflict). We use a pulse oximeter to monitor their heart rates to identify physiological changes that indicate flooding. We watch for positive signs, too, such as attempts to repair, expressions of affection, moments of shared humor, and attempts to compromise. Partners also fill out extensive self-report questionnaires that include standard measures of relationship satisfaction, sound relationship house questionnaires, family history, and individual psychological issues. In addition, we interview each individual to collect their psychological history, information about their family of origin, and their point of view on the relationship. A full report is then generated from these data, and the assessment ends with a session focused on feedback and treatment planning.

In our first conversation with Nicole and Martin, we learned that they had been married for 30 years and had two adult children. They told us that they'd been living parallel lives since their children had grown up and left their home. During the course of Martin's work, he developed a close mentoring relationship with a young woman and eventually began to experience deep feelings of connection with her. When Nicole discovered inappropriate, secretive text messages between Martin and this young woman, she was extremely hurt and made plans to separate from the marriage. Nicole believed Martin hadn't been sexual with this person, but she still experienced a deep sense of emotional betrayal. Her experience of being betrayed created symptoms of trauma that often accompany the experience of discovering a partner's betrayal (Glass & Staeheli, 2004; Gordon, Mitchell, Baucom, & Snyder, 2023). Martin expressed a high level of sorrow and regret for having gotten involved with this other woman. He hoped to persuade Nicole to give him the opportunity to repair the damage he had done and work together with her to find a path forward.

The initial assessment indicated that the marriage had a strong and happy beginning. During their history interview we learned that, while raising their children, Martin's work demands created a dynamic wherein Nicole began to resent him. She frequently felt alone raising the children and taking care of the home. She lost her sense of self and felt a great deal of anger about this. Unfortunately, when she sought to address these feelings with Martin, the conversation would frequently degenerate into an escalating pattern of negativity. Nicole's pleas frequently came out as criticism and were met with high levels of defensiveness from Martin. As this pattern became more entrenched, they became increasingly distant from one another. This often occurs when couples are unable to manage gridlocked conflicts in a satisfactory way. The result is disconnection from each other to avoid the unpleasant feelings that come with the arguments. Gridlocks begin as differences of viewpoint or opinion about an issue, such as the role of each member of the relationship in terms of parenting or housework. The differences of opinion about an issue can become a source of pain, distress, and eventually distance. Over the years, Nicole and Martin had developed several other gridlocked issues, including a significant separation in their sexual relationship. By the time they came into treatment, they hadn't had sex for years.

Gridlocked issues, such as the ones Martin and Nicole were facing, lead to ever increasing levels of negative feelings. This negativity became the defining feature of their relationship. The positive emotions that initially brought them together were nowhere to be found. It was in this context that Martin's feelings for his coworker began to grow. We made it clear to both Martin and Nicole as we were discussing this dynamic that in no way does the negativity in their relationship justify an inappropriate connection with someone else. However, the distance and negativity can contribute to the tendency of a partner to make the harmful choice of allowing themselves to get involved with someone else.

BEGINNING PHASE OF THERAPY

We began by asking Martin and Nicole what they wished to accomplish by the end of our time together. Couples usually have an internal list of what they want out of therapy. Nicole wanted to understand the problems in their relationship that led to his "betrayal" (her word) and to know what to do when she got emotionally triggered. She also wanted better communication tools, so that she could be less emotional. Finally, she wanted Martin to notice her. (We reframed this in our minds as a desire for Martin to turn toward her.) Martin wanted communication tools that he could use, so that they could have successful conversations. He reported that when Nicole gets triggered, he retreats. Both Martin and Nicole believed that the expression of any emotion was irrational and therefore harmful to their relationship. They wanted to eliminate it from their relationship. Don explained that emotions have their own logic and inform us of what we need. We hoped that Don, as a male, affirming the validity of emotion, would help each of them accept their own feelings.

We knew that they needed to process the betrayal before they could begin to rebuild their relationship. Unprocessed incidents continue to circle around in our memory until there's a sense of closure. Nicole needed to understand the full extent of Martin's feelings for this person and the nature of his involvement to move forward in their relationship. The Gottman method for healing a betrayal follows an "atone–attune–attach" approach we describe below.

We began the first phase of therapy with an atoning conversation in which the partners talk directly to each other. In this conversation, the uninvolved partner needs to be able to both ask any unanswered questions about what happened and to share all the emotions that were evoked through their experience, as well as hear remorse from the involved partner. This conversation is necessary to begin reestablishing feelings of trust. The involved partner is encouraged to answer all the questions fully and completely in the spirit of complete transparency. Trust has been destroyed when there's an inappropriate outside involvement and is built back by being open and honest. It's also important that the couple refrain from slipping into criticism or defensiveness during the atoning conversation. That can be a balancing act for the therapist, who typically can empathize with both partners to some degree. In addition, while it's important that the uninvolved person get answers to their questions about what happened, the question "Why did you do it?" is intentionally deferred because, at this juncture, the involved person may criticize or blame the uninvolved person by saying something like, "You never had time for me," or "You didn't seem interested in me anymore."

Nicole told Martin what she knew about his relationship with his mentee. She noticed that when Martin mentioned this woman, he seemed excited and began to speak of her often. He seemed very attentive to this woman. Nicole became concerned that he was getting too close to her and had told him so many times. He insisted that he was just mentoring her, nothing more. He suggested that Nicole meet the woman, but she refused. In the end, Nicole sent an email to the woman to inquire about the extent of her relationship with Martin. The woman replied that she wasn't romantically involved, nor was she interested in a romantic relationship with Martin—their relationship was professional and platonic.

In the atoning conversation in our office, Nicole asked Martin whether he was infatuated with this person and whether he fantasized about her. Martin responded that he had strong feelings of connection and felt energized and excited around her. She expressed admiration toward him for what he had accomplished in their field. He acknowledged that he shared too much personal information with her, and that he had become emotionally connected to her. He fantasized about building a business with her but stated that he didn't have sexual fantasies about her. (We both wondered about the veracity of this and discussed it together outside of the session. We concluded that Martin was likely minimizing the extent of his fantasies. However, Nicole didn't question his statement, so we decided not to push that issue.)

There are times when uninvolved partners don't know what questions to ask, so we helped Nicole generate questions to help facilitate a more complete understanding of the situation. We encouraged Nicole to ask questions about the nature of their interactions since she found out about the situation. Martin reported that he was able to make some changes at work so that they didn't have to engage with one another much and, if they did, it was strictly by email. He gave Nicole access to his email account so that she could read the content of those emails in the spirit of transparency and to build trust. Nicole then asked, "What was it about her that attracted you to her?"

Martin responded, "I felt a kinship with her because we were like-minded. We were both frustrated with management, and we talked about starting our own business together." He stated that he enjoyed sharing his knowledge with others, and she listened to him and seemed to admire him.

Next, it was Nicole's turn to share how the betrayal had deeply affected her. There's a tendency for the involved person to minimize the consequences of their actions on their partner, and it's important for the involved person to connect with the depth of their partner's pain. When the uninvolved partner believes the involved person has heard their pain and is truly remorseful, then, slowly, the hurt partner can begin to heal. Nicole shared with Martin that she experienced anger, resentment, emotional pain, and fear about his involvement with his mentee. She expressed her anger about the extent that this person was allowed into their personal lives. A stranger had personal knowledge about Nicole, their children, their home, their extended family, and had even been introduced to some of their friends in an effort to help her career. Nicole imagined that Martin spent all of his time thinking about this woman and trying to find ways to engage with her, all the while she had been trying to get his attention.

At one point, Nicole stated, "She seemed to be all that you talked about. You were forcing her down my throat so, no, I didn't want to meet her. You had already decided how you were going forward, and I just had to accept it." We knew that it was important that Nicole share how she felt about the betrayal, but she needed to be able to express herself in ways that would help rather than hurt the relationship. While we empathized with Nicole, we also knew we needed to protect Martin. Criticism, defensiveness, and contempt are always destructive. We create emotional safety for each partner, so we intervene when we hear these creep into the conversation. Martin needs to witness the full impact of his actions on Nicole, but he can only do so if he feels emotionally safe. Carrie recognized that it was important to reconstruct this exchange and used body language to indicate she wanted to say something in the moment. She leaned forward and shared with Nicole, "Careful, when we say things like 'you were forcing her down my throat,' it can feel like criticism and blame. When someone feels blamed, they have a hard time listening. Let's try that another way. Talk about how you felt about the situation and what you needed." This is called a "softened startup."

Nicole was able to reframe, "I felt powerless. I had no control over this woman being let into our personal life, and I need to be able to have a say in who is let into our lives." Nicole later told Martin that resentment built as she felt abandoned by him emotionally and physically through the years. When she needed his assistance physically due to a recent injury, he was preoccupied with his job and engaging with his mentee, and Nicole was left to her own devices.

At one point Martin began to get defensive by stating that he has fears of losing relevance and was excited about his work, so that's why he engaged with her. We gently encouraged Martin to just take in the information for now and reminded him he'd have a turn to speak as well. We didn't step in with the antidote to defensiveness, which is accepting some responsibility at this point, because we wanted to keep Martin in the listener role and keep the focus on Nicole. We would ask Martin to take some responsibility for his behavior later. Martin successfully summarized what Nicole said and validated her emotional pain. He appeared sad as he said, "I know that my focusing on her like that really hurt you. I'm sorry that I did that. I know I've said that before, but I am. I want to change so that I'm actively thinking about you." Nicole teared up, looked at Martin for a moment, then reached out and put her hand on top of his. She told him that his acknowledging her pain meant a great deal to her. It was the first time he'd expressed empathy for what she'd been going through. She finally believed that he understood the emotional toll on her, and she accepted his apology.

Many individuals become emotionally triggered by certain events after there's been a betrayal. For example, every time Martin picked up his phone to check for text messages or email, Nicole became tense and imagined that he was receiving a text or email from his mentee. The very mention of Martin's company by name, or the other woman's name, evoked feelings of anger. We encouraged Nicole to let Martin know when she was getting triggered, and they discussed what would be helpful to her during those times. She needed Martin's understanding and empathy. She also needed Martin to understand that these strong emotional reactions were beyond her control.

Finally, we checked in with Nicole to see if she had any other unanswered questions. She and Martin had had many conversations about his relationship with the other woman before they entered treatment; however, these usually devolved into frustrating, tearful, exchanges in which both felt defeated. Nicole said that she was now satisfied that she knew everything that she needed to know, and it was clear to us that they were much calmer at this point. They also indicated that they understood Nicole's emotional triggers and what to do when those occurred. They expressed that the atonement process, which had lasted about 6 hours, had been completed. Since people often need to review parts of the atoning conversation, we told them that if Nicole had more questions or negative feelings arose, that's okay. These phases aren't completely linear.

INTERMEDIATE PHASE OF THERAPY

The main part of Gottman therapy for betrayal is the attunement phase; it focuses on improving the couple's relationship, which had been deteriorating over time. After Martin and Nicole worked through some of the issues directly related to the betrayal, it was time to help them face the fact that their marriage had degenerated almost to the point of complete failure prior to Martin's becoming involved with another woman. It's sometimes difficult to know when a couple is ready to move from the atonement phase to the attunement phase. Fortunately, there are clues that helped us know that it was time to move forward in the therapy. With Martin and Nicole, as with most couples when there's been a betrayal, the involved partner is motivated to get to the second stage and move beyond the conversations about the betrayal itself. Those conversations are uncomfortable, and most involved partners want to shift the focus from the betrayal itself to the larger context of the problems that existed prior to the betrayal. However, we can't assess the readiness to move forward based on the desires of the involved partner; instead, the hurt partner has to be the one to tell us when they're ready to begin dealing with the problems and events that had driven them apart. We began to hear Nicole describe how she knew their marriage was in trouble before Martin had ever gotten involved with his mentee. She began to say things like "I know not everything was your fault" and "I know I was part of the problem, too." Statements like these indicate that perhaps it's time to introduce some of the interventions that we use to help couples understand their conflicts better, and to begin to make changes in the way they relate to one another.

Of course, there are times when moving from atonement to attunement requires more therapy than is offered in a marathon session. For example, the uninvolved partner may need additional therapy to deal with their trauma from the betrayal, especially if they've had similar experiences earlier in life. Other moderating influences include the duration and extent of the betrayal. One of the most difficult issues arises when the involved partner has developed a deep connection or feelings of love for the person with whom they've been involved. The grieving process over the loss of that relationship can't proceed within the couple sessions. Moreover, either partner may feel anxious about reentering a relationship that has felt bad for a long time. Indeed, some of this dynamic was present with Martin and Nicole. Before proceeding to the attunement phase, we (Carrie and Don) privately discussed that we'd need to facilitate a structured conversation about those anxieties at the beginning of this next phase of therapy.

As with many couples, we found it necessary to address the dynamic of flooding. It comes as no surprise that many people have little understanding about how intense negative emotions can make it impossible for them to have safe, productive conversations. We use different terms to identify this state. Sometimes we refer to it as "flooding," other times as "diffuse physiological arousal." There are times in a couple's interaction when their bodies react to what's going on at a hormonal and neurological level. The amygdala senses danger, the heart rate accelerates, and stress hormones such as cortisol and adrenaline are released into the bloodstream. There are many changes that occur when these hormones rise—including changes in the frontal cortex of the brain, reducing one's ability to hear and see clearly what is occurring. Nicole and Martin both identified how much they hated the feelings that come when they're flooded. They had developed a pattern of avoidance years earlier to prevent or escape moments of flooding. This approach typically leads to stonewalling—another element of destructive patterns for relationships. Often, when someone begins to sense that they're getting flooded, they seek to shut it down. They break eye contact, stop speaking, and stop listening. Usually, one person goes into stonewall mode, while the other person tends to escalate and become louder, attempting to break through their partner's withdrawal (also known as the demand–withdraw pattern). This had happened with regularity in Nicole's and Martin's past. We decided on explaining the process of flooding, with the goal of creating a safe response as a primary intervention.

We introduced Martin and Nicole to a simple time-out procedure. We asked each of them to identify a simple gesture or word that would signal to their partner the request for a 30-minute break in the interaction. We discussed how best to use those 30 minutes to calm down and restore a sense of normality within their own bodies and brains. We also emphasized how to reconnect at the end of the 30-minute break. Like so many other couples, they had attempted a similar process to calm down negative exchanges but without a clear ending to the time-out, and they ended up feeling more distant. Since we know that a heart rate of over 100 beats a minute indicates flooding for most people, we asked each of them to wear pulse oximeters during our therapy conversations. Our hope was to interrupt any flooding that might occur in the session, as well as to train them to become more aware of their own autonomic processes that lead to a state of diffuse physiological arousal.

Martin and Nicole had been living in a pattern of discussing problems in the two-speakers and no-listeners model for years. We asked them to converse about why they thought they had fallen into such an extreme parallel lifestyle. They immediately began to point to one another, attributing the problem to the other's mistakes—a classic criticism–defensiveness pattern. We interrupted the conversation and introduced them to a structure that enables both partners to feel heard, understood, and validated. In this technique, each person is given the opportunity to be the speaker and the listener. The listener is asked to postpone their own agenda, jot down some notes about what their partner is saying, and then summarize and validate their partner when they've finished speaking. Validation is an important part of the process—accepting and understanding the partner's feelings and point of view without necessarily agreeing with them. Martin volunteered to take the listening role first. We encouraged him to ask Nicole open-ended questions about her feelings related to the distance between them.

We instructed Nicole to speak directly to Martin about the way she felt, which was difficult for her at first. One of our goals is to strengthen partners' ability to converse directly with one another about their experience rather than through us. Nicole expressed her feelings of frustration and loss as Martin's work demanded more and more of his time and energy. She saw that he was intentional about making time with the children a priority, but not time with her. After a few moments, Nicole began slipping back into the language of blame and criticism. When that happens, we pause the conversation, gently point out the language of criticism or defensiveness, and coach the couple into a more positive way of expressing their feelings and needs. Criticism has at its heart a desire for something to change for the better. However, when that desire is expressed as blame, the situation doesn't improve. After a few unsuccessful attempts by Nicole to express herself without using criticism, Carrie decided that Nicole needed some extra help. She drew on her own empathic skills to speak in the first person as if she were Nicole (a technique described by Wile & Kaufmann, 2021) to model for Nicole a way of expressing her deepest feelings and needs without the language of attack. Carrie helped Nicole express her fears that the changes they might make would only be temporary, and that she couldn't face the pain of continuing to live in a disconnected marriage. Carrie asked Nicole if this was what she was trying to say, and she affirmed Carrie's reframing of her experience and feelings. Carrie then asked Nicole to express these to Martin in her own words. Nicole then stated, "I need to be seen and engaged with. I would love to do that with you. I've felt abandoned and unfulfilled in life. I crave love, intimacy, and joy. We've fallen off of the horse and need to figure out if we want to get back on. If we do want to get back on, we need to figure out how to get on and stay on." This created a sense of apprehension for Martin, and he expressed that he was wondering about Nicole's commitment to their future together. We helped him understand that Nicole was pleading for a new relationship with Martin rather than simply patching up the old one. This helped them create a common narrative for what it was that they both were seeking.

Martin summarized notes that he'd taken and validated Nicole's needs and feelings to her satisfaction. He said, "You've been feeling so alone and left out for a long time. My work seemed to trump everything, and you were left to handle everything to do with raising the kids and running the house. I spent time with the kids, but not with you personally. You lost who *we* were, but maybe more importantly you lost a sense of who *you* were along the way." Martin softened and said, "How sad, and lonely, and scary."

Then we reversed roles and asked Nicole to listen to Martin. He identified that the distance between them grew so much wider after their children left the home. He teared up and paused at times to collect himself. He said that he felt that his role had degenerated to one of simply providing money for the family and that he wasn't loved or desired for himself. More tears began to flow. He shared that his father never offered him any sense of admiration for his accomplishments, and Martin had worked hard his whole life just for some acknowledgment. Those feelings were repeated for him in his relationship with Nicole. Whenever he brought up what he had accomplished, he felt that Nicole minimized it. He was also hurt by Nicole when he expressed similar feelings about being discounted at work and she seemed not to care about the pain that caused him. He expressed admiration for Nicole's caretaking of her own mother but, at the same time, felt that he wasn't a priority for Nicole anymore.

At one point, as Martin slipped back into criticism, Don looked at Carrie and prompted, "Dan Wile?" Carrie then asked Martin if she could try speaking for him, similar to the way she had with Nicole. She moved over to sit next to him, and spoke as if she were Martin—adopting more emotional and metaphorical language. Carrie wanted to paint an emotional picture of Martin's loneliness, his longing to be loved and respected by Nicole, and to feel worthy of that love in a way that he'd never experienced before. Carrie checked in with Martin to see if that was accurate, and he replied that it was exactly how he felt. Carrie then asked him to share that message to Nicole in his own words. As he did so, they seemed to move past criticism or blaming.

Nicole asked, "How did that affect you?" and Martin explained that he sensed her tacit approval for him to intensify his independence. Martin had drawn from the message that what gave him a sense of identity had no value to Nicole, who seemed involved in her own journey of discovering new interests and passions. As Martin spoke, he seemed careful to avoid saying anything that might upset Nicole, and we encouraged him to speak honestly about his needs and feelings. Finally, Nicole was able to hear Martin's deep sense of hurt, sadness, and loneliness. Nicole summarized notes she'd taken and validated Martin's feeling of loneliness, being left out, and longing to be acknowledged and loved. She was silent a few moments and then continued, "What a wonderful feeling that you would actually want to partner with me to find my interests."

Don said, "You seem surprised." She stated that she was surprised that Martin was interested in her. This was new information. This conversation proved a pivotal interaction for this couple. It softened them toward one another and allowed them to voice their feelings about the parallel lives they'd been leading, and their need for things to be different.

A major goal of our work is for couples to process and repair arguments or other negative moments from their past. An intervention drawn from the Gottman method for addressing "the aftermath of a fight or regrettable incident" was designed to help with this process. It's a five-step approach that helps the partners (1) express the feelings they had during the incident, (2) understand one another's subjective reality of the incident, (3) explore past emotional triggers that contributed to the argument, (4) take responsibility for their own part, and (5) discuss ways that might help in a similar situation. Often, this intervention is introduced in the initial phase of therapy but, when there's been a betrayal, as in this case, it's best to wait until the conversation about the affair itself (the atoning step) has been completed. We never use this intervention to talk about the betrayal itself since, by its nature, this intervention prompts each partner to take some responsibility for the event and would be counterproductive in the event of a discussion of betrayal.

During breaks in our sessions, we frequently consult with one another about what we think would be the next helpful step. Then one of us asks, "Do you want to start this next conversation, or shall I?" We believe it's best for couples to experience us alternating in the lead role when we introduce an intervention, as modeling for how to interact as equals.

There are times during the session that we ask the other out loud what they think is the best course of action. We want to model how to seek and accept influence, as well as how to be respectful toward one another. So we say things like "May I step in here?" or "May I say something here?" We notice that couples intently watch us as we interact with one another.

Don introduced Nicole and Martin to the need for repair by explaining that miscommunication is the norm in relationships. We're all frequently distracted and not giving our partner our full attention, so misunderstandings occur often. We need some way of repairing when things go off track to regain our sense of emotional connection. We asked Martin and Nicole to tell us about an argument they both remembered that was painful for them. They recounted a conversation they had had about who would get what if a divorce occurred. Nicole had presented Martin a list that she thought was supportive and considerate of them both. However, he got the message that she'd already given up on the marriage, and a fight erupted.

They took turns listing many negative feelings that were associated with this event. It was striking how many of their feelings were similar, especially the feelings of loneliness and rejection. Listening to one another's subjective reality can be very difficult. Like most couples, Nicole and Martin initially tried to convince each other that their own version of the story was correct and that their partner's version was flawed. Using our five-step structure for processing negative events, we stepped in anytime they began their criticism and defensiveness dance as they discussed their own experiences of the earlier exchange. In Nicole's subjective reality, she had given a lot of thought to how their possessions would be divided. When she presented Martin the list and heard him say, "It's all mine! Lawyer up!" she became enraged. She followed him into the bedroom and brought up a lot of old wounds that she knew would hurt him.

But in this conversation after we paused her, she shared, "I crucified you. I saw you in agony as you left the room. I wasn't proud of myself." She felt abandoned and thought to herself, "It's going to turn really ugly, which is my worst fear."

We encouraged Martin to ask her, "Why was that your worst fear?"

Nicole tearfully responded, "Not only was our marriage over but also our family would be torn. We were role models for our kids." Martin summarized Nicole's reality. We asked him to imagine being in Nicole's shoes, to feel the pain of tearing their family apart, envisioning what that might look like. Martin looked at Nicole, nodded, and said that he could understand her feelings of hurt and abandonment if that's what she experienced.

Then it was Martin's turn. He stated that, in his reality, it seemed that Nicole was making a unilateral decision to end the marriage and he had no say. He was going to fight to keep them together. He felt attacked—shocked, hurt, confused—when Nicole came into their bedroom and brought up all of his prior misdeeds. At that point, he thought to himself that maybe he would be better off on his own. Martin recalled saying, "It's as much mine as yours—lawyer up!" Nicole softened as she realized the full emotional weight of Martin's belief that he was powerless over the loss of his family, his possessions, and her. She validated how his feelings of loss, defensiveness, and powerlessness must have seemed like his whole life was being taken away from him, so his emotions made sense given his perspective.

Exploring their triggers may have been the most helpful part of this experience for the couple. Martin stated that he felt excluded and that he was being thrown out of his own home. Initially, he wasn't able to identify a story related to this trigger. However, Carrie recalled that Martin's mother had left the family, and his parents had divorced when he was a child, so she said, "Think about your mother."

Martin's facial expression changed to sadness. He said, "Mom made unilateral decisions. There was no discussion. Then she just left us." He felt helpless. Nicole also had a trigger associated with this fight. She had favorite aging relatives who had no children, to whom she very close. Her sister had been caring for them, but it became too much for her. They hired a caretaker, a woman they knew and trusted to take good care of the elderly couple. Her relatives then changed their will and left everything to the caretaker. All of her beloved relatives' possessions and home were taken without so much as a small memento by which to remember them. Nicole had felt caught off guard and powerless. During this discussion, both Martin and Nicole were able to take in their partner's emotional stories, have greater empathy for one another's triggers, and understand how they were activated in this situation.

Martin then apologized for attacking Nicole and causing her to feel threatened and abandoned. In kind, Nicole expressed regret and apologized for having said things to Martin that she had known would hurt him. We then encouraged them both to ask for what they need in positive terms. Many couples state only what they don't want or need, which leaves their partner clueless about how to be successful with them. As they discussed a plan to make similar events better in the future, Martin stated that he could recognize when he's flooded, remove himself, and go calm down. He said it would be helpful if Nicole did the same. Nicole stated that she could also take a moment to calm down and use the word "Gottman" to encourage them both to calm down. (We were amused by her choice of this verbal prompt, and smiled at one another.)

Nicole and Martin found this processing of the prior critical incident helpful. They reported that they understood why things went off track in that discussion, and they felt more emotionally connected to one another. We discussed ways they could use this approach on their own by checking in with each other on a weekly basis to see if anything had occurred that needed to be processed in this way. We also told them about additional resources available on the website *https://gottmanconnect.com* and encouraged them to watch videos there demonstrating the process we'd just used together.

As Martin and Nicole continued to explore ways to create the marriage that they both desired, it became apparent that they were struggling with a number of gridlocked conflicts. Gridlocked conflicts begin as normal, ongoing differences of opinion. However, when they become so difficult to manage that every conversation about that issue leads to feelings of extreme negativity or a sense of hopelessness, they're destructive. Martin and Nicole had developed a painful gridlocked conflict around the idea of giving praise and acknowledgment and the role that acknowledgment should play in their interactions. Each of them had developed extreme negative reactions to the way their partner would ask for or withhold acknowledgment. In fact, this was a central contributing factor in Martin's involvement with a woman outside the marriage who provided the praise and acknowledgment that he wanted. We sometimes share examples from our own relationship of differences, and how we negotiate them, to illustrate that all couples have differences, so partners need to collaborate in managing them rather than becoming entrenched in fixed positions (e.g., we have ongoing perpetual differences around what it means to be "on time"!).

We used an intervention we refer to as "dreams within conflict" to help Martin and Nicole understand the nature of their gridlock and to resume a dialogue about the issue.

This intervention provides a structure for a conversation that enables each person to gain a deeper understanding of their partner's feelings, needs, and core values. Often, partners also gain insight into their own deep values as they go through this conversation. The goal is not only to go beyond the expression of their feelings and needs, but also to gain insight about *why* they feel so strongly about the issue and defend their position to the point of gridlock. As each partner understands the other's deepest dreams, the hope is that they'll find ways to honor that dream, even when it differs from their own.

Nicole and Martin took turns as speaker and listener. Martin was the speaker first—and Nicole, as the listener, was given a list of nine open-ended questions that she was to ask in order—for example, "What are your core ethics, beliefs, or values that are part of your position on this issue?" and "Is there a story behind this, or does it relate to your childhood history in some way?" We want partners to be introspective and try to answer these questions as specifically as possible. We encouraged Nicole to ask any additional questions as long as they helped to enhance her understanding of Martin's feelings and dreams. Martin began by talking about how important he believed the role of both giving and receiving acknowledgment is in all relationships. He believes that doing so is a sign of both humility and respect. He was strongly affected by his father's and infrequent acknowledgment or praise. His father created a competitive environment between Martin and his siblings that made him feel inferior. Martin's only experiences of his father's approval came secondhand from what others told him his father had said. While discussing his feelings about this, Martin said that he feels a great deal of anger when others seek to take credit for something that he's said or done. He's careful to offer credit to others and finds himself quite upset when that isn't reciprocated. In addition to anger, Martin identified feelings of sadness, frustration, and even powerlessness when acknowledgment is withheld. He shared that his dream would be to have a greater sense of sincere praise and acknowledgment from others, especially from Nicole. In this exercise, we typically don't ask partners to summarize or validate what the other has said, but simply to take in at an emotional level their partner's sharing.

After switching roles, Nicole then answered these same questions posed by Martin. She described a core belief that one should do things for others without a sense of reward or recognition, and that receiving recognition for herself creates a sense of discomfort. These beliefs were rooted in ideas she had learned from her family growing up. For Nicole, being a team player and not needing to be recognized was the proper approach. She had struggled with a learning disability and, therefore, her family had focused on the effort that went into the work rather than its outcome. She was taught that bragging and seeking admiration was the opposite of being humble. She has strong negative feelings about people whom she sees as self-promoters. Nicole's dream was to be gracious and humble, and she hoped to find a way to balance this difference with Martin. She wished to become more gracious in the giving and receiving of acknowledgments, as well as to honor her own values around humility.

This dreams within conflict exercise proved to be central in helping Nicole and Martin begin to tune into one another in a new way. Their deeper understanding of one another's core values related to this issue and their individual histories that helped shape those values opened the path to discussing their feelings and needs without negativity and blame. At the end of this intervention, we asked them what they had learned about themselves or their partner, and if they felt that their partner had heard and understood them. Each reported that they had learned a great deal, as they had never tied their past to the current problem.

After they understood one another's core needs, the next step was to help them develop a temporary compromise that considered both partners' needs. Nicole and Martin developed a compromise around the issue of acknowledgment and praise. Nicole could look for opportunities to share Martin's accomplishments in the company of others, and Martin could be patient and wait to engage until the subject had been introduced. They both agreed that Martin was good at giving recognition and praise to others. However, he would try to wait for others' acknowledgment of his accomplishments rather than seek it out. He also agreed to let Nicole know in private if he felt slighted or overlooked.

CONCLUDING PHASE OF THERAPY

The final phase of therapy when betrayal has occurred is attachment. We introduce this phase of therapy when the negativity within the relationship has subsided and the couple is ready to build back positivity in their relationship. This is an important step. However, there are times when the negativity remains high, even at the end of the marathon sessions, and follow-up sessions are needed. Fortunately, Nicole and Martin were able to begin working on the attachment phase during the marathon therapy. We used several specific interventions to help them restore a deeper friendship: (1) development of rituals of connection, (2) drawing on a positive adjective checklist, and (3) use of the "state of the union" method to create regular check-ins.

One specific ritual of connection we proposed is a stress-reducing conversation, in which partners talk with each other as friends about stressors that are external to their relationship. We ask them to use the speaker–listener format. The speaker shares their external stressors, and the listener remains curious and empathic. The listener avoids solving the problem or any attempts to introduce another point of view. Don explained that when this conversation is done well, it can be a binding force in the relationship, as it builds trust that one's partner will be there for them emotionally in times of need. We suggested that they practice this in the session.

Martin began by describing how his colleagues keep ignoring his proposals even though he has more experience than they, so he has a strong feeling of not being heard or valued at work. He also struggled with what to do about some mediocre employees in several locations. Nicole listened, empathized, and asked some insightful questions. She asked, "What's the worst that could happen in that situation?" He responded that all of the work would fall on his shoulders.

Nicole then shared her stressors. Her mother's health is deteriorating and Nicole doesn't live nearby, so she relies on others for information. Martin asked about her fears. She replied that she feared not understanding the issues and what to do about them. She needed to feel like she's ahead of the learning curve. Nicole was also concerned that someone else would become the caregiver for her mother and she would be cast aside. Martin listened and empathized. He was aware of the prior family situation in which Nicole's aging relatives had changed their will to give everything to a paid caregiver and cut out the family. Martin asked if this factored into Nicole's feelings, and she replied that she didn't believe her mother would do that, but the feelings of being cast aside were similar.

One of our favorite interventions for building positivity is to provide partners with a positive adjective checklist, ask each of them to identify five positive adjectives from the list that are qualities that their partner has, then tell a specific story about a time when the partner displayed that characteristic. In describing Nicole, Martin chose "generous," "considerate," "good friend," "warm," and "intuitive." And in describing Martin, Nicole chose "playful," "organized," "interesting," "intelligent," and "great partner." Both of them shared a specific story connected to each characteristic in a way that emotionally touched their partner. We watched Nicole and Martin smile, tear up at times, and laugh with each other. We asked what this experience was like for them. They both loved the exercise and wanted to continue to incorporate it into their lives. We suggested that they create a morning ritual in which they would share an appreciation and story daily.

Another intervention aimed at maintaining changes a couple has made is to ritualize a weekly "state of the union" meeting. "What is the state of our union?" The partners discuss how they're doing with respect to positivity in their relationship. They also ask each other if there were any moments during the week that didn't go well. Did any of those moments rise to the level that they need to be processed further now? If so, they're encouraged to use the previously described five-step method for processing negative incidents. Finally, each partner asks what the other needs to make the next week better.

We revisited the boundaries that the couple had discussed earlier in the atoning phase. Nicole needed Martin to limit his interactions with the other woman. The consequences of any deception would devastate their marriage. To continue to develop trust, she needed access to Martin's emails and text messages, and these were not to be erased. Martin's phone would be in plain sight. Nicole also needed to be able to share triggering moments and have Martin be supportive of her needs at those times. This could be as simple as asking the question, "What do you need?" Martin agreed. He said he wanted to have more "frontal lobe" or intentional thinking about Nicole.

As our work with Nicole and Martin ended, we gave them online access to the Gottman Relationship Builder, which offers a series of videos on how and why to do specific exercises. We hoped they would refer to these videos to reinforce the learning acquired during therapy. We followed up with Martin and Nicole 3 weeks later to see how they were doing. They reported that they were pleased with how diligent they'd been with their weekly check-ins and stress-reducing conversations. They had remained curious about one another. They reported some tense moments, mostly in dealing with friends who could be a bit stressful. Each told the other what they needed during those times. Martin acknowledged that he encountered some "Dad" triggers in feeling devalued around that group of friends, and he asked Nicole to use her diplomacy skills to intervene on his behalf. She graciously had agreed to do so.

FURTHER REFLECTIONS AND IMPLICATIONS

Our work with Martin and Nicole went well, and they expressed deep gratitude as we said our good-byes. As we reflect on our work with this couple, questions we've asked ourselves include the following: What were the pivotal moments for this couple? And what are the strengths and limitations of this type of therapy?

We recognized several pivotal moments. We knew we needed to get Martin and Nicole to be softer with each other, which meant we had to keep them out of the criticism and defensiveness dance. We interrupted them every time they launched into a criticism and helped them describe how they felt about the situation and what they needed. We helped each of them take responsibility for their part in the problem rather than defending themselves from perceived attacks.

It was also important that each of them felt that their partner heard their emotional pain. One of the pivotal moments occurred when drawing on the intervention described by Wile and Kaufmann (2021) in which Carrie modeled empathic responding for Nicole. We use metaphors to paint a graphic picture of what the partner's emotional pain is like, taking care not to blame the other person. We're firm believers in keeping the experience within one's own body. So instead of saying, "I felt like you didn't care about me and what I needed," we reframe it to "I felt totally invisible. I was desperate for some sense of connection. In a sense, it's like I was drowning. I was screaming at the top of my lungs for someone to save me, but no one could hear my screams." When Nicole was able to share with Martin her emotional experience without attacking him, he softened toward her. He leaned in toward her and reached for her hand to console her. His gesture indicated that she did matter to him a great deal.

The dreams-within-conflict intervention had a big impact on Nicole and Martin as well. They'd never considered how their childhood histories had impacted their struggle regarding being explicitly acknowledged or affirmed. We suspect some therapists would have seen Martin's need for acknowledgment as some narcissistic need and judge it negatively. While we didn't fully understand his need for acknowledgment at the outset, rather than judging him we trusted the process of this intervention and learned that there was never a sense of fairness for Martin as a child. He loves mentoring young adults because he wants to give them something that he needed. He was committed to righting an injustice from his past, and one of his missions in life is to motivate others. An important recognition for them both was that Martin's overinvolvement with the mentee was mostly rooted in his feelings of loss of attention and specialness from Nicole. She was able to recognize her role in his feeling unimportant. The more he seemed to demand recognition, the more she felt the urge to withhold it. They were able to discuss this without making that dynamic an excuse for his overinvolvement with the young woman. The takeaway from this new understanding became the basis of their compromise plan for Nicole to look for opportunities to share Martin's accomplishments in the company of others, and for Martin to be patient and wait to engage until the subject had been introduced.

An additional pivotal moment was when Nicole and Martin learned to work with their physiological flooding. Psychoeducation helped them understand what was happening both within their own bodies and between them in their interactions. They learned how to reconnect with one another after the time-out to avoid their tendency to drift apart when things felt negative or out of control.

What are the strengths of marathon therapy compared to more traditional formats of pacing sessions across weeks or months? Marathon therapy allows a therapist to delve deeply into the couple's struggles and work toward deeper insight and understanding. Time in each session is limited in traditional weekly therapy. A couple comes in and may complain about a current problem that gets discussed, but deeper underlying issues often don't get addressed. Marathon therapy, on the other hand, provides sufficient time for the couple to process their major gridlocked issue thoroughly and completely.

One limitation of the marathon format is that although there's enough time to explore some gridlocked issues, other gridlocks may need to be processed by a couple on their own or in follow-up sessions. We've found that once couples have successfully worked through their major gridlock, they've often gained necessary skills to manage remaining gridlocked issues on their own. For example, we wish we had had time to explore Nicole's and Martin's struggles with their sex life. We knew that we had to clear the debris of the betrayal and then reduce their gridlocked conflict before we could delve into their sex life, and there wasn't enough time to do a thorough exploration. On occasion, certain comorbidities make it necessary to modify our marathon therapy format—for example, issues of substance misuse, intimate partner violence, unresolved grief, or major mood disorders. Sometimes these issues appear prior to beginning therapy, and other times they appear during the assessment process. We remain flexible in the marathon therapy process to make sure that those issues are addressed in the most helpful way. We often refer partners to individual therapy in these situations. Although some individuals are more psychologically minded than others, the structure of the interventions can help most partners learn to identify and express their emotions. We've found that the main predictor of successful marathon therapy is the partners' desire to create a new and better relationship.

We addressed each of the three systems essential to a healthy relationship (friendship, conflict management, and shared meaning) in our work with Nicole and Martin. After dealing with the pain of betrayal, we worked to promote more effective conflict management. Interventions to enhance their friendship and sense of togetherness followed, and we were pleased that Martin and Nicole were able to use these successfully after struggling through the negativity of betrayal. Addressing these three systems—and following an explicit sequence of interventions addressing atonement, attunement, and attachment—guided our work and helped Nicole and Martin rebuild the marriage they each so desperately desired.

We enjoyed working with this engaging couple. One of the things we really like about marathon therapy is the depth at which we get to know our couples. We also love working with each other as cotherapists on the rare occasions that we get to do so. Each time, we find that we develop a new respect for the gifts that our partner brings into the therapy room. Sometimes we feel completely in sync about what direction the therapy needs to take or which intervention to use. At other times we're surprised at what our cotherapist partner suggests. It's often brilliant, and we may not have thought of it on our own! Carrie has high empathic intuition and is strongly attuned to partners' emotions, and Don has a gift for synthesizing information and conveying this in a way that all fits together. This blend of talents enlivens our work and seems to provide a therapeutic experience that our couples connect with as well.

REFERENCES

Glass, S. P., & Staeheli, J. C. (2004). *Not "just friends": Rebuilding trust and recovering your sanity after infidelity*. New York: Atria.

Gordon, K. C., Mitchell, E. A., Baucom, D. H., & Snyder, D. K. (2023). Couple therapy for infidelity. In J. L. Lebow & D. K. Snyder (Eds.), *Clinical handbook of couple therapy* (6th ed., pp. 413–433). New York: Guilford Press.

Gottman, J. M., & Gottman, J. S. (2018). *The science of couples and family therapy: Behind the scenes at the love lab*. New York: Norton.

Gottman, J. M., & Gottman, J. S. (2023). Gottman method couple therapy. In J. L. Lebow & D. K. Snyder (Eds.), *Clinical handbook of couple therapy* (6th ed., pp. 362–386). New York: Guilford Press.

Wile, D., & Kaufmann, D. (2021). *Solving the moment: A collaborative couple therapy manual*. [Published by Dorothy Kaufmann and available on Amazon.com at *www.amazon.com/solving-moment-collaborative-couple-therapy/dp/b08ydb69wf*]

CHAPTER 6

An Integrative Relational–Neurobiological Approach to Transforming Couple Vulnerability Cycles

MONA DEKOVEN FISHBANE

Editors' Comments

In this enlightening case narrative, Mona Fishbane offers a unique approach to integration—drawing on the best findings from neuroscience to complement a sophisticated blend of well-established psychosocial methods. Among the various implications of neurobiology for couple therapy, Fishbane emphasizes two in particular: first, the importance of early experiences in "wiring" emotional reactivities that persist and generalize well beyond their original acquisition; and, second, the importance of mindful intentionality governed by the prefrontal cortex in disrupting and regulating the "automaticity" of old habits fueled by long-term emotional memories associated with the limbic system and, specifically, the amygdala.

    Notice how sensitively Fishbane interweaves this neurobiological perspective into her overall therapeutic approach. She astutely avoids a reductionistic emphasis that focuses exclusively at the neural level of behavior but, instead, draws on neurobiology to promote partners' understanding of their own (and each other's) disproportionate or displaced emotional reactions to promote a softened empathic joining and, as importantly, alternative response strategies. In this way, Fishbane facilitates partners' choice, intentionality, and value-driven responses to previously unrecognized or underregulated emotions. This neurobiological perspective also promotes compassionate views regarding the difficulties of change and the likely reemergence of emotional reactivities under stress—thereby reducing risks of despair and facilitating renewed efforts consistent with partners' higher goals and values.

    Illustrating her integrative method, Fishbane also demonstrates how she draws on systemic, intergenerational, emotion-focused, and related approaches. Listen to how she carefully encourages partners to consider their enduring vulnerabilities, frequently rooted in family-of-origin experiences or other early trauma, and how she helps partners

> to understand their interlocking vulnerability cycles. Observe how Fishbane implements her own commitment to "multidirected partiality"—building a safe context and alliance with each partner. Notice also her thoughtful flexibility in briefly including other members from the family of origin in the service of helping one partner expand her understanding of her parents' own struggles and limitations. This case narrative offers a broad range of perspectives and specific interventions, delivered sensitively by an experienced therapist.

Some therapists love doing couple therapy; others find it intimidating to work with two people in conflict, especially if they are emotionally dysregulated, blaming each other, and looking to the clinician as judge. For therapists who as children were caught between warring parents, this dilemma is particularly painful. I'm in the "love doing couple therapy" category. I was born and bred to be a couple and family therapist. While not caught between warring parents (my parents had a loving marriage), I was highly tuned in to conflicts in my family of origin, wanting to make everyone happy. Of course, I learned that I couldn't do that—but I did connect with the claims and feelings of my parents and siblings, trying to see the merit in each person's perspective. Making room for multiple voices is key to my work as a systemic therapist.

My father was my first role model for working with people with conflicting claims. Whereas my mother and I were redheads, passionate, and at times tempestuous, my father endorsed the mantra "Be philosophical"—by which he meant calm down and see the bigger picture. When I was 8 years old, he asked if I wanted to know what an ancient Roman philosopher said about managing one's emotions. Intrigued, I said, "Sure." Dad shared these words from Seneca: "Most powerful is the person who has himself in his own power." I was blown away: I wanted that power! This wisdom has stayed with me all these years, informing my own ideas about power and emotion regulation as they apply to couple relationships (including my own).

When I was in psychology graduate school in the 1970s, I learned about the new contextual therapy of Ivan Boszormenyi-Nagy ("Nagy"). His approach highlights the ethical realm in relationships, with a focus on healing intergenerational wounds and cultivating "resources of trustworthiness" in families. One of contextual therapy's most significant ideas is "multidirected partiality" (Boszormenyi-Nagy & Krasner, 1986): The therapist sides with each partner in the couple or family, is partial to each. When clients feel that the therapist is on their side, they are more open to being challenged about unproductive behavior. Multidirected partiality applies as well to clients' extended families; Nagy was concerned with all the people in a client's life who might be affected by the therapy. I was immediately attracted to contextual theory and have devoted much of my professional life to teaching and expanding Nagy's ideas. Nagy was influenced by the dialogical philosophy of Martin Buber, as I was. My work with couples, demonstrated in this chapter, owes a great deal to both Buber and Nagy: How can we help couples in distress cultivate resources of trustworthiness and the capacity for dialogue? How can we side with each partner and earn their trust while challenging problematic behavior?

In 2004, I encountered the developing field of neuroscience, intrigued by research that shows what is going on neurobiologically when one falls in love, feels safe and secure, or is threatened or angry. Neuroscience sheds light on how to regulate emotions, and on the complex interaction of habits and change. Interpersonal neurobiology—the interplay of brain, body, and relationship—informs my approach to couple therapy (Fishbane, 2013).

My work is integrative, incorporating interventions from psychodynamic, systemic, intergenerational, narrative, and emotion-focused approaches. At the center of my therapy with couples is the "vulnerability cycle" (Scheinkman & Fishbane, 2004). Therapist and clients together map out the couple's dance, identifying feelings and behaviors that contribute to mutual reactivity. The couple is invited to shift from linear, blaming views to a circular view, each exploring responsibility for their part in their dance.

Couples come to therapy discouraged and disempowered, not knowing how to get through to each other, at times emotionally dysregulated and trapped in recursive cycles. Allying with both partners, I make room for multiple perspectives and explore core relational issues. In drawing the vulnerability cycle with the couple, we consider factors fueling each partner's vulnerabilities and self-protective survival strategies—often stemming from old wounds from the family of origin, or from injuries due to sociocultural traumas or oppression (e.g., racism, homophobia, migration, poverty, war). I help each partner to speak from vulnerability rather than react from survival strategy, and to "grow up" their survival strategies so they are more adaptive and less damaging to the other (e.g., negotiating a time-out to calm down rather than storming off in a huff). I offer techniques to increase empathy, respect, voice, and listening, encouraging couples to consider the impact of their behavior on each other. Clients are helped to identify their higher values and operationalize them, cultivating skills of empathy, respect, and repair.

Neurobiological research shows that humans are wired for care and connection as much as for fight or flight. In addition to ensuring safety and healthy boundaries between partners, I help couples cultivate habits of respect, compassion, and mutual care. This includes learning to "make a relational claim," speaking in a way that honors one's own concerns while at the same time holding concern for the partner and the relationship.

Therapists are in the business of change. Clients come to treatment to change (or sometimes hoping to change their partner!), yet may resist therapists' suggestions. Clinicians have long pondered how to deal with "resistance." I put this word in quotes because, informed by neuroscience, I understand that both the desire (and capacity) to change *and* the fear of (and difficulty with) change are built into the human brain. On the one hand, we are habit-driven creatures. Our habits are reflected in circuits of neurons in the brain; the more we repeat a habit, the stronger the circuit becomes. Clients' survival strategies are self-protective habits, often stemming from childhood; it is hard to change these ingrained ways of being.

At the same time, humans are capable of change and adaptation. Research shows that neuroplasticity, the ability of the brain to change, can continue throughout life. But it is harder to change old habits in adulthood; couple dances and survival strategies reflect habitual ways of interacting that have become automatic. Understanding how hard change can be helps me feel compassion for clients who are ambivalent about change. Rather than viewing them as "resisting" my therapeutic suggestions, I see clients' struggles with change as legitimate: Letting go of old habits of self-protection can be terrifying. Working collaboratively around the change–no change dilemma is crucial. There is no room for power struggles in the client–therapist relationship.

Most of the time, humans function on autopilot, enacting deeply ingrained patterns of thought and behavior. This automaticity is adaptive; the prefrontal cortex requires a great deal of energy (in the form of glucose) to function, and that energy supply is limited. The automaticity of daily life relies on lower brain regions that require less energy. But this very automaticity fuels couple distress. Partners react habitually, enacting behaviors and cycles that are not in keeping with their higher goals or values. I help clients cultivate *choice* and *intentionality* in their daily interactions, bringing prefrontal thoughtfulness to emotional reactivity and habitual interactions.

INITIAL ASSESSMENT AND CASE FORMULATION

Ron calls seeking couple therapy for himself and his wife Monica. As I take his call, I reflect on how, early in my career, with different-sex couples it was usually the woman who initiated therapy; men tended to see therapy as something for women or crazy people. But these days, it's as likely that the man makes the call. In this case, Ron is eager for couple therapy, since his long-term marriage with Monica is tottering on the edge of divorce. I ask what's prompting his call, and he briefly tells me about their marital difficulties since their daughters left home for college. We make an appointment for the following week.

As I prepare to meet this couple for the first time, I connect with my intention to be gracious to both partners, making room for each of their perspectives. Multidirected partiality is a core therapeutic value for me. Both partners need to feel I'm on their side if we are to work together. I also reflect on my concern that my office be a "shame-free, blame-free zone."

Like many couples, Ron and Monica are feeling a sense of shame and failure as they seek therapy. Sharing their difficulties with a stranger is embarrassing for them. I want to acknowledge their pain while also identifying their strengths, creating a space of safety and respect. As it turns out, these are two highly competent individuals who are struggling in their relationship. I've heard a bit of Ron's side of the story on the telephone; now it's time hear both of their concerns. I start with where they are now, why they're seeking help at this point. As I learned early in graduate school, "Why now?" is a key question to ask clients in the first session. In addition to hearing about their concerns bringing them to therapy, I inquire about the history of their relationship, what drew them to each other, and how they've evolved as a couple over the years.

As I learn in our first meeting, Monica and Ron are a White couple, married for 25 years. Their twin daughters are sophomores in college and doing well. Ron is an artist, Monica an attorney. Both report that they were a good team raising their children. Monica took off time from work when their daughters were young, then returned to full-time work once they were in school. She has always managed the practical aspects of the family's life. Once Monica returned to full-time work, Ron shouldered the main parenting role. Working from his home studio with flexible hours, Ron was a hands-on, devoted dad.

While the division of labor seemed fair in those days, since their daughters left home, Monica has become increasingly resentful over what she sees as lopsided responsibilities. She complains that she carries more than her share: taking care of the house, paying the bills, worrying about finances. She has a long-standing frustration over Ron's refusal to share cooking responsibilities. When their daughters were growing up, Ron nurtured their creative side, generating warmth and humor in the home. His involvement as a father assuaged Monica's sense of inequality in other spheres in their home life. But now that the girls are gone, Monica is frustrated and critical, accusing Ron of not doing his fair share. Ron, hurt, gets defensive and retreats to his studio.

Another long-standing difference between them has become increasingly contentious: Ron tends to be messy, leaving his stuff around the house, whereas Monica craves order and neatness. When Monica asks Ron to clean up (in a critical tone), he retorts that she should relax and live in the moment instead of constantly straightening up. They have similar fights about money; Monica worries about their financial future, while Ron believes in *carpe diem* ("seize the day") and tells Monica she is too uptight. Monica, feeling dismissed, gets angry, and Ron shuts down.

Listening to their story—really two different stories of how their relationship is so disappointing now—I wince as I feel their pain. Both are looking to me to validate their position, hoping that I'll judge their partner to be at fault. I sidestep the judge role. Guided by the contextual principle of multidirected partiality, I make space for each to speak their concerns, holding both with compassion and respect. Each must feel that I'm on their side. As we talk, it becomes clear that the girls' going to college has upended their balance at home and called into question their division of labor. In their upset, they become reactive and nasty. In their worst moments, Ron calls Monica "anal," and Monica retorts that Ron is a child, a "slob." I want to help them address their legitimate concerns—but they can only do that if they change the tone of their interactions, with less contemptuous name-calling. We will need to address their cycle of criticize–attack (Monica) and defend–withdraw (Ron). It's clear they are both hurting and, in the process, are hurting each other.

Before we get deeper into their cycle, I ask them how they met, and what drew them to each other. The tone in the room shifts as their eyes light up with the memories of their early love. "Ron was a free spirit," Monica recalls, "a breath of fresh air. He was funny, dashing, talented, and brought me out of my dutiful, 'good girl' self. He made me laugh! I felt so alive with him."

Ron smiles as he hears Monica's description of the young man who swept her off her feet. He is flush with memories of being adored and able to light Monica up. Ron recalls being immediately drawn to Monica: "She was beautiful, graceful, sexy, confident, practical. I loved how she navigated in the world, mastering the latest computer technology, understanding politics and the economy. She was so competent! She made feel safe. And she adored me, laughed at my jokes, and admired my paintings. I'd never felt so at home with someone in my life!" Monica's eyes are wide as she hears her husband recall his early infatuation and admiration of her.

I comment, "It's moving to see the two of you light up when you talk about your early love! I can see it in your smiles and shining eyes. Not every couple has that magical beginning of love, and your ability to recall that time so vividly suggests to me that your bond has been very strong." They nod in agreement as they shyly glance at each other. I indicate that while we'll be addressing what's gone wrong between them, we'll also bear in mind their love and care for one another. We'll work on ways to rekindle their connection. They tell me that they used to have a vibrant, mutually satisfying sex life. But now they have turned away from each other physically as well as emotionally.

I ask about their work lives. Monica, a partner in a big law firm, has labored hard to achieve status and security in her profession. While at times overburdened, she loves her work. Ron is a talented artist, an abstract painter with an international reputation. Over the years, his success has waxed and waned; when the muse visits him, he creates large, dramatic pieces, some displayed in major museums. He has been paid well for his work in the past. But the demand for his art is not steady, nor is his income. When bereft of his muse, he is less productive, and as he puts it, spends time "idling," waiting for inspiration. Monica rolls her eyes, suggesting that "lolling around" would be a better description. It drives her crazy to see him with no obligations or schedule, and no concern about earning money—while she "slaves away" every day and often into the evening on her law cases. Ron retorts that she is "bourgeois" and overconcerned with materialistic issues; she doesn't "stop to smell the roses."

Monica blows up: "How dare you call me bourgeois and materialistic?! I'm the one who pays the bills so you can wait for your muse to visit!"

I reflect to myself on how what I intended as a fact-based question about their work has sparked so much hostility in this couple, who just a few minutes ago were remembering their early love with a sparkle in their eyes. I say, "Clearly, my question about work touches on a painful issue between you. Can we look a bit more in depth at what each of you is feeling about your differences?" They nod. I indicate that I have heard each regarding their pain; I'm open to see if we can work together to improve their current relationship. Before we end our first meeting, I ask if they would like to meet a few more times and then assess whether they want to continue in therapy with me; they agree, and we make several weekly appointments.

BEGINNING PHASE OF THERAPY

As we continue our early sessions, I work toward a formulation of this couple's impasse—starting with their interactional dance (apparent in the first session), and then deepening our understanding through the vulnerability cycle diagram, as well as a genogram that explores intergenerational factors in each partner's stance and an exploration of larger contextual factors (culture, gender, power, financial resources, health, other concerns). I listen for strengths in each partner and in their relationship—what's working or has worked well in the past. I begin to focus on each one's vulnerabilities and survival strategies, and their impact on each other. Throughout, I identify painful feelings, as well as strengths and resources of trustworthiness.

All this exploration is done together with the couple. If I share a thought or observation, I do so tentatively, asking whether it makes sense to them. My stance is collaborative, including what I call "construal humility": I offer my ideas flexibly, not as dogma. While I have theories that guide my work, I am not wedded to them. Inspired by Martin Buber, I cultivate a "readiness to be surprised." Most importantly, as they share their pain, I hold both partners with compassion. They see me making space for two points of view—which is what I will help them do with each other. Indeed, I encourage *them* to adopt a stance of construal humility, open to multiple perspectives.

I don't draw the vulnerability cycle diagram, or construct a genogram, in the very beginning of therapy. I first listen to each partner's story, resonating with their pain and struggles. This is multidirected partiality in action, listening respectfully and empathically to their different narratives. Each partner needs to "feel felt" by me. I love this idea, which I learned from Dan Siegel (Siegel & Hartzell, 2003). With this stance, I am also role-modeling for the couple, facilitating curiosity and empathy between them—antidotes to blame and judgment. After three sessions, I ask if they want to continue our work: Do they think I can be helpful? The choice is theirs. Ron and Monica decide to continue.

The couple's dance (Monica's criticism, arising from her frustration; and Ron's withdrawal in hurt) is clear from the first phone call and first session. I see her criticism and his withdrawal as survival strategies, self-protective behaviors. As we continue to meet, the vulnerabilities that trigger these survival strategies start to emerge. I wonder to myself, "Why is Monica so angry?" Clearly her criticism pushes her husband away—so why does she stick with this strategy? And why does Ron keep shutting down and running to his studio in the face of Monica's criticism? Why can't he see the pain behind her anger and reach out to her? Did they learn to protect themselves in these ways long ago, perhaps in childhood? I am curious about their experiences growing up, which likely shaped their vulnerabilities and prompted survival strategies that were perhaps adaptive then but are so unproductive now, even threatening the marriage.

Drawing the Vulnerability Cycle Diagram

By the third or fourth session, I have a sense of their survival strategies and some hunches about vulnerabilities. I ask Monica what it's like for her that Ron doesn't help more in the house, especially since he has so much free time while she works long hours. She talks of feeling alone and overwhelmed. I ask Ron how he feels when Monica criticizes him. He sags in his chair, and says, "She makes me feel worthless. I'm already feeling badly that I haven't sold a painting in a long time, and her anger breaks my heart." As each shares these tender feelings, vulnerabilities underlying their reactivity, the mood in the room softens. They don't usually confide in each other like this, and something is starting to shift.

I suggest that we draw a diagram that illustrates what they're describing, their interactional pattern. Intrigued, they agree. We draw their vulnerability cycle diagram together, identifying each one's vulnerabilities and survival strategies; here is the result (see Figure 6.1).

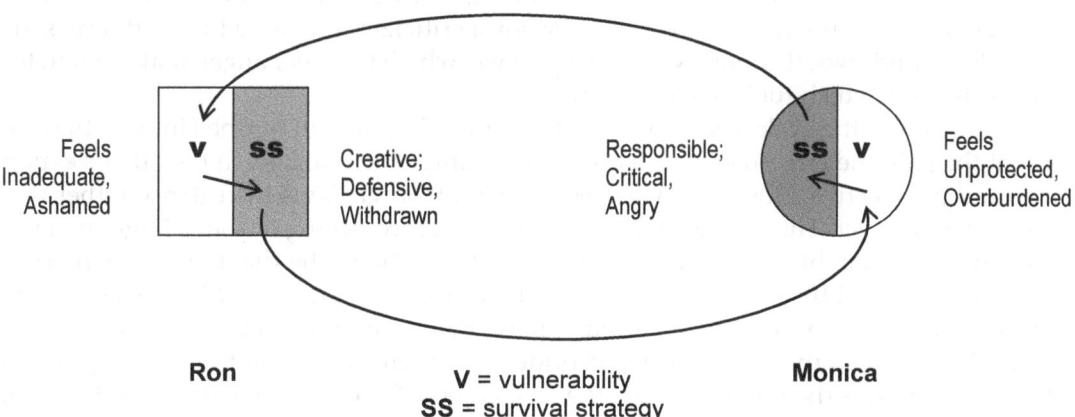

FIGURE 6.1. Vulnerability cycle diagram for Monica and Ron.

It's important that we draw the diagram in a collaborative manner. I don't impose my view of their dance; conjointly, we identify the components and process of their cycle. I explain that V stands for vulnerabilities, the tender feelings most of us carry, often from childhood; and SS stands for survival strategies, the self-protective mechanisms that get triggered automatically when our vulnerabilities are activated. I normalize this process: Self-protection ("survival strategies") when we feel threatened is instinctual; the particular survival strategy we use often stems from childhood.

I ask each to share their experience of being hurt in the relationship, and how they react in these moments to protect themselves. As unfolds in our exploration together, when Monica feels overburdened or unprotected (her vulnerabilities, which she experiences frequently with Ron these days), she can become resentful and critical (her survival strategies). When Ron feels a sense of inadequacy or shame (his vulnerabilities), especially around not being productive in his art and not earning money, and when Monica's criticism heightens these tender feelings, he resorts to defensiveness or withdrawal (his survival strategies), retreating to his studio, at times even sleeping there at night. When Ron withdraws, Monica feels more alone and unprotected. (They also have survival strategies that are not necessarily activated in their dance: Monica's responsibility, Ron's creativity. But even these positive traits can get caught up in the dance, for example, when she feels overresponsible and resentful, and he is creative to the point of being oblivious to the mess he is creating.)

Drawing the vulnerability cycle diagram, if done collaboratively and sensitively, can be a powerful intervention in couple therapy. Ron and Monica are wide-eyed as they see their dance laid out in front of them on paper. They see the circular nature of their interactions, and how each one's attempt at self-protection is hurting the other. It's crucial that I don't shame them for their vulnerabilities or survival strategies. I convey my compassion for their vulnerabilities and my respect for their survival strategies forged in childhood—even though they may be problematic now in the relationship. Something starts to shift in the room; instead of blaming and insulting each other, arms crossed in a defensive manner, they are leaning over the pad of paper, seeing their dance "out there." Drawing the diagram externalizes their cycle (Scheinkman & Fishbane, 2004). Rather than blaming each other in a linear fashion ("She's so controlling!"; "He's so inconsiderate!"), they see the circularity of their interactions: The more Monica criticizes, the more Ron withdraws; the more Ron withdraws, the more Monica feels alone, which fuels her anger, making Ron feel more ashamed, which fuels his withdrawal.

As we draw the cycle, their "who's the bad guy?" argument morphs into mutual sorrow at the pain they're causing each other. I encourage them to take in the other's experience and perspective. Slowly, they are becoming a *team* vis-à-vis their dance rather than blaming each other. They're "getting meta" to their dance, seeing it from a larger perspective, no longer caught up in it. Ron suggests that they hang the diagram on their fridge at home, to remind themselves, "This is the dance we've co-created." Monica agrees, and says that reminds her of how they used to hang their young daughters' drawings on the fridge. They did so then with glee and pride; now their vulnerability cycle diagram on the fridge reminds them that they are the co-creators of this unhappy dance. Rather than being victims of each other, they see they are coauthors of the dance, and that they can coauthor a new dance that is more in keeping with their values. This is our work. They leave the session with a bit of hope.

Neurobiology of the Cycle

In unpacking a couple's dance, I sometimes share insights I've gleaned from neuroscience about reactive cycles and emotion dysregulation. I ask Ron and Monica if they'd like to know what's going on in their brains and bodies when they get reactive with each other. Intrigued, their answer is "yes."

As part of this "neuroeducation," I demonstrate Dan Siegel's "Hand Model of the Brain" (Siegel & Hartzell, 2003). I ask each to hold up their right hand and make a fist, thumb folded inside fingers. I explain that the fist symbolizes their brain, the arm their spine, with the vagus nerve carrying information between brain and body. The fingernails represent the prefrontal cortex—the part of the brain behind the forehead that allows for thoughtfulness, reason, emotion regulation, and perspective. This is the most recent part of the brain to evolve, and it is unique to humans.

Like other animals, deep in our brain we have an amygdala that scans for danger; when it senses threat, it sets off the "fight–flight" response (or "freeze" in life-threatening situations). With the fight–flight response, stress hormones are released, priming the body for action. The amygdala's job is to keep us safe; it is biased toward the negative. Raising the fingers in our hand model of the brain, I explain that the thumb represents the limbic system, with the amygdala, the source of the fight–flight response. With the fingers closed over the amygdala/thumb, the prefrontal cortex is active; the middle prefrontal cortex—represented by the middle two fingernails—regulates the amygdala. But, as Siegel notes, when we "flip our lid" (lifting the fingers, exposing the thumb), our higher brain goes offline, and the amygdala is left running the show. Ron and Monica laugh, recognizing their own "flipped lids" when they get reactive.

Part of our work, I explain, is to improve communication between the prefrontal cortex and the amygdala, so they can *choose* their own responses rather than be driven by knee-jerk reactivity. This neuroeducation is normalizing and deshaming for Monica and Ron: We all have an amygdala and can get dysregulated. Intrigued, they ask how they can bring their prefrontal cortex back online when they have an emotional meltdown. I tell them that we'll work on techniques for emotion regulation to help them bring prefrontal thoughtfulness to amygdala reactivity.

I share a bit more "news from neuroscience" in terms of habits and change. I note that the vulnerabilities and survival strategies that fuel their vulnerability cycle have become "wired" into their brain as circuits of neurons that are reflected in long-standing relational habits. It's hard to change these habits as an adult—but it *is* possible. I relate the wonderful, relatively recent news that neuroplasticity—the ability of the brain to change—is possible throughout life. But it takes work to make changes in habits as an adult. Ron and Monica are reassured that they can change their long-standing patterns, although it will take a lot of work and repetition of new behaviors, so their preferred interactional patterns will become "wired" into the brain as new habits. Eventually, the new behaviors will themselves become less effortful and more automatic.

When offering neuroeducation to clients, I don't give long lectures about the brain. But for many couples, learning a bit about what makes them reactive and how they can become more thoughtful—and the neuroscience behind it—is intriguing and empowering. Ron and Monica are committed to trying to utilize the capacities of the prefrontal cortex to make better choices and regulate their emotions. They are reassured to see that they're not doomed to be victims of their own reactivity. They are shifting from trying to change each other to working on their own issues.

INTERMEDIATE PHASE OF THERAPY

Having identified the interactional dance, drawn the vulnerability cycle, and discussed the neurobiology behind their reactivity, we now deepen the work, identifying roots of their vulnerabilities and survival strategies and exploring ways to transform the cycle. By this point in our work, they trust me and are willing to explore some of the historical roots of their individual experiences and modes of self-protection.

"The Magic Question"

I am curious about the origins of each partner's vulnerabilities and survival strategies in their families of origin, as well as the larger sociocultural context. For clients who have experienced sociocultural trauma—racism, homophobia, poverty, war, or migration—the origins may lie in this larger contextual realm. Ron and Monica are White, different-sex, cisgender, and privileged in terms of socioeconomic status. They have not known sociocultural trauma. However, as I now learn, both come from intergenerational histories of poverty, which shaped their family-of-origin experiences. Their current impasse, especially around work, is informed by the role of poverty and other dynamics in their intergenerational families.

I ask Monica, "Is it familiar to you, this feeling of being unprotected and overburdened that you feel with Ron? Have you felt that way before, maybe as a child?" I call this "the magic question," since it often deepens the conversation as we explore each partner's dynamics fueling the dance.

Monica replies, "As a child and teenager, I had to care for my younger brothers while my parents were at work all day and into the evening in their small grocery store. I was expected to make dinner, supervise my brothers' homework, and get them ready for bed. I had to clean up after them. I had no time for myself. If I ever protested, my parents talked about their own histories growing up in utter poverty in eastern Europe, and their difficult immigration journeys. I learned to do the work and not complain. But inside, I was frustrated, watching my friends being indulged, having playdates, their moms cooking dinners for them, while I was left to do it all with my rambunctious younger brothers. I became highly organized, a good student. I vowed that when I grew up, I would have enough money, so my kids wouldn't experience the deprivation I did. I worked my tail off to get into law school and rise in my law firm so I could have money, status, and job security."

Ron and I are moved as Monica tells her story in a rush, all the words she hasn't spoken before tumbling out. Ron knew that Monica grew up with little money and was a very responsible daughter and older sister, but Monica had never confided in him the price she paid for her parentified role in the family.

I ask Ron, "Is it familiar to you, feeling disconfirmed and inadequate, as you sometimes feel with Monica? Is this an experience you had growing up?" Ron clears his throat, fighting off the painful feelings rising inside. I wait patiently, as does Monica. He says that his mother saw his creative gifts and encouraged him to become an artist. He thrived with her affirmation. But she died of cancer when he was 12 years old, and everything changed. His father focused on keeping a roof over their heads and making ends meet. He, too, came from poverty; not having a higher education or profession, he worked two jobs. Determined that Ron, his only child, would be financially secure, he urged him to become an accountant and was dismissive of his son's dream of being a painter. After attending college on a scholarship, Ron dutifully went to accounting school but dropped out after a year; he couldn't bear it. Shrinking from his father's disappointment, Ron distanced from him, a rift that has not healed in all these years. Ron was determined to prove that he could make it as an artist and worked very hard. He put himself through art school, achieved a respected reputation and, in good times, was able to live off the sale of his paintings.

This conversation is moving to both partners as they imagine each other as young children, doing their best in painful circumstances. I help them see the origins of their vulnerabilities (Ron's sense of shame and inadequacy; Monica's feeling overburdened) and survival strategies (Ron's withdrawal; Monica's overresponsibility and resentment) in their families of origin.

They are beginning to deepen their perspectives on their chronic fights. Their unhappiness is not just about their current relationship; it carries the weight of history and old wounds. At some level, Ron is still trying to prove his worth as a person and as an artist. Monica is still carrying resentment over being a parentified child with too much responsibility—now enacted in her relationship with her husband. As they witness each other's wounds, compassion starts to grow.

Speaking from Vulnerability

I encourage them to tune in to their bodies and identify when they start to feel vulnerable—Monica, when she feels overburdened and unprotected, and Ron, when he feels inadequate or ashamed. I suggest that when their vulnerabilities are triggered, they confide in each other about it rather than going automatically to survival strategies (her criticism, his withdrawal). I ask Monica, "Instead of angrily accusing Ron of never cooking a meal, might you invite him to chop and sauté the onions for the soup you're making?" Monica had never thought about that option. Ron, hearing this, agrees to help in food prep. He never saw himself as a chef, feeling outshined by his wife in the culinary world. But he's willing to be her sous-chef. Ron reflects on how, after his mother died, he and his father ate fast food, avoiding the creative cooking his mother had done. I suggest that Monica might confide in Ron when she's tired at the end of the day and ask for his company and help in the kitchen. I offer, "Coming *to* Ron with an invitation to make dinner together would feel very different from coming *at* Ron with your anger." Ron agrees and confides that he assumed he would have to prepare gourmet meals if he agreed to cook, a skill he lacked. I suggest that he could ask Monica what he could do to help, and they could cook together. They are willing to try.

I encourage Ron to confide in Monica about his vulnerability around not making great art these days, and not selling enough to contribute significantly to their finances. Speaking from this vulnerable position is very different from attacking Monica about her "materialistic" concerns.

As we discuss finances, Monica shares her worry that she'll have to support her parents as they age. She explains that her parents have been giving more money than they can afford to her middle brother, a musician who has never been able to earn a living.

Monica worries that her parents will run out of money. As we explore this, a parallel emerges between the musician-brother who can't support himself and Ron's difficulty earning money from his art. Ron starts to get defensive, but I invite him to simply witness the burden Monica carries, with her fear that she will have to support three generations and will never be able to cut back at work. It takes a while, but with my help, Ron starts to see the burdens his wife is carrying with more empathy.

Somewhat reluctantly, Ron offers to revisit skills he learned in accounting graduate school before he dropped out. I make it clear that we're not fencing Ron into an identity or behaviors that limit his artistic inclinations. He agrees to go over the budget with Monica.

"Growing Up" Survival Strategies

As each partner becomes more aware of how their vulnerabilities trigger self-protective reactions, we work on the survival strategies themselves. I have rarely met a survival strategy I don't respect, once I hear the backstory of how it evolved in the person's family of origin. It makes sense that Monica is overresponsible and resentful given her position as a parentified child in her family of origin. And it makes sense that Ron learned to self-protect in the face of his father's disconfirmation by withdrawing. But these behaviors aren't working for the couple now; they're threatening the marriage itself. I work to help these clients modulate or "grow up" their survival strategies, so they are more adaptive and appropriate in their current relationship.

I suggest to Ron that when he feels inadequate or ashamed with Monica or hurt by her criticism, and particularly if he feels emotionally flooded, he might negotiate with her a time-out, revisiting the issue when calmer. Rather than feeling abandoned when Ron stalks off to his studio, Monica (with my help) sees Ron taking some time to collect himself *so he can come back to her in a more constructive manner.* This is not Ron abandoning Monica; it is Ron collecting himself in order to reconnect with his wife. I suggest to Monica that she might invite Ron to share household responsibilities not by calling him names, but by confiding her sense of burden and asking him to think creatively with her about ways to approach the challenges of their practical lives. Monica is intrigued that Ron might be a resource, a sounding board for some of the decisions she has on her shoulders. I note that criticism and contempt—the name-calling she reverts to when upset—don't get her the partnership she craves, but rather push Ron further away.

Ron's muse has stubbornly kept a distance in recent times, leaving him bereft in the creative process and unable to contribute to the family finances. When their daughters were growing up, Ron nurtured their creativity, drawing and painting together. This mentoring stimulated Ron's own creative juices. But, lately, there has been no one to mentor. As we discuss this issue, I wonder aloud whether Ron would consider mentoring other youngsters. Ron had avoided becoming an "art teacher," viewing this as less sublime than producing his own paintings. But now he reconsiders and lets people know he is available for private lessons. He reframes his professional journey to include sharing his creative expertise with younger aspiring artists.

Rethinking Power

Like many couples, Ron and Monica get caught up in power struggles, holding a win–lose view of their interactions. Buying into the values of the dominant U.S. culture—competition and individualism—they vie over who is right, and who will prevail in their disagreements. This "Power Over" mode of interacting diminishes both partners and weakens their bond. While dealing with power disparities and addressing behavior that is domineering or violent, I have developed more nuanced ways to address power in couple therapy. Influenced by feminist theory and my own experience, I explore with clients the dynamics of "Power To" and "Power With."

"Power To" is the ability to live according to one's own higher values and reach for one's best self, regulating emotions and choosing how to respond thoughtfully rather than with knee-jerk reactivity. "Power With" is the ability to co-create a loving, safe, fair, respectful relationship, cultivating empathy and making room for multiple perspectives. Framing these capacities as relational empowerment, and operationalizing ways to live these values is intriguing to Monica and Ron. Becoming more adept at Power To and Power With makes it less likely that they will revert to Power Over tactics such as power struggles or demeaning behavior.

Emotion Regulation

When Ron and Monica came to therapy, they were quite dysregulated emotionally. Monica would become angry and demeaning; Ron would shut down, withdrawing to his studio, leaving Monica feeling abandoned. I offer to teach them skills for managing their emotions. They agree, though a bit hesitantly. Ron is afraid I'll take away his ability to protect himself in the face of Monica's anger, and that he'll have no way to defend himself if he can't run away to his studio. Monica fears that I might try to silence her, or have her "make nice," as she had to do as a child. Expressing her anger has been a part of the freedom she embraced as an adult, unlike the disempowered, silenced role she had in her family of origin.

I validate their concerns, indicating that I have no intention of taking away their means of self-protection. Rather, I want to offer them some tools for emotion regulation that might be more effective and less harmful to their partner. But first I address their fears of change. With their permission, I introduce what I call the "giant exercise."

I ask Monica to close her eyes and imagine that a giant comes along and takes away her anger all at once. How does that feel? Monica says that she feels tiny, like a bug, unable to protect herself. I thank her for her honesty and ask her to open her eyes. I say, "Monica, fortunately, there is no giant. No one will take away your means of self-protection. Certainly, I have no intention of trying to do so. Your anger has served you well for much of your life, and it has propelled you to success as a lawyer. But your anger is pushing Ron away at just the moments when you want him to be closer and more caring. Can we work together to devise a more successful way of getting Ron's attention and conveying your needs?" Monica agrees that her anger and derision, while self-protective, are alienating and hurtful to Ron. She sees how her sarcastic comments stir up memories of his father's belittling him as a boy who wanted to be an artist. We work on her ability to speak assertively to Ron without veering into derision or sarcasm.

I ask Ron to close his eyes and imagine that a giant comes and takes away his tendency to withdraw or shut down when Monica is upset with him. He lets this image sink in, saying he would be completely defenseless to attack if he can't shut down or escape. I respond that it makes sense that he runs to his studio when Monica is upset with him. I then indicate that there is no giant; no one will strip away his self-protective mechanisms.

But might he choose to modify his response to Monica, so she is not feeling so abandoned by him? Ron is intrigued.

With the "giant exercise" I access partners' worst fears of what would happen if they don't use the survival strategies upon which they have relied for so long. No giant—and no therapist—will force them to give up what they've relied on for self-defense. Rather, *they* can choose to modify their own responses to be both self-protective *and* protective of the partner. This is a key moment of change in this therapy, one that promotes empowerment and thoughtfulness.

We explore techniques for emotion regulation, so they don't have to revert to attack or withdraw when stirred up. I explain that mindfulness meditation has been found to be very helpful in calming down and is associated with good mental and physical health. We practice some simple mindfulness meditation and breathing techniques. These "bottom-up," body-based means of regulating emotion are easy and effective. We also explore "top-down" cognitive techniques such as naming one's emotion (which activates the prefrontal cortex and calms the amygdala), reappraisal ("She's tired from a long day, not out to get me"), or identifying one's higher values. In addition to individual techniques for emotion regulation, we explore ways they can help each other calm down when upset. A gentle touch or hug, empathy, and sex are all positive ways partners can co-regulate and soothe each other. These loving interactions release oxytocin, "the love hormone," which lowers cortisol, the stress hormone. Since their daughters left home, Ron and Monica have been awash in cortisol, with little oxytocin flowing. They talk about how much they miss their sexual connection and discuss ways to reconnect.

Relational Ethics

In recent times, Ron and Monica have not been functioning well as a team, as they did when raising their children. Each feels wounded and unsupported, instinctively protecting self at the expense of the other—and hurting each other in the process. I invite them to explore who they want to be in this relationship—how do they *want* to impact each other? I share with them an intriguing article on narrative ethics in couples (Carlson & Haire, 2014), which explores the ways partners impact each other's identity and well-being for better or worse by how they treat each other. This is a new way of thinking for this couple—exploring relational ethics, the balance of give and take, and the consequences of each one's behavior on the other's well-being (Fishbane, 2023a).

Making a Relational Claim

I address how Monica and Ron raise concerns with each other. They've now moved past the name-calling, blaming, and withdrawing that characterized their interaction when they first came to therapy. But at times, they still get confused about how to state their concerns in a way that takes the other into account. I share my idea about "making a relational claim"—speaking one's own concerns, while holding concern for the other partner and the relationship at the same time. When Monica is fed up with too much on her plate, how will she raise this with Ron? In the past, she would just "let it rip," which felt great for a few seconds as she got her frustrations and anger off her chest. But soon after, seeing how her words hurt Ron, who then abandoned her, spending the night on the couch in his studio, Monica would feel guilty and unhappy. I coach her on how to formulate her concerns to Ron in a way that holds him with respect and considers how their relationship will be affected by how she speaks. Making a relational claim entails slowing down and thinking about priorities. Monica balks, worried that I'm asking her to silence herself. I make it clear I have no intention of silencing her; her voice deserves to be heard. Rather, I encourage her to be more effective in getting through to her husband. I invite Ron to think about how he responds to Monica when she's disappointed. Stalking off to his studio is abandoning her; is this his intention? Seeing it this way, Ron is open to finding new ways of responding.

Automaticity versus Choice: The Fork in the Road

Changing old habits is hard. Monica and Ron periodically fall back into their prior patterns and come to therapy disheartened. Will they ever really be able to make the lasting changes they want? I acknowledge the difficulty of transforming old habits, explaining that most of the time, we humans are acting on automatic pilot. On the other hand, we can learn to *pause* and *choose* how we want to respond. I invite each to imagine a fork in the road, anticipating a time when they're about to get reactive or revert to their automatic critical or withdrawal behaviors. Ron goes first, picturing how he might respond the next time he feels criticized by Monica. His typical go-to reaction is to get defensive and withdraw, avoiding her anger—which, of course, only fuels her hurt. I encourage Ron to think about what he could do instead in such a moment, asking him to literally picture a fork in the road, as if he were hiking in the woods. One path represents his usual knee-jerk self-defensive response. What might the other path look like? Ron thinks, looks at Monica, and says that it would have something to do with hearing Monica's concern more empathically and less defensively. We try out various options of what he could say or do in such a moment. Ron offers, "I could say, 'Monica, I want to help, but you're impossible to please!'" Monica rolls her eyes, and Ron sees this is not a new path after all.

I suggest that Ron could perhaps let go of the accusations and defenses for a moment, and just look at his wife when she shares with him her feelings of being overwhelmed. And even if she doesn't do so perfectly, he can try to look "behind the scenes" at the pain that is fueling her criticism. I offer, "Behind an angry Monica is a hurt Monica." This is a new idea for Ron. He remembers our work on the vulnerability cycle and gets the point. I encourage him to see the hurt and yearning behind Monica's criticism—a tall order, but one I think he may be able to accomplish. My belief in his ability to change fortifies his commitment to trying. At times I lend hope to my clients when they themselves can't see new possibilities for themselves.

Now it's Monica's turn. Her fork in the road entails being more thoughtful about how she asks Ron for help or addresses their division of labor at home. I suggest that dropping her eye-roll habit might help. I share John Gottman's (2011) finding that eye rolling is a classic sign of contempt; and that contempt is one of the most toxic habits of an unhappy relationship. Instead of criticizing Ron, might Monica be more inviting in how she conveys her needs? Monica is open to exploring other ways to get Ron's attention. She is aware that inviting rather than criticizing Ron is the way to go.

Healing Intergenerational Wounds

Early in our work, we explored the family-of-origin roots of this couple's vulnerabilities and survival strategies. Ron and Monica have made good progress in transforming their dance but, periodically, they still get reactive around core dilemmas that trigger vulnerabilities and survival strategies forged in childhood. As I do with some clients, I broach the topic of addressing unresolved intergenerational wounds (Fishbane, 2023b). I explain that one of the functions of the amygdala (in addition to scanning for danger and setting off the fight–flight response) is to hold emotional components of old memories. In an amygdala-dominated reactive moment, memories of childhood wounds are triggered beneath awareness. If Monica feels abandoned by Ron, upset that she's carrying more than her share in the household, her childhood feelings are activated, and she has an intense reaction to her husband. When Ron feels criticized by Monica for not contributing to the family financially or practically, Ron is back with his father, who pressured him to "live in the real world" and make a living as an accountant. Ron's reaction to Monica is intense; his withdrawal from her mirrors his pulling away from his father, an intergenerational rift that has never healed.

As we discuss the replication of family-of-origin issues within the couple relationship, I raise the possibility of revisiting their views of, and current relationships with, their families of origin. They are both distant with their parents. Ron has kept his father at arm's length for years. Monica is a dutiful daughter, visiting her parents regularly, but remaining emotionally distant. Both see their parents through the lens of a hurt child. They haven't "grown up" their views of their parents, or worked to create a more authentic relationship with their families of origin in the present.

We explore their childhood wounds a bit more fully—Monica being put in an overresponsible position with her siblings, with no room for her feelings; Ron's artistic light dimmed by his father's economic worries. The wounds were real and still haunt this couple—Ron feeling disconfirmed, Monica feeling overwhelmed with responsibilities.

As we consider these overlaps between the present and the past, *I am careful not to blame their parents*. It's tempting for therapists to judge parents for clients' wounds. However, inspired by Boszormenyi-Nagy, I extend multidirected partiality to parents as well as my clients. Ron's and Monica's parents didn't intentionally hurt their children; they were carrying their own intergenerational burdens of poverty and leaned on their children to do what was necessary to survive. I think about how to affirm my clients' pain while holding compassion for their families of origin. How can I help Monica and Ron heal old wounds, so they're not continually reenacted in the couple relationship? And how can I invite this couple to explore intergenerational issues when they came to work on their marriage, not their relationships with their families of origin?

Both Ron and Monica are replicating old issues from the past in their interactions. Seeing the connection between how they felt as children and how they feel with each other, they're open to exploring their current family-of-origin relationships.

I ask them to share more about their experiences growing up, and what they know of their parents' own stories. Ron talks about the pain of losing his mother, his biggest cheerleader, at age 12. He and his father never processed the death or Ron's feelings of loss. When Ron was in high school, winning recognition for his painting, his father worried that Ron wouldn't be able to support himself as an artist. His father never got an education past high school because of the need to work to support his family. He pressured Ron to become an accountant, a solid profession that would ensure financial stability. Ron acceded to the pressure, but found accounting crushing to his spirit, so he dropped out and went to art school. His father was disappointed. Ron achieved considerable success as an artist, but he never invited his father to an opening of his gallery shows. To this day, Ron harbors resentment, keeping a distance from his father. He doesn't know much about his father's own history growing up, only that the father's parents were immigrants who struggled to make a living.

Monica is more sympathetic to her parents, understanding that they worked hard to keep a roof over their children's heads. But she is angry that her parents were oblivious to the parentified position in which they put her. Her voice was silenced; she was to be a dutiful daughter. She has never considered talking with her parents about this. Monica is also worried and resentful about the current drain on her parents' resources from her musician brother who doesn't earn a living.

As we talk about their strained relationships with their families of origin, I sense how each is burdened by the past. Given the parallels between their marital dynamics and intergenerational wounds, I gently propose the idea of getting to know their parents as "real people" on their own journeys, with their own vulnerabilities and survival strategies from *their* childhoods. I mention that some of my clients choose to invite their parents in for a session, to explore old family dynamics, as well as current intergenerational relationships. Others prefer to have a meeting with their parents on their own, with some coaching from me on how to have a productive conversation.

Ron takes me up on my suggestion; he invites his father to lunch and a visit to a local gallery showcasing Ron's paintings. In coaching Ron, I encourage him to leave his anger at home and come to the lunch with as open a heart as he can muster. I ask him to think of his father's limitations in light of his own life journey, especially around poverty, lack of education, and the early loss of his wife. Our work in couple therapy has increased Ron's capacity for empathy, and he musters this capacity as he readies for the lunch meeting.

Ron is surprised by how old and frail his father seems; they haven't seen each other in years. His father is grateful for the reunion as they catch up over lunch and says he has followed Ron's artistic successes in the press, sharing photos of his son's artwork with his friends. He apologizes for not expressing faith in Ron's artistic ability; he feared his son would be a penniless painter, unable to support himself. Ron asks his father about his childhood; his father speaks of dropping out of high school to help support his parents, and his lifelong regret at not getting an education. He wanted better for his son. Ron is moved that his father was celebrating his artistic successes from a distance and appreciates his father's apology and sharing of his own history. They decide to meet a bit more frequently, and Ron feels some release of his long-standing burden of resentment toward his father. Feeling confirmed by his father eases some of the vulnerability to criticism Ron has been carrying that has negatively impacted him in his marriage.

Monica opts to invite her parents to a joint session with me. I ask her to try to leave her grievances at home and come to the meeting with curiosity and openheartedness. In our session, Monica asks her parents about their own childhoods and hears new stories. Her parents both grew up in poverty in eastern Europe—her father's family barely scraping by, her mother's family not able to stay together, as relatives took in various of the children when the parents were too impoverished to maintain a home. They came to the United States with little support, met each other here, and married. They shared a fierce determination to have children and to keep their family together at all costs. They succeeded in this, but one of the costs was the burden placed on Monica as responsible older sister. Monica is getting a bit of the backstory of her parents' struggles out of poverty, and their commitment to keeping the family together, even at Monica's expense.

Without overwhelming her parents with accusations, Monica shares some of her experience as a child who carried too much responsibility. Her mother starts to get defensive; I step in, gently noting how helpful adult children find it when their parents can hear their pain, and that it would be a great gift to her daughter for her to listen compassionately to Monica's experience. To her credit, Monica's mother is able to step a bit more into empathy, dropping some of her defensive reaction. I make it clear that the point of this conversation is not for Monica to dump on her parents, but rather to see whether they can build a closer connection by being more open with each other. With this frame, Monica and her parents edge a bit closer toward dialogue. Monica feels that finally there is some room for her experience in this family. She also raises her concerns about the parents' support of her brother. In a follow-up meeting, Monica and her parents devise a more realistic plan for helping the brother without impoverishing themselves. Monica's ability to voice her concerns respectfully with her parents through these conversations strengthens her growing ability to have voice in her marriage. For both Monica and Ron, there is a synergy between these limited family-of-origin meetings and the couple work. I find that when clients are less burdened by resentments toward their parents, they are able to be more generous and empowered with their partner.

I don't invite parents into sessions with all adult clients who have family-of-origin issues. In most couple cases, it's not necessary to do family-of-origin work that entails actual meetings. When I do think it might be helpful, I only initiate such meetings after clients have grown beyond anger at parents, to a place of some compassion and curiosity. Not all parents are open to a dialogue with their adult children; some are too defensive to make such a meeting productive. In other cases, it may be dangerous or counterproductive to host a parent–adult child meeting. Some cultures frown on explicit exploration of family issues. Even if I don't facilitate intergenerational meetings, I do encourage clients to "grow up" their views, with an appreciation of the parents' own journeys, struggles, and limitations. This process enhances the couple work, empowering partners to go beyond constraining perspectives and patterns forged in childhood.

CONCLUDING PHASE OF THERAPY

Ron and Monica's personalities are not transformed by our work. She, highly organized and responsible, still craves order. He is still more of a free spirit, doesn't see the mess on the table, and is not on top of family finances. But they are less polarized around their differences. They have softened, seeing each other as human beings with their own proclivities and struggles. They are better able to take responsibility for their own part in their interactions, are less reactive and more compassionate, addressing concerns and differences more effectively and kindly. When Ron holds Monica in mind and cleans up his mess from the kitchen table, he is rewarded with an appreciative smile. When Monica invites Ron in a loving way to partner more in household affairs, Ron feels affirmed and useful rather than demeaned.

These changes do not emerge from a single "aha" moment in therapy. Identifying their interactional pattern and the roots of their vulnerabilities and survival strategies are powerful interventions, helping them shift perspectives. But it takes a great deal of practice for new views and behaviors to become firmly rooted. I explain that new habits require a lot of practice to become "wired" into the brain. I also indicate that in the future, they might find themselves falling back into their old dance, and not to be alarmed if that happens. Old habits don't disappear; they can get reactivated in times of fatigue or stress. Knowing this ahead of time gives my clients perspective, so they aren't thrown if occasionally they revert to old behaviors. We start spacing out our sessions to every other week, then once a month.

We agree it is time to end our regular meetings, as they have largely achieved their goals. I make it clear that my door is open in the future. I don't spend time on elaborate terminations. I see myself as akin to a family doctor, available in the future if something comes up or they need a refresher meeting or series of meetings. I am a resource for the future.

FURTHER REFLECTIONS AND IMPLICATIONS

Ron and Monica are privileged in many ways; they do not carry scars from sociocultural oppression or trauma. But, like most of us, they carry residues of issues from their own families of origin, which in their case includes multigenerational anxiety about poverty. Privilege does not mean one is not impacted by painful issues in one's family of origin. Their impasse was also shaped by gender socialization and expectations: Ron, who as a man would be expected to be the primary wage earner, was struggling to provide. Monica, a woman who felt trapped as the primary wage earner, was resentful. We addressed these expectations and disappointments in our work.

This couple was educated and able to grasp the "news from neuroscience" I shared; it normalized their reactivity and helped them chart a course for change. They were decent people who cared for each other and had a strong bond early in their relationship; it mattered to them that they were inadvertently hurting each other. They had enough perspective and generosity of spirit to explore their own responsibility in their vulnerability cycle, and were able to transform their blame–defensiveness dance into a more productive mode of interaction in keeping with their values. I worked to elicit their strengths—kindness, compassion, responsibility. These resources of trustworthiness were waiting to be discovered and cultivated. Not all clients have the resources and capacities of this couple. But I have found that most clients are open to developing greater empowerment, including awareness of how their knee-jerk reactivity is driven by the emotional brain. Offering specific tools for emotion regulation, making a relational claim, and connecting with one's values is helpful with most couples.

It's an honor to work with a couple like Ron and Monica, helping them transform reactivity into opportunities for connection. I've invited you into my internal process as I do this work, hoping it may encourage and guide some of your own work with couples. Thank you for joining me.

REFERENCES

Boszormenyi-Nagy, I., & Krasner, B. R. (1986). *Between give and take: A clinical guide to contextual therapy*. New York: Brunner-Routledge.

Carlson, T. S., & Haire, A. (2014). Toward a theory of relational accountability: An invitational approach to living narrative ethics in couple relationships. *International Journal of Narrative Therapy and Community Work, 3*, 1–16.

Fishbane, M. D. (2013). *Loving with the brain in mind: Neurobiology and couple therapy*. New York: Norton.

Fishbane, M. D. (2023a). Couple relational ethics: From theory to lived practice. *Family Process, 62,* 446–468.
Fishbane, M. D. (2023b). Intergenerational factors in couple therapy. In J. L. Lebow & D. K. Snyder (Eds.), *Clinical handbook of couple therapy* (6th ed., pp. 199–224). New York: Guilford Press.
Gottman, J. M. (2011). *The science of trust: Emotional attunement for couples.* New York: Norton.
Scheinkman, M., & Fishbane, M. D. (2004). The vulnerability cycle: Working with impasses in couple therapy. *Family Process, 43,* 279–299.
Siegel, D. J., & Hartzell, M. (2003). *Parenting from the inside out.* New York: Penguin Random House.

CHAPTER 7

Integrating Common Factors in Couple Therapy

SARAH E. GRIFFES
ADRIAN BLOW

Editors' Comments

Sarah Griffes and Adrian Blow provide a striking case narrative illuminating the importance of common factors in couple therapy. Common factors provide a scaffolding for various theoretical approaches to therapy, and specific strategies for harnessing these are incremental, if not essential, to treatment effectiveness. As the authors note, couple therapy presents unique challenges to creating and maintaining a strong therapeutic alliance—shown repeatedly to influence both therapeutic process and outcomes. It's striking from their narrative how the same couple—seen as stuck and resistant by a prior therapist—forges a strong alliance and achieves positive outcomes with a different therapist. Note as the narrative unfolds how this new therapist (Griffes) draws strategically on specific interventions throughout the therapy to foster connection with both partners.

    This case study also calls into focus other important aspects of common factors, including both client and therapist characteristics and their congruence or divergence. Here, tuning in to the unique qualities of this couple and their struggle was essential. So was generating some realistic version of hope and positive expectation (to combat hopelessness), adapting the therapy to the clients (to allow for a sense of progress), holding a systemic perspective (to move them out of blaming each other for the problem), and attending to the cultural context of the therapy (to acknowledge and integrate those aspects of their experience). The positive impacts of harnessing such factors in this therapy demonstrate the incredible difference the person of the therapist can make, reminding us all to consider carefully any information about previous therapies and not to preordain the outcome of this next segment in a couple's journey.

    Notice too how Griffes strategically interweaves common factors within well-established couple interventions—for example, teaching foundational communications skills, exploring developmental narratives from family history, promoting emotional disclosure and empathic responding, and attending to experiences of systemic discrimination and marginalization. Observe the interplay of common factors and specific

> models—how at times common factors evolve from a specific intervention and how the couple's response to the intervention is facilitated by the common factors. This case narrative provides a rich example of an integrative–pluralistic approach—with techniques from different schools of couple therapy adopted harmoniously in pursuit of the best possible outcomes.

The two of us were drawn to common factors in couple therapy at different times over the past decades. One of us (AB) began his work in this area decades ago in the 1990s as a doctoral student at Purdue University. In my professional writing course with Fred Piercy, I worked on my first common factors article focused on personal agency in family therapy theories (Blow & Piercy, 1997). Soon thereafter, I began working with Doug Sprenkle on other common factors articles that included my dissertation on common factors across theories of couple and family therapy. Since that time, I've written more articles and two books on the topic, and have been particularly interested in the role of common factors when working with couples. I've come to realize that even though there are many excellent approaches to couple therapy with evidence for their effectiveness, all punctuate common factors in important ways, starting with building strong therapeutic alliances with each partner, building hope and expectancy, and including a liberal amount of reframing in the work.

The other of us (SEG) became interested in common factors more recently. One of the first books I read in discerning whether to pursue further degrees in marriage and family therapy was *Escape from Babel: Toward a Unifying Language of Psychotherapy Practice* (Miller, Duncan, & Hubble, 1997). In the earliest stages of my career, I loved that—when in doubt—I could rely on the common factors of the therapeutic alliance and instilling hope and expectancy to help my clients. I harnessed these basic skills before I could successfully implement the specific models that I was learning. In my continued practice of therapy, I return to common factors time and time again. Working with couples is my true passion, and I love the challenge of maintaining a strong relationship with each partner.

In this chapter, we describe a common factors approach to working with couples. In adopting a common factors approach, we emphasize therapist flexibility, because our approach with any given couple varies depending on specific partners, presenting problems, and contexts. Drawing on common factors doesn't mean that our work does not also include specific models. We both use models to guide our work, but we emphasize and punctuate the common factors as we illustrate below. One of us (AB) utilizes an integrative approach that is heavily influenced by emotionally focused couple therapy, whereas the other of us (SEG) uses an integrative approach drawing on theories of family differentiation, emotionally focused couple therapy, and cognitive-behavioral therapy. We never assume there's only one correct way to help couples, and we build on the foundation created in the therapeutic alliance.

COMMON FACTORS IN COUPLE THERAPY

Common factors have long been recognized as influencing the course and outcome of couple and family therapy (Sprenkle & Blow, 2004). Common factors include broad factors, such as the therapeutic alliance, hope and expectancy, client and extratherapeutic events, therapist factors, and narrow factors such as changing the viewing (cognition), experiencing (feelings), and doing (behaviors) (Davis, 2023). There are also common factors unique to couple and family therapy—such as conceptualizing difficulties in relational terms, expanding the therapeutic alliance, expanding the direct treatment system, and interrupting dysfunctional sequences or patterns of behavior (Sprenkle, Blow, & Dickey, 1999; Sprenkle, Davis, & Lebow, 2009).

The Therapeutic Alliance

The therapeutic alliance is a foundation of all therapies and comprises three key components. The *bonds* of the alliance refer to the emotional connection between the therapist and the clients. Do the clients feel understood, cared about, and connected to the therapist? In working with couples, the bond of connection needs to exist between the therapist and each partner. The *goals* of the alliance refer to agreement between the clients and therapist on the aims of therapy. In working with a couple, does each partner and the therapist agree that they're working toward the desired outcomes? This creates a challenge when partners have different goals. The third component of the alliance refers to *tasks* used to achieve the couple's goals. Some people are more comfortable with certain therapy tasks than others, and it's important that they buy into specific tasks used to pursue desired goals. For example, if one partner has greater comfort with emotional processing than the other, a breach in the alliance can occur if the therapist insists on focusing exclusively on emotions. In recent years, the use of formalized feedback (in which partners complete brief measures at the end of each session regarding the therapy process) has grown as a means of strengthening the therapeutic alliance. Discussing and responding to such feedback has been shown to have positive effects on the therapeutic alliance specifically and on therapy as a whole.

Hope and Expectancy

Therapists can use hope and expectancy to increase clients' engagement in therapy both within and outside of sessions. With couples, this is particularly important, because partners often have different levels of hope that things will improve, or they may have different expectations about how the therapy or therapist can help them achieve their goals. Engaging the couple in therapy may be particularly difficult, and the risks of attrition higher, when one partner feels hopeful but the other feels hopeless. It can be equally challenging if partners have different expectations regarding the work of therapy or specific roles of the therapist. Differences in partners' hope, expectancies, and motivations are often hidden or covert and can hinder both therapeutic process and progress (Karam & Blow, 2023).

Client Factors and Extratherapeutic Events

Various characteristics and events in the life and context of the client can affect therapy. These may be traits or characteristics unique to the clients (e.g., a disability) or either negative or positive factors in the larger socioecological context. Examples of the former include poverty, neighborhood violence, or unemployment, whereas the latter might include social support systems, a supportive employer or supervisor, or an uplifting religious community. Such contextual factors can be utilized by the therapist as a therapeutic resource or leverage point.

Therapist Factors

Strong evidence affirms that therapists contribute significantly to variability in therapy outcomes—whether in working with individuals, couples, or families. Mindfulness, flexibility, and emotional attunement are important factors. Couple therapy can be especially challenging, requiring the therapist to attend and respond both to overt interactions and covert dynamics at all times—facilitating the couple's work but not getting in the way of their own processes. Couple therapy includes multiple decision points guided by theory and principles of intervention, and the therapist needs to tailor interventions based on observations or feedback on how things are going or on new information that's acquired, often in a volatile emotional context.

Changing the Experiencing, Viewing, and Doing

Across both theoretical approaches and treatment formats, therapists typically intervene across domains of emotions, cognitions, and behaviors (or experiencing, viewing, and doing). For example, various approaches to couple therapy emphasize the importance of helping partners to soften and deepen their emotional experience of each other. Thoughts and feelings are inextricably linked, and a common factor across approaches involves interventions aimed at helping partners to change how they think about each other and the influences impacting their relationship. Challenging attributions and reframing partners' beliefs or explanations for various events or interactions are ways of promoting changes in viewing. Changes in experiencing and viewing often lead to changes in doing, but at other times, couple therapists use various interventions to alter behavioral changes directly. For example, it's common for therapists to suggest activities for couples to engage in outside of therapy (going on a date together or engaging in connection conversations). Other interventions aim at preventing specific negative behaviors at home (e.g., arguing in front of children) or interrupting recurring negative interaction patterns (e.g., the demand–withdraw cycle typical of many distressed couples).

Conceptualizing Difficulties in Relational Terms

A key component in systemic therapies is that the therapist conceptualizes problems in relational terms; that is, the focus is on partners' ongoing recursive dynamics of influencing and being influenced by each other. Systematic assessment of couples' interaction patterns facilitates a conceptualization of these patterns as reflecting the interplay of both partners' contributions and guides interventions aimed at the couple as a dyad rather than focusing on either partner separate from the other.

Expanding the Direct Treatment System

Regardless of modality (individual, couple, or family therapy), therapists may expand either their assessment or interventions beyond the client to include other individuals or entities who may be affecting the client or therapy, such as other family members, medical personnel, court officials, and the like. In couple therapy, significant others (children, extended family members, former spouses) may be included either incidentally or on an ongoing basis as they impact or are impacted by the couple's relationship.

In the case narrative that follows, we illustrate how the common factors described earlier were harnessed in working with a couple. As the therapist, I (SEG) drew from specific theoretical approaches and techniques throughout our work, but consistently viewed these through the general lens of the common factors approach. From this framework, I began with an emphasis on building the therapeutic alliance and careful assessment activities that would facilitate conceptualization of the couple's difficulties in systemic terms.

INITIAL ASSESSMENT AND CASE FORMULATION

A colleague who was moving out of state referred a couple to me whom he had seen for over a year. My colleague considered this one of the most challenging couples he had encountered and shared that he and the couple had often felt that change was slow and laborious, if existent at all. He also reported difficulty in maintaining a healthy alliance with each partner, although they both attended sessions consistently throughout therapy. He reported that the male partner was often combative toward him, the therapist, and that he hadn't found good footing in any of his typical couple therapy models. Given my colleague's reports, I was apprehensive about taking on this couple. As we collaborated before the first session, my colleague and I decided that the essential first step was for me to establish good rapport through validating and challenging the clients more equally than my colleague had been able to manage due to his tough relationship with the male partner.

I scheduled the first appointment on the phone with Trey, who had Cara with him in the car when I called. Upon first meeting them at my office, what struck me most was their contrasts in size and style: Trey was a tall Black man who carried himself confidently and spoke decisively, whereas Cara was an average-height, White woman who wrapped her arms around herself, seemingly trying to take up as little space as possible. They sat on opposite ends of the couch, never touching and rarely looking at each other, and only addressing each other when I requested. As I usually do with clients, I discussed with them from the get-go the ways that our various identities differed from each other (they had reported things like race/ethnicity, age, and gender in their intake paperwork). I discussed how my identities impacted my lived experiences and, as such, I knew that their identities did as well. They seemed to appreciate me acknowledging these differences and welcoming further discussion on cross-cultural impacts throughout our work together.

During our first session together, Trey reported, "We made small steps with our previous therapist and now we need to make some bigger ones, if that's even possible." He sounded frustrated and exhausted in his "this might be as good as it can get" attitude about their relationship. When asked about his hopes for therapy, his primary desired outcomes revolved around more cohesive co-parenting, so that their teenagers had a better experience than their adult children. Cara indicated that she was interested in seeing the changes that therapy could continue to bring to their relationship. She was more optimistic about the changes that had occurred with their previous therapist and those that could occur if they continued therapy with me.

I pursued my typical assessment process, which included the joint first session, followed by an individual session with each partner to further establish the therapeutic alliance and to see things from each person's perspective, and then another joint session to present my initial formulation, collaborate on therapeutic goals and plans, and provide structure for sessions and further treatment. This couple had experienced many problems during their 18 years of marriage, as had each partner from well before. Both of their families of origin were characterized by abuse, neglect, addiction, and physical and mental health problems. Trey was 55 years old, and this was his first marriage. Cara was 49 years old, had been married twice before, and had one adult son from each previous marriage (raised mostly with Trey). Trey and Cara had two biological daughters together, ages 12 and 17. They reported numerous difficulties in co-parenting—with Cara being more lenient and Trey being the enforcer of rules and consequences. Neither liked the way the other parented, but their respective parenting styles had persisted since they married. Trey described their children as being a major reason for his staying in the marriage and sometimes spoke about only viewing his wife as "the mother of my children."

Trey and Cara both identified as Christian, and their belief system was a vital resource in their relationship. Their commitment to their family and to attending therapy were also valuable resources. They had been in couple therapy previously both voluntarily and, once, as part of a court mandate related to their kids temporarily being removed from their home a number of years before due to neglect allegations. They reported that therapy had never been especially effective and believed that sometimes it had led to greater problems and disagreements.

Building trust and intimacy were primary goals that Trey and Cara wanted to work toward. During this marriage, each partner had been involved in an extramarital affair: Trey at the beginning of their relationship and Cara about a year before they began therapy with my colleague. Although infidelity was important to their lack of trust, it was rarely spoken about with emotion or grief—it was simply a fact of their relationship that they seemed to ignore or avoid discussing. A few months before seeking therapy with my colleague, Cara had begun the process of filing for divorce, although she hadn't completed the necessary procedures to finalize the divorce. From what I gathered, Cara had reached a breaking point, believing that their life together would never get better and feeling desperate to end the marriage. Anytime they discussed their potential divorce, both would immediately emotionally escalate, indicating to me that this issue had never been fully processed. Both partners recited numerous grievances beyond the obvious breaches of trust that kept them from obtaining closeness in their relationship. Both reported times in their relationship when they felt lonely, abandoned, and unlovable, based on their partners' words or actions (e.g., sleeping in separate rooms, forgetting special events). Each reported a complete lack of physical intimacy (no sexual intimacy, kissing, hand holding, hugging, etc.) for several years and only inconsistent patterns before then. I noticed that only Cara mentioned an interest in having any sort of physical relationship again and, when I asked, Trey responded that he believed that part of their relationship was over.

I couldn't help but be moved as I listened to their stories. This was a couple who'd been through some of the biggest storms of life—both in their chaotic families of origin and their own relationship—who'd been knocked over many times and, yet, still managed to get up. I was impressed with their perseverance as individuals and as a couple but recognized that their endurance had come with a cost to themselves and their relationship. They lacked a basic foundation of trust, which resulted in consistent patterns of miscommunication, difficulties in coparenting, rigid roles, and low investment in their relationship.

In the fourth session, we discussed their being stuck in rigid patterns in their relationship and in parenting that resulted in neither feeling satisfied with outcomes and both being frustrated with the other. We discussed the importance of skill building around communication and working on trust to mitigate their current issues. We also talked about progress that they had seen in their relationship so far (there was less yelling and stonewalling, they viewed themselves more as a team) and I complimented them for the hard work that they had done despite their difficult circumstances and their commitment to further work.

Given their difficulties in prior therapy experiences, I expected that our alliance would be both difficult and crucial to maintain. I was careful to attune to both partners during the initial assessment. Our two individual sessions enabled me to express understanding and concern for their unique histories and relational desires, and through this process deepened my alliance with each of them. Throughout our work together, I was especially attentive to important life events and would ask about their work, teenage or adult children, families of origin, and so on, and strived to remember specific details such as holidays or birthdays. I was always looking for additional ways to connect with this couple and be sure that they knew I cared about them as a way to maintain our alliance even through difficult disruptions. I expressed care and concern while also maintaining lightheartedness in our casual interactions just before and after sessions. It became common for the three of us to joke together or playfully poke fun at each other. Through these alliance-building actions, we felt connected to each other and developed a deeper trust that sustained us through difficult times in therapy.

BEGINNING PHASE OF THERAPY

Most of our meetings began with my asking about the relational highs and lows from the week. Trey would often respond first: His answers were often long-winded and confusing to follow, ending far from the original prompt. Cara would typically look at the floor, making eye contact with me if she was especially bothered by something Trey said, her facial expressions clearly conveying her negative reactions. When Cara spoke, Trey would nod if he agreed and shake his head if he disagreed, always looking up toward the ceiling. When I asked either partner to reflect on what the other said, Cara would often respond with her feelings and thoughts regarding a specific phrase that Trey had used, and Trey would note ways that he disagreed with Cara's assertions, not delving into emotions unless prompted and pushed. They seemed to misread each other constantly. Each was so wrapped up in their own interpretations of the other that they seemed unable to listen and understand in the moment. I discerned that part of my role would be to help each of them slow down and more accurately decipher what the other was trying to communicate. I also anticipated that the connection I was building with each of them would be essential to gaining influence over their processes.

Within the first few sessions after assessment, I could see how my colleague had had such a hard time with this couple. It was difficult to maintain my position as the provider of structure in therapy as each fought for it in their own way. After ending a few sessions with me feeling bulldozed by the couple, I decided that I needed a new approach. Instead of allowing Trey to meander, hoping to gain insight into his inner thoughts and feelings from his words, I would interrupt earlier and ask for his inner thoughts and feelings. When I noticed Cara's facial expressions, I would directly ask her to share how she was feeling or what she was thinking with Trey and me. I also carefully shared my own feelings regarding these actions, guessing that each also felt similarly to me. Cara agreed that she often was lost when Trey gave long responses, and Trey agreed that he was always trying to guess how Cara felt based on her expressions. Through this process, I was able to successfully interrupt one of the pervasive negative interactions of their relationship.

As a result, we spent many months at the beginning of therapy working on the skills of listening, summarizing, and then responding. I'd lead them through enactments in which they'd sit across from one another and discuss hot topics in their relationship, with me as a coach helping them navigate difficult issues. During these enactments, strong emotions were invariably stirred up, and I helped them practice regulating these to avoid escalation and instructed them on how to do the same at home. During these sessions, we focused on their experiencing of deep emotions in the here and now, with the goal of creating a new (and better) experience of their relationship with each other in session. Throughout this work, I continually interwove interventions targeting each partner's experiencing, viewing, and doing. This was slow work, as there were many hot topics to discuss. I'd invite them to come in with topic ideas, and we'd then work through them each session.

> ME (SEG): What have you decided on for this week?
>
> CARA: We had an incident with our older daughter this week. We were shopping for Christmas gifts, and Em was being rude. She'd sit on her phone instead of looking around, would try to stay in the car while the rest of us got out, things like that. Eventually, Trey yelled at her.
>
> TREY: That's not what happened! You know that . . . [the escalation was immediate]
>
> CARA: Yes, it is! You did yell at her!
>
> ME (SEG): Okay, we're going to slow down right here. I want you to practice using reflective listening like we talked about . . . I'll walk you through it and interrupt as needed. Let's go back to Cara's point of view. Trey, remember that you're just listening to what Cara is saying and you'll repeat back to her what you heard and understood. Go ahead, Cara.
>
> CARA: Okay (*takes a deep breath*), like I said before, Trey, Em, and I were out on Saturday doing some gift shopping. Em was spending a lot of time on her phone, which was frustrating for me and Trey because we had other things to do that day. I'd already asked her a number of times to put the phone away while we were out. As we were getting out of the car at the second store, Em just stayed in it without moving, watching a video or something. I could tell that Trey was completely done with what was happening and he totally exploded, just yelling at her. He grounded her from her phone for a week, which I thought was ridiculous and too harsh.
>
> ME (SEG): Okay, Trey, I just want you to reflect back what you heard.
>
> TREY: Cara told us about our outing and how Em was on her phone. I didn't know that she had asked Em to put it away a few times already, that was new for me. I thought she was just ignoring Em and ignoring my frustrations about the situation. Then, I got angry and took Em's phone away.

Me (SEG): So, earlier you thought that Cara did nothing, but now you found out that you didn't know that Cara had asked Em to put the phone away. How does it feel knowing that at that moment you were on the same team as a parental unit? [I hoped at this moment that my reframe could change his interpretation and reactions to this incident.]

Trey: Well, that feels good, I guess. Sometimes I feel like Cara just ignores it and waits for me to be the bad guy, but I like knowing that she was on my team. I have no idea when she did that though. I didn't hear or see her do that.

Me (SEG): Cara, how does it feel that Trey appreciated that you were on the same team? [I was hoping she'd experienced the slight shift in Trey's perspective and response.]

Cara: I mean, that's what we're going for, right? I'm glad that he saw it that way.

Trey: (*looking at Cara*) I wish I would've known earlier. I don't think I would've been so upset if I knew you were talking to her about it.

Cara: But you know this is how I work. I do things in the background. I've always preferred to have these types of conversations one-on-one. I don't think it needs to turn into a big blowup. (*She was starting to get frustrated, and her volume and tone were escalating.*)

Me (SEG): Let's pause here. I think this is a really important moment for you two. You were on the same team in a parenting matter. You didn't know it at the time, but your goal was the same and you were both addressing it with your child, just in different ways.

Trey: Yeah, it *is* important. I never feel like we're on the same page. I usually feel like she's undermining me. But I was wrong in this instance. (*looking toward Cara*) Thanks for working on Em in your own way.

Cara: I want the same things that you do in parenting. I want our girls to learn responsibility and respect better than the boys did. We both do.

Me (SEG): I want to highlight an important change here. From the beginning of our work together, parenting has always been a taboo topic for you two—something that nearly always led to escalation. But today you did it! You talked about a parenting issue, and you both were able to calm down when you felt escalated. You even discovered a time when you were working on the same team. [I was hoping that by highlighting this difference from their usual pattern and reframing this exchange I could deepen their experiencing and empathic joining in this moment.]

This example highlights just one of many times when we worked together to interrupt a negative pattern or sequence of behaviors. Their conflict pattern of escalation, especially any discussion about parenting, was strong. Using reflective listening and encouraging self-regulation for each partner in session helped Trey and Cara to have these same types of conversations between sessions as well. I taught them many skills (emotional recognition, time-outs, grounding techniques, etc.) and they practiced these at home with intermittent success and failure. But when failures occurred, they would suspend their exchange and bring that conflict to me the next week for us to work through together.

Although progress was slow in skill building, the small steps helped me to have more hope for change in the therapeutic process.

These weekly discussions required a lot of intentional effort on my part toward balancing alliances with both Trey and Cara. Maintaining strong and balanced alliances was difficult when one partner presented the other as fully to blame for the situation. Sustaining alliances with both of them required alternating my roles in validating versus challenging each partner's perspectives. If I was too validating of Trey's experiences of being undermined by Cara in parenting, Cara would defend herself. If I challenged Trey too often or too strongly, he'd become defensive. If I was too validating toward Cara, Trey would shut down—but if I was too challenging toward her, she would shut down. It was a constant balancing act each session. I benefited from them each trusting me—my commitment to their relationship and to treating each of them fairly and with respect—and this enabled me to gently confront each of them with different perspectives. Having learned much about each of their histories, being able to remember and relate their current experiences to previous family-of-origin or other relationship experiences also helped to build our alliance. They trusted me to guide them through difficult things, and that trust helped our progress in therapy.

One procedure that helped me maintain my alliance with both partners was to collect feedback at the end of sessions when I was worried that alliance ruptures occurred. I invited Trey and Cara to each complete a brief rating scale assessing four aspects of the alliance: bonds, tasks, goals, and overall. This allowed me to understand more about how I was connecting with the couple, but more importantly, it provided an opening for me to discuss our relationship with each other and respond in real time to their identified concerns. As we began our next session, we'd discuss their feedback from the previous week and also identify both a high and a low point in their relationship in the time since then. Sometimes they would report the same situation or fight as their low and other times one would describe a relationship strain that the other felt was unimportant. This provided me opportunities to listen, understand, and validate both the positive and negative things that had happened. It also provided me the opportunity to listen when things may not have been going well, validate their perspectives, and repair any perceived missteps in the therapeutic alliance. Finally, these discussions at the beginning of a session also gave me some clues about potential topics or goals for that meeting, although I encouraged the couple to set their own agenda for each session.

INTERMEDIATE PHASE OF THERAPY

As we approached a point where Trey and Cara could discuss hot topics without escalating either in sessions or at home, I checked in with them about evolving goals and what was next for therapy. In my initial conceptualization, I worried about unresolved issues each partner brought in from their families of origin and previous relationships. From a systemic perspective, I considered that these life events likely would affect their relationship and that we'd have to work on these events together at some point. While our initial work served to stabilize their relationship, both partners recognized that there were parts of their personal and shared histories that disrupted their trust and connection, sometimes seeping into their conflicts and detracting from collaborations in various other areas of their lives including co-parenting.

I emphasized common themes and vulnerabilities that seemed present across interactions. Trey and Cara each had a core vulnerability that was present in many of their interactions. For Trey, it was a consistent feeling that he didn't belong. We discussed how his childhood experiences with foster care, as well as experiences of racism and discrimination, led to these feelings. As we discussed race, I was careful to acknowledge how these sociopolitical influences impacted his life in ways that I had never experienced, that I valued hearing about his unique experiences, and wanted therapy to feel like a safe space to share.

In his marriage to Cara with her two sons from previous relationships, he felt like he was never really a part of the family. When Cara would disagree with him on parenting matters and seem to side with the youngsters, he felt that she was actively trying to push him out of the family. Cara felt that she and the children all had to tiptoe around Trey. She also viewed her siding with the children as a way that she enacted her protective "mama bear" role—a role she'd felt compelled to adopt during her time as a single mom.

Trey's feelings of not belonging played out in other areas of his life as well. In his workplace, he was the oldest worker and was rarely invited to spend time outside of work with others. In his family of origin, he was only contacted when he was needed—for example, to fix a car or give someone a bed in which to sleep. He never felt close to his family of origin, though he was in contact with a few members consistently.

Cara never felt like she was good enough. She described being a parentified child who had to perform well in school and in other activities while caring for her three younger siblings. This experience led to her tend toward perfectionism, as well as anxiety and depression when she couldn't achieve that perfection. She described how her earlier relationships included emotional abuse and being told she wasn't good enough. Being divorced twice before made her believe she wasn't good enough for a long-term relationship. As a parent, Cara believed that the only way that she would be good enough was if she avoided conflict with her children—designating Trey as the disciplinarian, so that her children would offer her the acceptance she so desperately needed. When Trey complained about their co-parenting relationship, this only reinforced for her that she wasn't good enough as a parent which, therefore, meant that she wasn't a good enough person.

ME (SEG): I think we've gotten to a really good place of understanding here. I see a pattern emerging throughout many of your experiences that you've shared with me. What I see is that you each start from this vulnerable place. Given your feelings of not being good enough, Cara, you don't make efforts with Trey because, based on past experiences, you expect to fail and worries about how that will impact both of you. Then, without her effort, Trey feels like he doesn't belong with you. This leads you, Trey, to reach out for connection in some way, but Cara doesn't always respond to that well. When she doesn't respond exactly how you had hoped, she again feels like she isn't good enough, which further increases her distance, which then reinforces your feeling you don't belong. Does that sound right to you?

CARA: (*after a pause*) Wow. I just . . . I just never saw that we could possibly be hurting each other like that. On my end, you're totally right. I'm always terrified that I'll fail, so I just never even try to connect. And when he tries, I worry even more about failing because he's already tried. So, I just do nothing. [I could see tears in her eyes. We'd touched on some deep emotions, and my gentle formulation had impacted how she viewed these.]

ME (SEG): Cara, thank you so much for sharing that—especially for owning up to some of your faults and being open about your scared feelings. That was very vulnerable and brave of you. What about you, Trey, does what I said earlier feel like it fits for you, too?

TREY: I mean . . . maybe, I guess? [He responds without any overt emotion here, as is his usual pattern.] I do get angry when she doesn't try, but I don't think I actively think about not belonging. That feels really dumb and childish. Of course, I feel like I belong with Cara—we're married for heaven's sake!

ME (SEG): I want to reframe the idea that "feeling like you don't belong" would be dumb and childish. Like we've talked about before, these core vulnerabilities can show up even in times when it doesn't make sense to you. You've had hard experiences in your life that made you feel like no one wanted or loved you, so, of course, there's a part of you that's just never sure that you're loved and wanted. It's not dumb and childish, it's protecting you from hurts from before. [Trey continued to look at me without evident emotion. I wondered if I had met or missed the mark in trying to normalize his experiences.]

CARA: I think I'm always on alert for how Trey's doing. Even now, I feel totally ashamed for not making him feel loved and like he belongs. It's my fault—I should have done something better! (*She's crying at this point, and Trey passes her the tissue box in a gesture of comfort.*)

ME (SEG): Cara, I just want to take a minute to breathe here. (*I lean forward, resting my elbows on my knees, speaking softly.*) Can you take a few deep breaths? (*She does.*) Cara, you can't fix Trey's past. You can't make his family care about him. You can't change that he had hard relationships and that his family, even now, doesn't seem to seek closeness. These things are facts of his past, and you're not responsible for them. You're responsible only for you and for how you interact with others, including Trey. This history predates your relationship, so, of course, it comes up in your relationship.

TREY: Yeah, well, I'm tired of it. And I'm tired of her feeling like all the stupid things that happened in my life are her fault. I'm just screwed up, and that's it. Cara can't fix it. [I was surprised by how Trey was viewing the formulation and the emotional spillover.]

ME (SEG): Hold on there, Trey. You're not screwed up. I think that anyone in your circumstance would have a hard time feeling like they belonged. You've had so many instances of people telling you, both literally and figuratively, that you didn't belong. We're just working on helping you know that you belong with Cara, and helping Cara know that she's good enough in your relationship, even when things don't go perfectly.

TREY: (*He sits further back in his chair and lets out an exasperated sigh.*) It's too hard. I just think it's too hard to work through all the problems from my whole entire life.

ME (SEG): You're feeling exhausted. We've done a lot of hard work together already, but this mountain feels even bigger than the others.

CARA: (*Without my prompting, she shifts in her seat to face Trey.*) Trey, I want this to work. I care about you, I want you, I love you.

TREY: Sure you do, Cara. [His tone sounds dismissive and concerns me.]

ME (SEG): I'm going to pause us right there. Here it is again—this same cycle. Trey, if you don't allow yourself to belong with Cara here, right now, you'll open yourself up to being even more hurt in the future. It's like a self-fulfilling prophecy. You don't let yourself belong because you might get hurt even in the moments when Cara's trying to reassure you that you do belong with her.

TREY: (*closing his eyes and exhaling in exasperation*) I really hate this. I don't like how I feel inside when we talk about this. Can we just stop?

At this point, we'd reached Trey's emotional wall. He hated feeling any sort of hard emotion. We'd get down to an emotional place and he'd jump right back out almost immediately upon feeling the discomfort. In these moments, it was hard for me to know if the emotional work was the way to go. I wholeheartedly believed that Cara benefited from it but was never sure that Trey did, and I continually feared a breach in the tasks component of our alliance if I pushed too hard on this issue. He often talked about feeling emotionally stunted, as if his emotional experience was much more limited than other people. He discussed feeling unable to relate to Cara's emotions and consistently stayed on the cognitive side during discussions in therapy.

Given Trey's retreat from emotional work, it was hard for me to know what was best for our work together. In the next session, I asked him about it and what he thought about doing the emotional work.

ME (SEG): Trey, I wanted to check in with you about something from last week. We got to this emotional spot, and you asked us to stop.

TREY: Yeah, I really hate it when we talk about those things. But I know that Cara loves it, and it helps her.

ME (SEG): So, you hate it, Cara loves it. What do we do with it?

TREY: I'm not sure. Isn't that your job to know? [I chuckle in response, because his query was offered in a playful jousting way—consistent with some of our previous banter before and after sessions that had nourished our alliance.]

ME (SEG): In some ways, yes. In other ways, no. I want therapy to be helpful for both of you. If talking about your emotions just shuts you down and you don't want it at all, I don't see that as a way for us to work together well.

CARA: But I do really like it! I need it. I just think that Trey isn't used to it yet.

ME (SEG): You think Trey isn't used to talking about his emotions. What do you think, Trey?

TREY: I guess so. I mean, look at me. I'm a large, intimidating Black man! I was taught that emotions are weaknesses. No emotions means I'm strong and powerful. I'm safer that way.

ME (SEG): I think that makes a lot of sense both from your family and from your position as a marginalized person. You want to be strong, but is this a safe place to have emotions and not be seen as weak? [I wanted to affirm his experiences as a Black man, especially as a younger White woman. I knew that his identities impacted every part of him and his lived experiences, especially given his experiences with discrimination and his socialization around his race and gender.]

CARA: It *is* safe! I'm safe for your emotions—I want to hear all of them!

ME (SEG): Hold on, I want to hear from Trey about this one.

TREY: Hmm . . . I guess. I want it to be. I worry that Cara will throw my emotions back in my face like other people have.

ME (SEG): That's a valid concern, especially if others have done that. How can she be different in this?

TREY: She can just not talk about them again. Ever again! [He chuckles—again using a playful joust to make his point, but in a deliberately softened way.]

ME (SEG): [I laugh along with him.] I don't think that sounds realistic. If we're going to open up the floor for more emotional talk, emotions are going to be a more consistent part of your conversations.

TREY: Fine, you're right. She can ask about them and talk about them. It's only fair.

ME (SEG): Yes, but how can that feel safer for you?

TREY: If she shares too, I think. I think because I don't share, she doesn't share. But if this is supposed to be a safe space for me, then it could be safe for both of us.

ME (SEG): I like that idea. She can ask about your feelings, and you can share. You can ask about hers, and she can share. This seems good for both of you.

This exchange offered further evidence of the softening and emerging trust that seemed to be developing between Cara and Trey. Their mutual caring and capacity for empathic joining seemed especially strong in this session, and I was proud of the progress they'd made in this area. I was especially glad that Trey was open to continuing being vulnerable, though it felt difficult and unnatural for him, and that Cara was willing to support him in this discomfort.

Given their important therapeutic gains, I decided it was time to address sex in their relationship. They'd reported to me at intake that they hadn't been physically intimate (sexually or otherwise) for several years, but the details were unknown to me. I knew that work in this area would invoke strong emotions, challenge exaggerated thought processes, and require behavioral tasks—bringing to the fore the narrow common factors of "viewing, experiencing, and doing" discussed at the beginning of this chapter.

ME (SEG): Since neither of you identified an agenda item for today, I'm wondering if now is a good time to discuss sex in your relationship. [Phrasing it this way invited them to codefine our goals, and I hoped that would promote more engagement.]

CARA: Well, it'll be a short discussion. There *is* no sex in our relationship. [I see Trey roll his eyes as she says this.]

ME (SEG): (*inquiring gently*) How long has that been going on? When's the last time you had sex?

CARA: It was . . . 5 . . . 5? . . . yeah, I think it was 5 years ago.

ME (SEG): Wow, that's really a long time. What kinds of other physically intimate things do you engage in? Hugging, cuddling, hand holding, kissing? Any of those?

TREY: Absolutely not. We hardly get close to each other.

ME (SEG): I've noticed that. Through all of our sessions, it's like you two want to sit as far away from each other on this couch as possible. [I gesture to their seating arrangement.]

CARA: I feel like I'm not allowed to be close to him, like he's gotten so far away from me that I can't possibly bridge that gap.

TREY: When's the last time you even tried to?

CARA: (*sadly*) Years. It's been years since I tried.

TREY: Well, there's your problem. You haven't even tried. [I worried they could slip back into their familiar blame–defense pattern, so I redirected the conversation to see whether I could promote more empathic joining or an alliance between them to improve this part of their marriage.]

ME (SEG): Trey, if Cara did try, would you allow it? Would you welcome her closeness?

TREY: For the past few years, no, absolutely not. I always felt like she only wanted to be close so that she would feel good enough . . . or, at least, I realize now through therapy that's how I felt about it for so long.

ME (SEG): Okay, so, can you blame her for not trying then? Of course, she hasn't tried if she expected that you would reject her. It's very vulnerable to initiate and be rejected over and over, so many couples just get to a point where no one initiates and then there's no physical or sexual intimacy.

CARA: Exactly, I was tired of being rejected. I felt for a long time like you were disgusted by me—repulsed even—like you didn't possibly want me close to you. It felt like I was supposed to wait for you to initiate.

ME (SEG): Trey, do you see it that way? That it's your responsibility to initiate when you're ready?

TREY: Not really. I just assumed that that part of our relationship was over.

ME (SEG): Do you still feel that way? Like you'll never have that again?

TREY: Hmm . . . I guess I haven't thought about it. We haven't had anything for so long, I'm just used to this now.

ME (SEG): [He had softened a bit, and I hoped that I still might be able to move the partners toward a shared goal of restoring physical closeness.] Is it what you want though?

TREY: I don't want to be physical unless there's trust and safety. It was too difficult before, and I don't want to be in that space again.

ME (SEG): I wonder if you could try some nonsexual types of physical closeness to start and then work up to sex? Would that feel safer for you?

TREY: Maybe.

CARA: I'd love to try.

TREY: Of course, you would! Cara has always been more interested in sex than I have. [He said this with a playful chuckle, indicating his readiness to move from a defensive stance to a more collaboration.]

ME (SEG): Nearly all couples have one person who's more interested; it's just normal. And it's not wrong to be more interested or less interested; both are okay. You just have to navigate the differences. [By reframing their discrepancy in sexual desire as normal and acceptable, I hoped to change both their attributions and feelings (their viewing and experiencing) of the difficulties in their sexual relationship.] Trey, I don't want to work on this unless you both agree that improving your physically intimate life is something that you both value. I'm sure there's already been pressures around sex in your marriage, and I don't want to add to that pressure.

TREY: No, I think it's okay. I think this can be one of our shared goals. I just need it to move really slowly.

I introduced them to David Schnarch's (2011) program for progressing toward physical and sexual closeness. Progress was slow, and there were weeks when they reported feeling they had regressed. Each time, we would return to the basics of trust and safety, pursuing conversations promoting emotional connection until they felt comfortable being close again.

Given Trey's initial ambivalence toward sex, each time they had a setback, I worried that they would give up. I was surprised at their perseverance given their lack of physical and sexual intimacy throughout their relationship. I was also impressed with their openness in discussing sex and physical intimacy with me. I saw that vulnerability as evidence that our alliance was strong and that they trusted me to continue to guide them toward greater connection. On occasion, they wanted to avoid the emotional intensity of this work. I reframed this impulse as normal—and doing so helped them view this through a different lens and stay focused on their efforts.

CONCLUDING PHASE OF THERAPY

My work with Trey and Cara lasted about a year and a half. As we approached the end of our work together, we transitioned to a biweekly format. Trey and Cara initiated weekly meetings of their own at home to discuss difficult topics. Together, we constructed guidelines for these conversations: having a set day and time, setting an agenda the day before with a limit of two items each, starting and ending by highlighting positive things about each other, and limiting the meeting to 1 hour. Their commitment to their relationship, grounded in part in their shared Christian values and commitment to their children, sustained them through difficult times.

A few sessions before therapy was scheduled to end, the couple brought with them a tension that I hadn't seen for months. I went through my usual "How was the week?"; "Tell me about highs and lows."; "How did homework go?" without either partner mentioning anything that I thought could lead to this tension. After about 10 minutes, I finally brought it up.

ME (SEG): Okay, something's going on here that we're not talking about. (*Cara starts crying, and tears form at the corners of Trey's eyes. I lean forward and soften my voice.*) Something really big and really painful, I can tell.

TREY: (*looking up at me*) I really screwed up. I yelled at her. I haven't yelled at her for months now. [His shame is evident from his face and tone of voice.]

ME (SEG): You yelled at her, and you really regret it. This hasn't happened in a while, so it surprised both of you.

CARA: (*with tears running down her face*) I thought we were past this and could talk about anything now! We've worked so hard and now it seems so useless.

ME (SEG): This was disappointing for both of you. (*Both nod in agreement.*) Can one of you fill me in on what happened?

TREY: (*sighing*) I'd had a hard day at work and wasn't doing well with that. When I got home, our daughter Soph was laying on the couch with the dog, which isn't allowed. I knew I was too frustrated to handle it well, so I go looking for Cara and she's in our bedroom with earbuds in listening to music. I started escalating pretty quickly. I was mad about Soph but also mad that no one had considered fixing dinner, even though I'd made it the past three nights. It was like everything came crashing down and I was screaming at Cara within minutes.

ME (SEG): Wow, it seems like you had a lot going on that day and you let it all out at Cara. How did it feel doing that?

TREY: Honestly, just awful. Cara didn't even yell back—she just looked at me and said that she wasn't okay with the way that we were communicating and asked to take a time-out. Then she left the room and made dinner, took the girls to dance practice, and came back to talk about it. I'd wanted her to blow up at me right then, but she showed nothing but kindness and good skills. That made me even more mad, so when she came back, I yelled at her again. Then she slept on the couch that night for the first time in . . . maybe 9 months? She's kind of been giving me the cold shoulder ever since. We didn't even have our weekly meeting yesterday.

ME (SEG): So, for you, it felt like you did this one thing, and it became a big thing that ruined all of your hard work in therapy?

TREY: Exactly. I'm still pissed about it.

ME (SEG): I think there's more there than just anger though. What do you think? What's below that feeling of being angry? [Even after all of our practice, dealing with emotions was still his least favorite part of our work together.]

TREY: (*taking a deep breath*) Disappointment in myself for messing up and continuing to be angry about it. Disappointment in us for letting this ruin our relationship for the rest of the week. Definitely shame for yelling. I also feel strangely proud of Cara for holding it together and asking for a time-out. That was a good move on her part. Maybe scared that I've ruined all our work of the past year. [I was struck by his ability to identify various feelings.]

ME (SEG): Trey, I'm glad that you can recognize all those different emotions. Cara, what's it like to hear Trey share emotions?

CARA: (*no longer crying, looking exhausted*) That was a lot for me to hear about. I feel like I've been barely keeping it together all week, and I was so sad about it. We were so close to being done, and now we have to start all over!

ME (SEG): Cara, I know you feel disappointed about how things went and fear you've lost all you and Trey have worked toward, but I still think that you're close to being done with therapy. Most of my clients have some sort of setback right before we end. It's a part of the process that can actually help you to solidify what you've learned and be even more connected to your partner. [I hope to reframe this setback to alter their interpretations of what happened and the despair linked to those.] Partners in strong relationships work through these types of setbacks, just like you're both doing now.

CARA: I feel so distant and alone, and don't know how to get close again.

ME (SEG): Trey, how does it feel hearing this from Cara?

TREY: (*turning to Cara*) You feel alone, and I feel like I've totally lost you. But I want you to come closer. I know I really screwed up. I promise to try harder and to talk to you early—like maybe giving you a heads up if I'm coming home from an awful workday?

CARA: Yeah, maybe that would help. But I don't want to tiptoe around you like I used to.

TREY: I'm not asking you to do that all of the time, just maybe give me some time and space when I've already had a lot of stress. I'm sorry and hope you can forgive me sometime.

CARA: I think I can—not right now, but sometime soon. [They're smiling warmly at each other and I choose to leave those emotions out there for a few moments before I then respond.]

ME (SEG): Wow, I'm so impressed with you two. Did you see how important that was for you to reconnect with each other?

CARA: It felt good for him to admit that he did something wrong and to ask for forgiveness.

TREY: I felt my shame growing throughout the week, but it's lower now. I think we'll be okay.

ME (SEG): I, too, think you will be.

When I checked in with Trey and Cara in our next session, both reported feeling the issue was resolved and that they'd moved on together. I was impressed with how quickly they bounced back. In our last session, we reviewed the ways that their relationship had changed over our time together. They reminisced about their increased connection and laughed at some of their early failings. We talked about what they'd learned that had been helpful and resources they could use when they needed additional help. I let them know that they could pursue a new season of therapy any time that they wanted. I offered a metaphor that therapy is like a revolving door that you can enter and exit as needed. Cara was emotional upon leaving the last time. Both expressed gratitude for our work together and I expressed gratitude for having been a part of their journey. It was one of those times when, as they left, I felt so proud of them—excited for the relationship they'd created and hopeful for their future. *They* did it and I was grateful to be a part of it.

FURTHER REFLECTIONS AND IMPLICATIONS

Though the narrative and dialogue offered here show progress in therapy over time, session-to-session change was very slow. Simply building communication skills took many months before these skills were used consistently and successfully. Along the journey, there were many setbacks and difficulties: The couple would often bring back to the table a breach that, to my understanding, we had already processed and resolved. The path of reconciliation and forgiveness was often long and laborious. This slow progress sometimes had me discouraged and wondering why this couple kept coming back week to week. When I would check in with them on how they felt things were progressing, they were often much more optimistic than I was, which helped me to persevere.

Given our diverse identities, this couple allowed me to apply much of what I knew about sociocultural attunement. I was able to learn from each partner about their various identities and families of origin, especially when they differed from mine. When asked, I was open in sharing about various aspects of my own life, including our differences in age, spirituality, race/ethnicity, and so on—and I openly discussed how I strived to stay attuned to their own values and relational desires. This personal sharing, while perhaps not necessary in every case, proved critical in my work with Trey and Cara, and enabled me to be a more effective agent of change.

Working with this couple taught me the importance of the therapeutic alliance in new and important ways. I'd had my share of challenging couples before, but Trey and Cara brought difficult individual and relational histories that sometimes made me feel uncertain about making any progress in therapy. Throughout many rough patches, we relied on our alliance to help heal wounds and reconnect. Hearing from my colleague about his difficulty with his alliance with this couple made me very aware of our alliance from the beginning. My work in balancing the alliance with Trey and Cara was vital to their feeling seen, heard, and understood, which helped both to stay engaged in therapy and the process of change. This required extra connections with Trey, as he was sometimes resistant to emotional expression in therapy, but the balance was crucial to our work. They also expressed appreciation for my willingness to share about myself while always maintaining our focus on their lived experiences, values, and relationship goals instead of imposing my own. Through our alliance, therapy was a place of safety even when change or my challenges were uncomfortable.

Furthermore, this couple's commitment to therapy always amazed me: They lived in a small town and, strongly preferring in-person meetings to virtual ones, drove over an hour each way every week for us to meet. They worked hard on weekly therapy homework but were careful in setting boundaries when certain topics risked escalation. Both partners remained engaged and vulnerable as we established mutual trust and respect. Looking back, I can see how my experiences with Trey and Cara tested me and helped me to grow as a therapist. It was a challenge and, in the end, it was a joy.

REFERENCES

Blow, A. J., & Piercy, F. P. (1997). Teaching personal agency in family therapy training programs. *Journal of Systemic Therapies, 16,* 274–283.

Davis, S. (2023). Common factors in couple therapy. In J. L. Lebow & D. K. Snyder (Eds.), *Clinical handbook of couple therapy* (6th ed., pp. 295–317). New York: Guilford Press.

Karam, E., & Blow, A. (2023). *Bringing common factors to life in couple and family therapy.* New York: Routledge.

Miller, S. D., Duncan, B. L., & Hubble, M. A. (1997). *Escape from Babel: Toward a unifying language for psychotherapy practice.* New York: Norton.

Schnarch, D. (2011). *Intimacy and desire: Awaken the passion in your relationship.* New York: Beaufort Books.

Sprenkle, D., & Blow, A. (2004). Common factors and our sacred models. *Journal of Marital and Family Therapy, 30,* 113–129.

Sprenkle, D., Blow, A., & Dickey, M. (1999). Common factors and other nontechnique variables in marriage and family therapy. In M. Hubble, B. Duncan, & S. Miller (Eds.), *The heart and soul of change: What works in therapy* (pp. 329–360). Washington, DC: American Psychological Association.

Sprenkle, D., Davis, S., & Lebow, J. (2009). *Common factors in couple and family therapy: The overlooked foundation for effective practice.* New York: Guilford Press.

CHAPTER 8

Discernment Counseling with a Couple on the Brink

WILLIAM J. DOHERTY
STEVEN M. HARRIS

> *Editors' Comments*
>
> Bill Doherty and Steve Harris describe here their widely acclaimed approach of discernment counseling for intervening with the many couples who experience the dilemma of one partner moving toward divorcing while the other partner leans toward preserving the marriage. Although this ranks among the most painful of couple dynamics, couple therapy as ordinarily practiced is poorly suited for these "mixed-agenda" couples, because it presumes both partners have at least some motivation aimed at improving the relationship. These couples provide a special variation on the well-known axiom that clients' stage of change is central to progress in therapy. With mixed-agenda couples, one partner may not only lack motivation to improve their marriage but also improvement of the marriage may be contrary to what that partner experiences as a present goal. As Doherty and Harris highlight in this case narrative, the circular coercive cycle about whether to stay together or not often becomes the central downward struggle in these couples, vitiating any opportunity for couple therapy to be useful.
>
> Through their extensive use of transcripts, Doherty and Harris illustrate the explicit focus, structure, and guidelines for this brief approach. The focus is fully on whether the partners can understand one another's point of view and move toward a collaborative decision about whether to move toward divorce or seek couple therapy as a fully engaged effort to improve the marriage. Note that although there are helpful steps toward improving each partner's ability to relate to one another in this difficult life situation, in discernment counseling the goal isn't about improving the couple's relationship. Instead, the emphasis is fully on being able to engage in an informed collaborative process—to either develop the understanding that the relationship is no longer viable for at least one partner or take the steps that might provide a foundation for an effective couple therapy if the choice is to work toward salvaging the relationship.
>
> Doherty and Harris are clearly the masters of this approach and provide a wonderful example of what to do and say in helping a couple engage in this process. The

> work is supportive—most especially in holding a stance that doesn't favor one partner or the other for the way they lean—while being direct in helping each person clarify how to better understand and respond to their partner, as well as possibilities for working on their own issues, whether they remain in this relationship or not. This chapter also illuminates how maintaining the relationship, while often preferable, is not the only useful solution for couples experiencing relationship distress.

Discernment counseling is a relatively new therapeutic approach we designed for couples on the brink of divorce (Doherty & Harris, 2017; Doherty, Harris, & Wilde, 2016). It is appropriate with "mixed-agenda couples," in which one person is leaning toward divorce and is ambivalent about trying couple therapy, and the other person wants to preserve the marriage and pursue couple therapy. Studies suggest that mixed-agenda couples might represent up to 25–30% of couples presenting for treatment (Doherty, Harris, & Wickel Didericksen, 2016). Because partners' goals usually differ so much in these couples, we believe that they need a different approach than launching directly into change-oriented couple therapy.

Bill drifted into doing couple therapy work after beginning his clinical and academic career in the 1970s doing family therapy with adolescents and parents. He learned that often the difficulties with adolescents stemmed from the parents' relationship issues, and the family therapy ended up with couple therapy. He developed discernment counseling out of frustration with "failure-to-launch" couple therapy when one of the spouses was ambivalent about the marriage and about working on it in therapy. It moved him from frustration to a place of actual enjoyment helping couples who were divided on their goals for the relationship. When Steve was in graduate school at Syracuse University and a professor asked him how he might consider specializing his practice, his response was simply, "I want to work with couples." The professor laughed and suggested it probably needed to be more focused than that. Fast-forward about 18 years and Steve is working alongside Bill at the University of Minnesota to fine-tune the discernment counseling protocol. He has also been involved in a nationwide research project on divorce decision making that empirically "feeds" the knowledge base for why this approach is so necessary.

The goal of discernment counseling is to help couples gain greater clarity and confidence about a direction for their marriage based on a deeper understanding of what's happened to their marriage and each person's contributions to the problems. (Throughout this chapter, we use "marriage" to refer to a relationship in which both partners once made a permanent commitment, and "divorce" to refer to dissolution of that relationship.) Note that this goal contrasts with the goal of traditional couple therapy approaches that aim to solve relationship difficulties and enhance bonding, connection, and problem-solving capacities. Discernment counseling deliberately focuses not on improving the relationship but, rather, on helping partners decide whether to try to improve it.

Discernment counseling is highly structured and short term (one to five sessions). It lays out three alternative paths for the couple's decision making: (1) keep the status quo; (2) separate or divorce; or (3) attempt to reconcile via a 6-month commitment to couple therapy, with divorce off the table for that time, and sometimes with other therapeutic referrals. An additional important focus is on helping each partner see the patterns in their relationship that have gotten them to the brink of divorce and their individual contributions to the problems. This exploration leads to identifying areas of personal work that each partner would commit to work on if they decide to pursue couple therapy.

The structure of discernment counseling reflects the fact that the partners come with different hopes. The "leaning-out" partner wants to decide whether to stay or leave, and the "leaning-in" partner wants to find a way to preserve the relationship. For this reason, most of the work occurs in individual conversations, with brief summaries that each gives to the other about what was learned in those conversations. (There are no enactments or problem-solving interventions when both partners are in the room together; the intensive work occurs one-to-one). The focus with the leaning-out partner is on making a decision on one of the three paths based on a deeper understanding of the problems and their own contributions to them. The focus with the leaning-in partner is on understanding (1) their partner's reasons for considering divorce (what has disturbed or demoralized the partner), (2) their own contributions to the problems, and (3) how to use this time of crisis to learn what they would need to change if they both choose to try and reconcile. The discernment counselor also helps the leaning-in partner avoid making things worse by pursuing or criticizing the leaning-out partner. In the roller coaster of decision making of couples on the brink, we sometimes see couples switching roles between leaning in and leaning out. We know from research that divorce decision making is dynamic (Allen et al., 2021; Galovan, Hawkins, Harris, & Simpson, 2021; Hawkins et al., 2017) and that what people think and feel at one time might be dramatically different than the next.

Prior to starting discernment counseling, there are separate screening phone calls with both partners to make sure they're candidates for this approach, to get an initial sense of their problems and concerns, and to screen for risks of violence or coercion. There's a limit of five sessions in discernment counseling in order to focus intensively on choosing a path forward instead of helping the couple try to change now (which would likely happen if the length of discernment counseling were open-ended). Couples commit to only one session at a time in order to maximize the leaning-out partner's freedom to choose to continue or end the process. We refer to this approach as discernment "counseling" rather than discernment "therapy" to emphasize that the leaning-out partner isn't committing to couple therapy. The first session is 2 hours in length and subsequent sessions are 90 minutes.

The first session begins with 40 minutes of joint interview with the partners to learn more about their goals and challenges, and to get a sense of how they relate to each other in the room. Then each partner is seen alone, with the other in the waiting room, and then that person does a brief summary of learnings to the other. Then they switch places. In subsequent sessions, there's a brief check-in with the partners together, but the bulk of the time is with each individual separately.

Although the discernment counselor accepts whatever decision the partners ultimately make about their marriage, the individual conversations have a special emphasis on painting a picture of what couple therapy might look like for each partner involved. The leaning-out partner knows why they're drawn to divorce, and their ruminations are usually about the pain of divorcing or the even worse pain of staying in a miserable marriage. Part of the job of the discernment counselor is to open up the possibility of another path, a temporary one that focuses on seeing whether change is possible via therapy. What does this path of reconciliation look like? What would I have to be doing? What can I expect my partner to be doing?

Discernment counseling ends when one of the paths is chosen, either by one person (someone decides to divorce) or by the partners together. If the couple chooses to pursue couple therapy, the discernment counselor can either become their couple therapist or refer them elsewhere for that work. If either partner decides on divorce, the discernment counselor helps the couple decide how to navigate the transition and may refer them to additional resources. If neither divorce nor therapy is agreed upon (i.e., maintaining the status quo), the discernment counselor helps partners decide how they want to be together for now with the things they've learned about their marriage. Success in discernment counseling isn't based on the path chosen but, instead, on whether partners have developed clarity and confidence about a decision for the future and have learned about their relationship dynamics and each person's contributions.

INITIAL ASSESSMENT AND CASE FORMULATION

When Pam brought up the idea of divorce to Mike, he was stunned. They'd been married for 30 years and had two grown children. Mike had been the breadwinner (a well-paid professional), and Pam stayed at home for most of their marriage after dropping out of graduate school. She currently worked part-time in health care. The couple was referred for discernment counseling by Pam's therapist after Pam disclosed she was seriously considering divorce.

Separate screening phone calls with each of them revealed that Mike was "leaning in" and that Pam was "leaning out." Like many long-term couples, they'd put everything into their kids and neglected their relationship. She reported growing up in a difficult family of origin and then making considerable personal gains through years of therapy, and that Mike couldn't or wouldn't empathize with her feelings. She became his emotional caretaker and felt she lost herself. He threw himself into his work, not understanding how his emotional neediness came across to Pam. Their conflict pattern consisted of her bringing up concerns and he would "treat them like a lawyer" (challenging her facts), and she would back down. Eventually sexual intimacy became infrequent (Pam had little interest), which was highly distressing to Mike.

They had done three rounds of couple therapy in the past, much of which seemed unfocused. Pam had pursued years of individual therapy for anxiety and depression. With so much couple therapy in their history, a challenge in discernment counseling would be to communicate how couple therapy could be different this time. As their discernment counselor, I (WJD) clarified during the initial phone screening that if they chose to pursue couple therapy, I'd refer them to a colleague for that work.

BEGINNING PHASE OF DISCERNMENT COUNSELING: SESSION 1

This is an abridged version of a transcript of Pam and Mike's discernment counseling conducted by Bill. We offer here a more detailed narrative of the first session in order to demonstrate the core approach to discernment counseling and to give a feel for the flow of sessions, and then we use briefer descriptions and excerpts showing key moments in the subsequent four sessions. The 2-hour first session begins with couple time, followed by individual conversations.

Couple Time

During the couple time, I (WJD) gather additional information and observe how Pam and Mike respond in each other's presence. I begin with the standard opener to make sure that their goals for discernment counseling are consistent with what discernment counseling is designed to offer.

> ME (WJD): I'd like to begin by asking you each to say what you hope to get out of discernment counseling. What would be a good outcome of this work?
>
> PAM: I'd like to know if the issues we have can be addressed with the hope of maintaining a very long marriage, or if it's time to end the marriage.
>
> ME (WJD): And Mike, how about you?
>
> MIKE: I think it's similar, just try to understand where we're at basically, and hopefully with better understanding, so we can arrive at a decision to move forward as a couple.
>
> ME (WJD): Okay, the goals of discernment counseling are consistent with what you both articulated—more clarity and confidence about a direction for your relationship, based on a deeper understanding of what's happened to your marriage and each person's contributions to the problem.

I then oriented the couple to what our time together will look like in this session, including time together and time separately. I organize the rest of the couple time around several questions we ask of every couple. We call these the "divorce narrative," "repair," "children," and "best of times" questions. Unless their conflict patterns are already clear, we ask an additional question to get at those.

> ME (WJD): So, what's happened to your relationship that's gotten you to the point where divorce is a possibility?
>
> PAM: During COVID we were together 24/7—it just really brought home a lot of the things that had been issues that we both knew we'd been able to avoid for a long time. And I kept thinking to myself, "Do I want to continue like this for another 30 years?" We've tried several different marriage counselors, none of which have really clicked or have really been successful for us.
>
> ME (WJD): Could you elaborate a bit more on those chronic issues you mentioned?
>
> PAM: For me, it was my own choice to be a stay-at-home mom. I kept very busy doing other things in school, but I never had a full-time job. Leaving behind a career was very difficult. I did it and enjoyed it, but always felt like I was sort of second. I made my life adjust to what Mike's needs were. It seemed to me that he did whatever he wanted, and I would adjust.
>
> ME (WJD): Thank you. So, Mike, what do you think has happened to your marriage that's gotten you to the point where divorce is a possibility?
>
> MIKE: Over the years, as the kids were growing up, there was more of a distance between the two of us. We even talked about it. I wasn't as supportive as I could have been in responding to the things that Pam identified. And then, a year ago, she just put it out there and said, "Hey, this isn't working, and I may want to go

in a different direction." After hearing that, I made a real shift and worked on trying to be more present and engage with her. I also made more efforts around the house, splitting up tasks in a fairer way. I think we've done a lot to repair, but the one piece that's just not clicking is our physical relationship. What's most important to me is that Pam finds something that makes her happy and I hope that's with me.

ME (WJD): Thank you. Let me ask you next about repair. What have you done individually and together, with help or on your own, to try to fix the problems you've identified?

Their responses made it clear that their prior couple therapists faded out of couple work after a few sessions and transitioned to working only with Pam. I always feel sad and angry when I hear these stories about how therapists bail out of couple therapy for people who show up to work on their relationship. Gathering this information about past couple therapy is important, because the third path in discernment counseling involves another round of couple therapy. I knew I had to make the case that couple therapy could look very different and be more effective than it had been for them.

ME (WJD): I realize your children are grown and living on their own, but what role, if any, do they play in your decision making about the future of your marriage?

They both indicated that their children didn't play a major role. This isn't always the case with couples who have grown kids; for some, breaking up a strong family unit is a big factor in their decision making.

ME (WJD): When you consider the entire span of your relationship, when would you say were the "best of times," when you felt the most connection and joy?

We ask this question at this point to see whether there were good times in the past, what was going on then in their relationship, and what they liked and enjoyed about each other. Pam and Mike both pointed to shared enjoyable times of physical activity and teamwork. In the midst of the heaviness of this first session, with so much on the line, I felt "lighter" when they described how much they used to enjoy each other. When one or both partners have a hard time answering this question and further queries result in no reports of connection, it can be a sign that there's very little keeping the couple together.]

ME (WJD): My final question for now is about what happens when you argue or have conflict. Can you paint a picture for me about what happens when a problem comes up, or you've got some big thing that you need to discuss?

We often ask this additional question when it's not yet clear what the couple's conflict patterns look like. In response to this query, Pam describes herself as conflict avoidant and tentative in bringing up concerns for fear that she'll be shot down by Mike's legalistic reasoning—and then she retreats in order not to upset him. Mike agrees that's what happens when Pam brings up issues. When he brings things up, mostly about sex, she retreats and he gives up.

Once we've addressed these standard questions we transition to individual meetings with each partner. We generally begin with the leaning-out partner to establish rapport with the person who's more ambivalent about therapy. At the end of the couple time with Pam and Mike, I felt that what they shared thus far was the kind of well-rehearsed story they had presented in prior couple therapy. I was hoping for more depth when I talked to them alone.

Individual Time with Pam

Like many leaning-out partners, Pam sees divorce as a sad but maybe necessary step, because she can't go on with the marriage as it is. I spend considerable effort in making sure Pam knows that I understand the depth of her concerns and really get that divorce is something she's seriously considering. Her main barrier to working on the relationship in couple therapy is her sense that Mike can't or won't change. Her skepticism comes from the fact that she's done a lot of personal therapy and Mike hasn't, and from the "failure" of previous couple therapy. Next, I encourage her not to focus solely on her husband's potential for change but rather on their joint interaction patterns that she's part of—and which could be changed with good couple therapy.

> ME (WJD): I really understand that you feel you can't stay married the way the marriage has been and so the second path—divorce—is a serious option for you. The question about possible couple therapy—what we call the third path—is whether you want to see if you can both make some changes that will help your marriage get to a healthier place. But you have your skepticism.
>
> PAM: Exactly. The things I've seen him do recently have really been different, and I think there's potential for there to be a depth that he and I aren't aware of . . . so I think I'm skeptically positive, if there's such a thing.

The discussion went into their 32-year marriage and how they settled into traditional gender roles, with her as a stay-at-home mom. I emphasized that their "settling" into these roles is now being challenged by both of them. We discussed their several attempts to get help, and I suggested that they never really seemed to get competent, consistent help for their marriage. For me, it's a delicate dance to point out limitations in prior couple therapy without throwing the previous therapists under the bus. I'm aware that I haven't always been helpful to the couples I've treated.

> ME (WJD): You've described a conflict pattern of multiple false starts. You'd bring up something and then Mike would "do his lawyer thing." And given your tendency to be cautious about conflict, you'd back off but, of course, you'd store it away. And then, the other dynamic was that Mike might get steamed up about something and bring it up, and you'd say, "No, this isn't a good time," but the two of you weren't able to find a better time, right?
>
> PAM: Because the topic was always the same—the physical part.
>
> ME (WJD): So with you not really feeling comfortable with conflict in general, sex would be really difficult to discuss. And you weren't going to say, "Well, if this isn't a good time, let's discuss it at later this evening." Because for you, this isn't going to get resolved, so let's not go down that path.

PAM: Right. It's just going to be another dead end, with me leaving the room.

ME (WJD): In good couple therapy, those issues come out, you get more of a sense of each of your contributions to them, and you get help learning to deal with less crucial conflicts as a practice ground. And then you build up to ones that are more powerful, but you can't go from zero to 10 if you don't have those abilities as a couple.

PAM: The only thing is that Mike doesn't really have any other issues than the physical part of our marriage.

ME (WJD): Well, okay. So let me suggest that as Mike makes changes in becoming a more emotionally well-rounded person—he's on that journey—I think he'll discover more issues. More things are bound to come up for him.

PAM: Ah, that's a good point. Yes, they may come up.

This is one of those key moments in discernment counseling when I help the leaning-out partner shift their storyline that it's mainly about the other's faults or limitations to seeing the problems in interactional terms that involve both of their contributions. This often requires direct challenge to this partner's well-practiced narrative, and I've learned to "go for it" in the first session. For me, discernment counseling is like emergency room work more than regular couple therapy—the immediate stakes are high and you may not see the couple again. The intensity is part of what I love about this work.

ME (WJD): Generally, for people who are attuned to their feelings and attuned to a relationship, there are issues. And then you choose which ones you're going to bring up and which ones you let go, but you know they're there. And so I think that may be the journey he's on. I'll talk more with him about that. By the way, if you do some more serious work in your relationship, you'll be challenged in other ways, not just about sex.

I have the sense that Pam was in accord with me on how she had to make changes, too. Our conversation shifts to exploring the sexual dimension of their relationship—thinking about choosing to pursue couple therapy in the third path would include exploring their sexual dynamic.

ME (WJD): Okay, it's time to finish up our individual time together. Reflect on what we talked about here. What would you like to say to Mike as something you're taking with you from our time that you'll maybe continue to reflect on? [Pam and I discuss what she learned in our conversation and I help her decide what to share with Mike when he returns to the room.]

PAM: (*to Mike*) Our discussion really put in perspective why our previous attempts at couple therapy weren't effective or didn't really come up with any way forward for us as a couple. And that's a little bit clearer to me now how each therapy attempt digressed into a focus on me. I'd never really considered how that really left you out in the cold . . . and left us as a couple out in the cold. So, I'm beginning to see that there might be ways to get better help for both of us, not just me.

I felt a small sense of elation and cautious optimism when Pam nailed a core part of what I hoped she would get from our conversation. I also knew that this was just a door-opener to hope, one that Mike might feel more optimistic about than would be warranted.

Individual Time with Mike

My main goals in the time with Mike were to see whether he'd sign on to my helping him understand his contributions to the problems and to reduce the pressure he'd been putting on Pam around sex and whether she's going to stay in the marriage. I begin with empathy for what it's been like for him since Pam said she might leave him.

> ME (WJD): It's been quite a journey you've been on the last year or so since Pam told you that your marriage was on the line.
>
> MIKE: The challenge is the incredible uncertainty as to whether she still wants to be married to me and just dealing with that all the time. Emotionally, it's like we're just sort of roommates for a while, until we figure out whether we're going our separate ways or what's the deal. [After a few minutes of empathic support, I switch to the future.]
>
> ME (WJD): So in terms of the three paths that we discussed [I summarized them again], where are you on those?
>
> MIKE: So definitely not the first two. I've felt strongly that I want to figure something out to whatever extent possible that will continue to bring us more together. So, the third path.
>
> ME (WJD): My job with you then is to help you make your best case for that, to present yourself in a way that makes it more likely that Pam will want to work with you on the relationship.

I give Mike some things to consider regarding how to navigate differing levels of sexual desire within marriage. And I let him know that those are the types of things that can be discussed further in good, competent couple therapy. I'm always mindful during discernment counseling that we're not working directly on the problems; instead, we're identifying them and teeing them up for possible future work in couple therapy. Since leaning-in spouses are often eager to start therapy, it's tempting to coach them on how to begin the work now. But without a couple-level agreement to work on change, Mike's efforts are likely to backfire. Discernment counseling with the leaning-in partner is about identifying issues to work on in couple therapy and not creating unrealistic expectations of change now. Similarly, with the leaning-out partner, we caution against expecting relationship improvements during discernment counseling; those will have to wait for a both-on-board couple therapy process.

We shift our discussion to their couple process and Mike's role in their sexual interactions.

> ME (WJD): You said earlier that you'd sometimes raise your concerns about sex at inconvenient times, and she'd push back about the timing. What kinds of things did you raise?
>
> MIKE: Recently, it's more along the lines of trying to get a better sense of what I can do that would help her get more enjoyment when we're physically together. She actually described feelings of disgust when I was even just kissing her on the neck in the kitchen. And that was one of the things that was tough for me to hear, but it's good that she's feeling more confident to tell me. It's been probably 3 weeks since we were together physically, and we took our time and had a massage, and she

certainly seemed to derive more enjoyment out of that. So I asked, "Are you more on the side of disgusted or more neutral, or potentially there's some enjoyment there?"

ME (WJD): I want to try to help you see how that affects Pam. From your point of view, you're trying to get some clarification so you could put less pressure and have her be more into it and not turned off. Am I right? (*He nods in agreement.*) But the effect on her, from what I'm seeing, is of feeling pressure. She knows that for many years, you'd like more sex. As I mentioned to her, it's hardly ever the case that two people are equally matched in that regard, and this has been an area of tension for many years. And so, if you then ask her questions to clarify what works for her and what doesn't, she's inevitably going to feel pressure.

MIKE: That makes perfect sense.

ME (WJD): What I'm urging you to focus on at this point is lowering the tension level for her around this issue of sexuality. And then deal with this issue in couple therapy, because sex is often the hardest thing for couples talk about—particularly when you're a bit on the brink of breaking up. [In discernment counseling, this kind of "intervention" with the leaning-in partner generally takes the form of "do no harm, and prepare for the work ahead in therapy." I give Mike some very specific suggestions on how he can position himself during this time of uncertainly and give Pam some space to do her discernment work. Taking the pressure off her also signals that he's willing to change by being sensitive to her needs.] And while you're in discernment counseling, I also urge you not to ask Pam where she is in terms of her decision making—about staying together and working on the marriage. Let her bring it up if she wants, because if you pursue her on this, it's just going to make it harder for her. Just be available, be present. Don't pursue her like, "Hey, are you thinking more like you're going to stay with me?" Let her say it, if she wants to. But also don't distance yourself, saying something like "I'm going to go to my room and you know where to find me when you want to stop rejecting me." [In working with anxious leaning-in partners, we help them take a differentiated stance during a time of uncertainty and stress by neither pursuing nor distancing.]

MIKE: You've hit it . . . I've already made both those mistakes. Sometimes this past year I've been effusive in terms of attention and gifts, and all the rest of that. And that kind of worked for a little bit, but then at some point, it doesn't. And then, I'm sort of like, "Well, okay, whatever." I'm trying to get to a happy medium where I'm just available.

ME (WJD): Great, beautiful. I think you're doing it well in terms of showing up and connecting. So, we need to finish up here and have Pam join us. What have you taken from our time together that you would like to say to Pam? [I help Mike put what he has learned about himself into a brief form.]

Pam comes back into the room, and then Mike shares his takeaway statement. [The first part refers to something we discussed that is not in the previous transcript.]

MIKE: (*to Pam*) I'm starting to understand better that when you come to discuss something, I respond in an interrogating kind of way, and it's not particularly productive.

I need to work on responding more from what's inside of me and how I feel, so we can have more of a discussion instead of me setting the stage for a debate. And in terms of my approaching you about how we're doing, as well as about being physical together, that's not particularly productive or helpful, because just the fact of me posing those questions generates unnecessary pressure. And so it's better to just know there's things that I can work on and we can work on together, and just kind of let things begin to flow—hopefully in a positive direction.

This was a typical first session of discernment counseling, and I felt hopeful about the next steps in the process. Pam seemed open to looking at their problems in a more systemic way, and Mike was open to my input about how he might consider showing up differently in their marriage. My hope was tempered by a concern that Pam would hold onto her belief that she is the more "enlightened" partner because of her prior therapy, and that Mike is too limited as a person to meet her needs. I've learned not to make predictions in discernment counseling, because couples on the brink can lurch in different directions from week to week.

INTERMEDIATE PHASE OF COUNSELING

Session 2

We always begin subsequent sessions with a reminder about the goals of discernment counseling; otherwise, clients can start to feel as if they're in traditional couple therapy. This is followed by a check-in question pertinent to these goals.

> ME (WJD): My check-in question is: Where are each of you today in your journey toward clarity and confidence about a direction for your marriage?

Note that this check-in question is not about how they have gotten along in the past week; that would signal a therapy-type process. Pam responded that she was still uncertain, but it felt good to continue discerning a path. When Mike answered by stating that he felt more disconnected from Pam this week, I clarified that this check-in was about where each of them were regarding a future direction for their marriage, as opposed to how the week went between them. He responded that he was still on board for maintaining the marriage and doing couple therapy.

I decided to have the individual time with Mike first to try to get him on track with a constructive leaning-in stance. I was concerned that he was putting pressure on Pam by inviting her to reassure him.

> MIKE: I like when we're just lying together with our arms around each other. That physical contact feels nice, and there wasn't any of that from her this past week. Pam could sense that something was obviously bothering me and asked me about it yesterday. I told her, "I'm just wondering whether it's better for me to help you find someone that you actually want to be with." [As Mike disclosed this, his posture and facial expression suggested that this wasn't what he really wanted but had said it out of hurt.] Pam said she took that to mean that she wasn't fulfilling a responsibility or obligation of a wife, that she was failing in some way. I said I

didn't mean it that way, but that's just the way I felt—that there wasn't any connection there for her.

ME (WJD): Let's talk about this. Your goal for discernment counseling, as I understand it, remains working toward a process for making things better. You'd like to do some serious couple therapy to see if you could get your marriage into a healthier place.

MIKE: Yes, definitely.

ME (WJD): Then my job is to help you understand what's happened throughout your marriage, your contributions, and to help you carry yourself now in a way that makes it more likely that Pam will be open to wanting to join you in this. I think part of what happened there, Mike, is that you were responding to her as if you both were on the reconciliation path, as if you both had said, "Yeah, I want to get closer. I want to really make this marriage work."

MIKE: I want to restore our intimacy.

ME (WJD): Okay, but during this difficult limbo phase, when you approach her and say you're not feeling close, that inevitably puts pressure on her, because you don't really have a joint agreement that you *both* want to get closer.

I focused the rest of the individual time with Mike on helping him recalibrate as the leaning-in partner—that is, to focus for now not on regaining closeness but on a posture of learning and hope for the prospects of couple therapy. During this past week, he had been too encouraged by a good sexual encounter and then discouraged that Pam distanced afterward. I coached him on how to maintain his boundaries and also respect hers. Mike responded well to this input, although I was concerned about his follow-through at home. It can be really hard for an emotionally needy partner to take a more differentiated stance when fearing abandonment. But that's exactly what we challenge leaning-in spouses to attempt in support of the overarching goal of preserving their marriage. When they balk and say that it's too hard or unfair, we return to the question of whether they want to save their marriage and want our help for that to happen. Pursuing their partner is counter to their fervent goal.

It can take careful coaching of the leaning-in partner on how to frame their sharing points with their spouse after the individual conversation. We want them to be honest about their mistakes and compassionate toward their partner. After we finished and Pam returned to the room, Mike shared the following:

MIKE: (*to Pam*) As you know, I was feeling sort of disconnected for a good part of this week, although I really appreciated our time together earlier. What I'm beginning to understand is that sometimes I go too high or too low in reaction to things, and it's probably better to try to be more even-keeled in terms of being available to you and just supportive. I know this is a tough time for you, too, as we try to figure things out.

[I then met with Pam individually.]

ME (WJD): So how can I be helpful to you in your ongoing discernment?

PAM: It was helpful to hear Mike say those words, because that's something I've been feeling. It's as if certain things I say send him into a tailspin or if I'm not constantly reassuring him, he starts asking questions and pushing me about what's going on. [A key moment in the session occurred when Pam continued to express skepticism about the possibility of change—common in leaning-out partners in discernment counseling.] And then I get stuck again with that dilemma of whether to try to save the marriage or just pursue divorce. And my hesitancy of jumping into the therapy is the lack of confidence in our ability to actually change the relationship.

ME (WJD): That's what we should be talking about.

PAM: And when you talk about divorce being off the table, I'm reluctant. Because my confidence that this will actually bring about a change is small.

ME (WJD): We've had a good discussion about some of the patterns you two fall into. And the question is, are these things changeable? So tell me more about your skepticism about the possibility of change. [In asking this question I continue to honor Pam's leaning-out status, taking it seriously, letting her know I really want to understand her position because I know that otherwise I'll have no influence in helping her consider the possibility of pursuing a new couple therapy.]

PAM: So part of my skepticism is from things we've learned in the past and things I've tried to impress on him that are important to me. Then Mike's effort is maintained for a while, but only for a short time. It wouldn't stick after counseling ended. [I found myself struggling to get Pam to stop focusing on how Mike cannot change. This is probably the common presentation of leaning-out spouses and the hardest part of doing discernment counseling. I decided to join with her frustration and then directly challenge her about not focusing on her part in the relational dance.]

ME (WJD): I get that—your relationship's history, the lack of enduring change, his not changing—that's all real to you. We could probably speak at length about it. Now, your own contributions to the stalemate or the falling back—you're vaguer about that. So your lens and focus is on Mike. Sitting where I am, I see both of you creating your relationship at every stage, and both of you having a role. I'm not saying it's 50/50, but both of you having a meaningful role in reverting back into stalemate. The other thing is you never know how much your *partner* can change. Nobody ever knows. What I always try to do is get back to the question: "What could *you* change?" Because the only one you can change is yourself. And so, the extent to which you understand your own contributions to the stalemate, the stagnation, can give you hope because it's something you can work on. [This was a very direct challenge, one that Pam accepted, to my relief.]

PAM: I'm sure that I, too, just revert back to the behavior that then creates inaction in him—and then we fall right back into it. That's a good point. I need to keep an open mind that he might make some changes. I feel like he's acknowledged that there's a lot more on the line right now.

ME (WJD): Right, so can you identify things that you need to work on that would be healthy for you and this relationship? When we talk seriously about choosing to work on the marriage in the third path, what I ask people to do is to identify aspects of themselves that show up in any relationship. These are things that they want to work on that would make them healthier and, if the other person changes, would make this a healthier marriage. But if it doesn't work out in this marriage, they would have learned and grown in a way that would pay off in another relationship.

What I shared here is a key part of working with leaning-out partners—helping them focus on what needs to change in themselves that would be important in this or any other future relationship—and not just an accommodation to their current partner. I then asked where Pam was in terms of a choice about the future of their relationship. Returning the leaning-out partner to the decision process among the three paths is central to discernment counseling; otherwise, the exploration could go on indefinitely and morph into therapy.

> ME (WJD): So, what are your thoughts at the moment? No need for any decision right now, but just asking where are you?
>
> PAM: It's incredibly freeing, I think, to begin to think of it this way. The way you spun the idea that my focus on the need to change was based on my skepticism of Mike changing, which, of course, is silly. It's an idea from my childhood that I could control other persons' feelings. So, slowly letting that go brings ease.
>
> ME (WJD): Yeah. And the implications for your discernment about the different paths we've discussed, what would you say about that? [I was bringing her back to the goals of discernment counseling. Otherwise, she was relating to me as if I were her individual therapist. Partners who have had a lot of individual therapy can assume that these conversations are their personal therapy, with lots of empathy and support for personal change, rather than discerning about a future path.]
>
> PAM: I guess I definitely want to continue with discernment counseling, because I feel like it's almost like I've been in this wedge I've just been moving around in and then sort of like, "Okay, I feel more freedom to move." It's weird, because when you think you have control over someone else, obviously, you don't. And when you shift to control of yourself, then all of a sudden you're like, "Oh, I feel so empowered." So then I feel more optimistic about a possible way forward. I know I've made changes in the past, so can I apply that same thing now? Maybe my pessimism wasn't about Mike's ability to change, but my own ability to change Mike.
>
> ME (WJD): Beautiful. Intellectually most people get that "I can only control myself," but experientially, it's harder. So, why don't we schedule another session? You can be pondering how what we talked about here plays into your decision about these paths and we can meet again and see where you are. So what would you like to say to Mike in terms of your takeaway from our conversation?

We ask both partners at each session whether they want to schedule another one. This keeps the sense of agency in each of the partners. Even when someone has said they've decided to divorce, we encourage another session to talk about how they both feel about it and how they want to pursue the divorce process. If both people are on board with couple therapy, then we schedule one more session to discuss what that will involve. Rarely would we not be in favor of another session (up to five) unless the process is clearly not working (e.g., the leaning-out partner isn't willing or able to look at their contributions or the leaning-in partner is making life hell for the other partner and not able to use our input).

PAM: Just the relief of knowing he's going to be working on being the best version of him, and I'm going to be who I'm going to be . . . and not feel responsible for his feelings. That's kinda freeing.

ME (WJD): Yeah, and you might want to add, if it's true, that this realization makes you a little more hopeful. [After Mike returned to the room, Pam shared her new understanding.]

PAM: (*to Mike*) I realize that a lot of what I've been doing is being sort of a helicopter wife—not letting you be completely free to experience what you experience, to travel your own journey at your own pace without me trying to manage you. Just you doing you. It's not that I don't care. But when I say cutting emotional ties, I mean the less helpful emotional ties—the ones where I think I know what you're thinking and can control what you're feeling. Instead, I can let you stand in your own experiences, and I stand in my own experiences, and we can grow individually, and together and that makes me much more hopeful for our future together.

As is customary in discernment counseling, I had helped Pam craft her sharing statement and practice it with me before bringing Mike back into the room. I felt energized and hopeful by her powerful statement.

Sessions 3 and 4

We continued with themes illuminated in the earlier sessions, with Mike struggling not to be up or down based on how much affection Pam showed him, and with Pam feeling like a yo-yo from his moods. It was clear that it would take serious couple therapy to resolve these patterns, and it was important for me as the discernment counselor not to try to "fix them" during this process. We remind couples that discernment counseling is about identifying issues to work on in therapy, not about making progress on them now. (We sometimes tell couples explicitly not to look for change during discernment counseling.) Mike was fully on board for pursuing a new couple therapy, but Pam said she was "in the middle," neither leaning in nor leaning out. A key moment in the counseling occurred as I met with Pam individually:

ME (WJD): Say more about where you are. You say sometimes you're feeling more hopeful and sometimes less.

PAM: It's because he's listening more, understanding more, and that's improving our conversations. But then I still feel the same lack of attraction to him that I've felt, and part of me gets a little concerned. I feel like I should be shifting more to a positive feeling. It's almost like the more Mike leans in, the more I lean out. He's either really optimistic or, if things aren't going well, he gets really sad. He's still in that "yo-yo-ing" and that messes with my brain, because when he's sad, I feel the impulse to make things better. I've been fighting that and doing much better, but then I think it creates a distance between us. I tried to explain to Mike that the distance he may be feeling is my trying not to be enmeshed so much with his feelings, so I don't feel it's my job to intervene.

ME (WJD): Yeah, a couple things there. One is that you've been expecting that if your relationship improves, your sexual feelings for Mike would start to come back, and that's not happened at this point. Then the other part is the enmeshment—that you're fighting to not be his emotional caretaker. That's led you to back up, particularly when he seems sad or something like that. The backing up isn't going to lead you to feel attracted to him, because you're trying to not get too close at that point. Does it make sense that you're in that dynamic now and that would lead to you not feeling more attracted? Because for sexual attraction, you have to feel close, but there has to be enough separateness, too.

PAM: Yes, it does make sense. I still feel that somehow, I'm responsible for his highs and lows. Even though I'm trying to separate, it's really quite ingrained.

ME (WJD): Well, this is an example of an issue that discernment counseling isn't going to take care of. I think you're identifying it and seeing your own part in it. That's what we do in discernment counseling. So the question is whether it's something that you want to work on in couple therapy and feel that, potentially, if you both worked on it, you could make gains in this area. [In another key moment, I challenged Pam to get off the fence about making a decision on the future of their marriage. She seemed stuck, and I wasn't sure how long their relationship could sustain the limbo they'd been in for the past year.]

PAM: This counseling has been a sort of clarifier—the way you made me actually do the exercise of looking at what I have control of in this situation. What are my feelings, and what can I shift? Because that's all I can do. So I'd have to say it's really these discussions that have helped me come to that shift.

ME (WJD): And so let's go then to the implications for how you go forward in terms of moving toward divorce, or working on the relationship in couple therapy, or staying with the status quo. You don't have to make a decision just because we're in discernment counseling—you can end with no choice. But the ideal is that you'd get out of limbo. because right now, you two are just sort of in neutral, without a direction. So how do you take what we've just been talking about and apply it to the decision about whether to try the therapy or not?

After she expressed more skepticism about Mike changing, I decided to challenge her directly.

ME (WJD): Yeah, well I'm glad you're being honest about your skepticism. So let me ask you a bit of a challenging question. What does your being skeptical about Mike changing do for you?

PAM: It makes me feel very unsettled, and maybe it kind of lets me off the hook, because if I'm thinking he's never going to change, then I don't really have to go through this work.

ME (WJD): So what I can say is my sense that Mike is serious about wanting to make some changes in himself. Now whether he can, whether you can, that's all to be determined, but I'm not getting any kind of resistance from him. And certainly not from you about the desire to change. [What I said about Mike reflects an important part of discernment counseling in which we have access to both partners (as opposed to someone "discerning" in individual therapy). I was able to leverage my clear sense that Mike was serious about trying to make changes. With this being the fourth of a maximum of five sessions, I felt it was time to call the question with Pam. We had a good alliance, and I felt she could go on indefinitely with her self-exploration. But the marriage was on the brink, and I didn't think that Mike could hold out indefinitely without a direction (divorce or try to repair). Discernment counseling often has "crucible" moments like this.]

PAM: Yeah—it's kind of that idea that it would be interesting to do therapy with Mike, because I wouldn't have thought any change was possible. But now I can feel myself kind of shifting, I think that this could be interesting to see what's possible. So I'd say I'm willing to begin couple therapy with Mike.

ME (WJD): Okay—that's a declarative statement. You're off the fence. So when Mike comes back in, I encourage you to say that to him and to say why.

PAM: (*to Mike, after he returns*) So with what I have learned over the past four sessions, I've become more confident that I understand my responsibility for our issues in the marriage and have been able to make some shifts in my own behavior that I feel have been positive. So I feel empowered that I'd be able to do some positive work in couple therapy and would like to go forward with that with you. [I invited Mike to respond directly to Pam, something that we don't do in discernment counseling until a decision to pursue couple therapy has been made. My prior conversation with him in this session left me with confidence in his ability to respond well.]

MIKE: (*to Pam*) I feel wonderful about that, a real sense of relief, as well as looking forward to figuring out how to grow together instead of grow apart. I know now the next challenge for each of us is to come up with a handful of things that we can work on in ourselves. And the one thing I've been working on is to be receptive when challenged and not to respond immediately with argument or by just withdrawing and kind of melting away and expecting you to take care of my feelings. But instead of either one of those extremes, to just stay engaged and try to work productively with you.

CONCLUDING PHASE OF COUNSELING: SESSION 5

Because Pam and Mike had chosen to move forward by engaging couple therapy, this session involved preparing for the transition from discernment counseling to that couple work (in this case, a referral to a different therapist). We don't aim for a couple consensus on relational changes, because that could involve more therapeutic work than is appropriate for discernment counseling (e.g., bringing into harmony their goals for their sexual relationship). Instead, the focus is on individual agendas for change that, if they happen, would help the couple relationship become healthier.

ME (WJD): So, this is our fifth discernment counseling session, and for the check-in, I wanted to see if you're both in the same place you were last time, about wanting to proceed with couple therapy, or whether something has shifted. [Both indicated they were still opting for couple therapy.] So, what I'd like to do in this session is talk with each of you separately about your personal agendas for change and then have you actually write out three or four that you can share with each other.

We then have our separate individual discussions, and I help them each formulate a few areas of personal change that would not only be good for them and their marriage but also good changes to make even if their marriage doesn't survive. They then come back together to read and briefly explain their personal agendas for change.

> MIKE: (*to Pam*) The first change is to learn to be more receptive and engaged when challenged instead of, at one extreme, to litigate things and cross examine or, at the other extreme, shut down and retreat. I think that by staying engaged and truly trying to understand what's being conveyed to me could allow for more strengthening of our relationship rather than antagonism. The second change is to be more open and vulnerable with my honest feelings, whether that's just simply being sad, lonely, or fearful, and then just make this simple declarative statement of the feeling and then just shut up and not overtalk it. And then the last change is more specific. I need to take a step back and allow for input when I'm focused on some objective rather than pushing you or other people away from me and continuing with tunnel vision—oftentimes a tunnel vision with some anger—because that simply degrades the relationship with whoever I'm with.
>
> PAM: The first change for me is to speak my truths about my thoughts and feelings without feeling bad or ashamed, so that other people know how I really feel. The second one is to balance negative thoughts with positive ones instead of always focusing on fixing a problem. And so by not always focusing on the negative, then whoever I'm with doesn't fall into the trap of me always fixing problems and then the other person trying to make me see the positive side. Because then I wallow in the problems and begin to resent that the other person doesn't seem to see those problems. And the third change is to allow others to express their feelings without feeling as though I need to fix or change them—to just let them express their feelings and not feel like it's my responsibility to do anything about that.

The personal agendas for change emerge gradually in every session of discernment counseling through the process of helping each partner look at their contributions to the problems. For the final articulation of the personal agendas, we stress that these are issues that would come up in any future relationship if this one ends, as opposed to accommodations to this relationship. The process involves giving each partner a few minutes to write down some notes for three or four areas of change, then going over them and making suggestions for clarifying them.

This session ends with reading through a list of principles for the couple therapy ahead, such as committing to 6 months of therapy and to keeping divorce off the table for this period of time. I explain that 6 months of therapy is enough time to see if therapy can help to get them to where they want to be as a couple, although they may need more time to fully restore their marriage. I then told them that I had checked with a colleague, who could see them in couple therapy. A follow-up with the colleague several months later indicated that they were making good progress.

Most of the time, the discernment counselor transitions to become the couple therapist and uses whatever therapy model they practice. When discernment counselors make referrals for couple therapy, they generally tailor the referral to whomever they believe would be well suited for the couple. This can be challenging when there are logistical issues such as insurance reimbursement and geographical location, but the principle is to refer to an experienced couple therapist, because these are often difficult therapy cases.

I was gratified by my work with Pam and Mike. They "showed up" with intensity in each session. They let me do two things I love about this work: support them emotionally in what it feels like to be leaning in or leaning out, and challenge them to see their problems in systemic terms that involved both of their contributions. They also let me move faster with them than what they may have been expecting from prior therapy. I felt grateful for their trust and hopeful for their future.

FURTHER REFLECTIONS AND IMPLICATIONS

Pam and Mike reached a joint decision to pursue couple therapy, which is the outcome in about half our discernment counseling cases. When divorce is the outcome, the final session aims to help the still leaning-in partner to deal with their disappointment and distress, and to help both partners articulate the values they want to bring to their next steps in ending the marriage. We also refer them to mediators and collaborative divorce lawyers. The third alternative of maintaining the status quo—neither divorcing nor working in couple therapy to improve the marriage—usually happens when the leaning-out partner is unable to decide on divorce or couple therapy. In those cases, we help the couple decide how they want to be together for the near future until things become clearer.

Discernment counseling has been done with a wide range of couples in terms of sexual orientation, gender identity, race, and ethnicity. The common factor across these facets of identity or social location is that the couple once made a lifetime commitment to one another and that this commitment is now on the line with one partner, while the other partner wants to continue the relationship and do therapy. The process of discernment counseling is similar across these variations. However, certain demographics, such as the length of marriage and the presence of children, create different tones in the process; for example, a young, childless couple might have less worry about divorce. Contextual factors, such as strong religious convictions, may make considering divorce more painful. The presence of a serious psychological or addiction problem in one of the partners has to be addressed without holding that person entirely responsible for the marriage being on the brink; future treatment for those problems is generally included in the personal agendas for change if the couple chooses to do couple therapy.

Finally, discernment counseling is intense, high-stakes work. The therapist has to be quick in assessing couple patterns and be both supportive and challenging to the individual partners—without making couple therapy interventions. Sessions are quite focused, and the therapist can't let either partner spend the time complaining about the other person. We find it to be an altogether gratifying and fascinating process to work with couples in the crucible of determining their future.

REFERENCES

Allen, S., Hawkins, A. J., Harris, S. M., Roberts, K. R., Hubbard, A., & Doman, M. (2021). Day- to-day changes and longer-term adjustments to divorce ideation: Marital commitment uncertainty processes over time. *Family Relations, 71*, 611–629.

Doherty, W. J., & Harris, S. M. (2017). *Helping couples on the brink of divorce: Discernment counseling for troubled relationships*. Washington, DC: American Psychological Association.

Doherty, W. J., Harris, S. M., & Wickel Didericksen, K. (2016). A typology of attitudes toward proceeding with divorce among parents in the divorce process. *Journal of Divorce and Remarriage, 57*, 1–11.

Doherty, W. J., Harris, S. M., & Wilde, J. L. (2016). Discernment counseling for "mixed agenda" couples. *Journal of Marital and Family Therapy, 42*, 246–255.

Galovan, A. M., Hawkins, A. J., Harris, S. M., & Simpson, D. (2021). What are they doing?: A national survey of relationship-repair behavior of those thinking about divorce. *Journal of Marital and Family Therapy, 48*, 371–390.

Hawkins, A. J., Galovan, A. M., Harris, S. M., Allen, S. E., Allen, S. M., Roberts, K. M., & Schramm, D. G. (2017). What are they thinking?: A national study of stability and change in divorce ideation. *Family Process, 56*, 852–868.

CHAPTER 9

Therapy with Black Couples
The Intersection of Race and Class

ANTHONY L. CHAMBERS

> ### *Editors' Comments*
>
> In this narrative of therapy with a Black couple, Anthony Chambers poignantly reminds us that when working with couples of racial minorities, "sometimes race is in the figure and sometimes it's in the background, but race is never absent." Chambers's description of his work with Beth and Marcus wonderfully illustrates this point. On the one hand, some of the challenges confronting this couple could readily be observed with any couple—navigating transition from courtship into marriage, stresses of buying a home, strains from a high-powered executive work position, difficulties around pregnancy, enduring sensitivities from families of origin, and emotion dysregulation linked to difficulties in managing differences. The narrative exemplifies how Black couples in therapy are now often well educated and middle or upper class. However, each of these struggles assumes a unique character in the context of being a Black couple in a White-dominated world infused with the special history of Blacks in America, issues of gender disparities, limited role models for a healthy romantic relationship, conflicts around leadership and power, and historical challenges around trust and vulnerability.
>
> Note how Chambers draws on the principles of integrative systemic therapy to guide much of his work with this couple—for example, his emphasis on the sociopolitical systemic context, constraints that prevent this couple from resolving their problems, and the multiple recursive influences between the two partners and with the outside world. Note also how he harnesses his own identity as an African American to foster the partners' expanded perspectives of their relationship struggles and of each other—moving from polarized positions of blaming each other to more compassionate understanding of one another's histories that fuel their differences. This chapter reminds each of us—regardless of our own race or other facet of social location—of the imperative to incorporate sociocultural considerations in our work with every couple.

> Chambers also provides useful guidance for addressing two issues separate from race—specifically, struggles around infertility and the emotional substrate to conflicts around finances. He also offers an important lesson illuminating the value of helping partners gain the tools needed for a healthy relationship—even when the impact of those tools may not be realized until some point further along in their respective journeys.

I am an African American, board-certified couple and family psychologist. I've been married for over 20 years, with a beautiful daughter who attends a century-old private school. I grew up in an upper-middle-class Black family in the suburbs of a major Midwestern city. My parents sent my brother and me to an affluent private school from nursery school all the way through high school, where we were two of the few African Americans in our school. My parents have been married for over 50 years. When I was in high school, my parents were on *The Oprah Winfrey Show* as one of the 25 best couples in America. My father was a successful physician and my mother, who was a stay-at-home mom, has her doctorate in education. My younger brother, who is also married with two kids, is a corporate lawyer and banker.

I share this personal information because being reared in a family that placed a premium on family and education has clearly shaped my thinking and interests. I originally entered the field of psychology with an interest in couples and families, because during college, when I attended Hampton University (a Historically Black College and University), I was saddened by the statistics that consistently document the problems that disproportionately affect Black Americans. I was equally frustrated and perplexed that the statistics didn't seem to capture my experience. I began to hypothesize that the two protective factors that benefited my brother and me were being raised in a healthy family and valuing education. It is that family context that shapes my personal and professional passions centered on strengthening couple relationships, especially among Black couples.

I believe we're entering a golden age of behavioral health, when the stigma of receiving mental health services has never been lower and the need has never been greater. Couple therapy continues to be one of the most sought-after modalities of therapy (Lebow, Chambers, Christensen, & Johnson, 2012), and that includes more middle- and upper-middle-class Black couples being major consumers of couple therapy services (Chambers, 2019). As community leaders and power brokers, the stability and strength of their relationships will have a significant impact on the Black community and American society in general. Hence, it behooves couple and family therapists to integrate the issues and challenges facing this group into our understanding of couples and couple therapy in the United States. In this chapter, I describe a clinical example of an upper-middle-class Black couple as illustrative of the complexities and nuances facing this important population. I use the term "middle class" to refer to Black couples who have at least a college degree and who own or are on the path to owning their own home (whether condominium, single-family home, or similar). Although this chapter is focused on middle-class Black couples, it's worth noting that the needs for services are also high for less fortunate Black couples. Moreover, Black couple therapists are significantly underrepresented among couple therapists.

Conceptualizing couples' problems and intervening are challenging enough but become even more difficult when trying to conceptualize possible racial, ethnic, and cultural factors. Moreover, given the increasing heterogeneity within the Black population, it's important to have a guiding principle to conceptualize that heterogeneity. A central task of any committed, romantic relationship is the management of differences. Given the transitional status of Black couples in the rapidly changing U.S. society of today, it can be helpful to consider the management of differences as a major task facing Black couples.

The notion of managing differences and constraint theory come together for me in drawing upon integrative systemic therapy (IST; Breunlin, Russell, Chambers, & Solomon, 2023; Pinsof et al., 2018). Couple therapy is a complex endeavor, and adding in the constructs of race and socioeconomic status further complicates the therapy. I have found that integrative approaches provide a framework for distilling that complexity, while still delineating sophisticated explanations for the human experience (Lebow, 2014). IST focuses on problem and solution sequences and both individual and broader systemic constraints that hinder more adaptive interactions. IST attends closely to the multiple recursive influences between the two partners and with the outside world.

The notions of managing differences and IST are foundational to my conceptualization and treatment of couples. Beth and Marcus, the couple described in the following pages, epitomize the struggles and nuances of working with this population in ways that continue to motivate and excite me to do this work.

INITIAL ASSESSMENT AND CASE FORMULATION

The initial therapy request contains a fairly terse, yet compelling, presenting problem:

> "We're a Black couple and we both just turned 40 and would like premarital therapy focused on helping us navigate finances and fertility issues."

I'm immediately excited to see this couple, as I really enjoy working with couples around issues of money, and I've received training working with couples going through *in vitro* fertilization (IVF). Thus, I feel uniquely qualified to help this couple with their difficulties.

During internship, I had the privilege of working with Dr. Anne Fishel, who was the Director of the Couple Therapy Program at Massachusetts General Hospital and Harvard Medical School. It was during my time with her that I learned about a four-session evaluation approach for assessing couples. The approach includes an initial conjoint session in order to understand the couple's relationship problems, followed by individual sessions, and then a feedback session, during which the therapist provides the couple with an initial formulation and a treatment plan (Chambers, 2012).

Whenever you meet with one member of a couple in an individual session, it carries the risk of having secret information disclosed about their partner. I take the position that the risks of keeping secrets outweigh the benefits, particularly in terms of the alliance. When being the keeper of a secret, such as infidelity, it potentially places the therapist in an ethically compromising position of attempting to be an equal advocate for both partners while maintaining a secret. This can be particularly problematic for Black couples, who may already have a hard time trusting in general (Chambers & Kravitz, 2011), and especially struggle trusting a mental health professional. When working with

Black couples, I find that having a no-secrets policy quickens and deepens my alliance with both partners, as it helps them to feel more secure and less guarded.

I begin our first session by saying, "Before we jump into the details of what brings you here today, let me get to know the two of you. Tell me a bit about yourselves, your age, occupation, education, kids, hobbies, all that kind of good stuff." Marcus states that he's 40 years old, has a college degree, and works for himself doing information technology (IT) consulting. He loves the work, and he loves the flexibility and autonomy of working for himself. Beth, also 40 years old, is a high-powered C-Suite Executive with her bachelor's and master's degrees in business administration. She works 80 plus hours per week and does not like her job but enjoys the income it provides. They've been together for 5 years, engaged for 1 year, with no kids, but they have been going through IVF since they started dating 5 years ago, because she has a strong family history of infertility. They also report purchasing a house the previous week.

I had mixed feelings about the IVF and their not being married. On the one hand, she's 40 years old, with a family history of medical challenges, so she must be intentional if she wants to have a child. On the other hand, going through IVF is a big commitment, and having a child is an even bigger commitment. What impact has IVF had on their relationship? What are their levels of commitment to the relationship and getting married? And what are their levels of commitment to having children? I considered how they're dealing with a pileup of stressors and transitions between buying a home, going through IVF, her dissatisfaction with her job, and planning a wedding. I wondered why they felt the urgency to do all of this at once, and had they thought through everything? I also wondered about the financial impact of IVF and the purchase of the home given that finances were part of their presenting problem. I also wondered about their decision-making framework. Have they thought about the sequencing of these major decisions? Are they on the same page? I know that these are all questions I want to learn more about.

One of my favorite questions to ask couples is the "HDYFAB" question—or "How do you feel about being here?" I use this question to gauge their level of motivation or resistance to couple therapy. Beth states, "We tried couple therapy before, but it wasn't a good experience." Marcus states that he's "open to couple therapy" but doesn't want therapy to be a "crutch." I'm pleased that they're willing to try couple therapy again after such a disappointing experience. I can tell that Marcus is much more hesitant about therapy, so I'll need to focus on developing a strong alliance with him.

"Tell me about the sequence of events that led the two of you to decide to start couple therapy." Marcus replies, "She's given me a bit of an ultimatum. She said that our getting married is contingent on me paying off my debt, and she resents the fact that I have debt and she doesn't feel like she should have to deal with or be impacted by my debt. So, she doesn't want to get married until the debt is resolved. And to me, Doc, she has the money, as she makes more than me, and we're engaged, so why can't she help me out? I believe that marriage is a package deal and successes and problems are shared, which is a key benefit to being married."

Beth jumps in. "Money to me is loaded given what happened to me as a kid. My dad racked up six figures of credit card debt, which resulted in us becoming homeless multiple times when I was a child. His reckless spending put our family in harm's way. I also resent that Marcus has had years to take care of his debt; he could've gotten a second job or work more hours or find another job to pay off the debt. But now that he's with me, he wants me to just pay off his debt? That isn't right and is unfair! I work 12 hours a day to earn my money, and he works a fraction of that and wants me to pick up the slack. No!"

The temperature in the room is rising, as she's starting to get both angry and teary-eyed. Marcus then jumps in. "If you wanted someone with more money, then you need to find that person or accept who I am. I feel as though you accept all of my good but only some of my bad, but I, on the other hand, accept all of your good and all of your bad. Doc, she makes twelve times as much money as I do! I even brought up the idea of having each of us contribute 20% of our income toward my debt. Obviously, her 20% is a lot more and she resents it, so she doesn't want to contribute at all, which makes me feel as though we have completely different ideas about marriage."

I'm concerned about how polarized they are around this issue. Moreover, money to her isn't just about money and security, but it's wrapped up in feelings she has about her father. Her emotional reaction is visceral—almost like she's saying, "I was helpless as a child, but now I'm an adult, and I will not let another person take advantage of me." That perspective, though understandable, is entrenched, and I'm skeptical about moving her from that position. This seems to be about more than just the dollars, but rather that his paying off the debt represents his proving his love to her and demonstrating that he's a responsible person by embodying a "do whatever it takes" mentality. I also wonder if he finds her statements emasculating. This is a common dynamic that I've written about among Black couples, with the woman being the primary breadwinner and feeling resentment about being in that role, while the male partner is feeling emasculated (Chambers, 2019; Chambers & Kravitz, 2011). I also wonder whether he has the capacity to understand why this is so important to her and whether they each can have empathy for the other's perspective.

As the session is coming to an end, Beth says, "Before we stop, I think it's also important for you to know that having kids is a lifelong dream for me. We've been through *several* rounds of IVF with no success. I'm also paying for IVF, so I am contributing." Marcus rolls his eyes. I end the session by expressing my appreciation to each of them for not only sharing their perspectives and their willingness to share their vulnerabilities but also for letting me into their relationship.

In addition to the complexities of race and socioeconomic status described earlier, this first session also highlights the multifaceted, complex issues facing this couple—which bolster why I find taking an integrative approach to be helpful. This couple reports dealing with issues of fertility, finances, family of origin, race, and gender layered with process issues of poor communication and conflict resolution skills. Having a client-centered, problem-driven data collection process nested within an integrative framework helps me to conceptualize that complexity (Chambers, 2012).

Beth's Individual Session

I start off all individual sessions with a reminder about confidentiality by saying, "Whatever we talk about today, I'd like to have the freedom to be able to share when we come back together as a group." Beth replies, "No problem." She then starts off by saying, "The biggest issue we have is about money! I found out that his debt is tied to his brother, who mismanaged his finances and racked up $100,000 in credit card debt! Marcus told me this would be cleared up in a couple of years, and 3 years later, it's still not cleared up! Marcus says that I'm not willing to help, but that's simply not true. I've given him thousands of dollars to help with the debt! I don't believe he appreciates what I've done to help him. I don't want to be the solution to his problems. I'm repulsed by the idea that he thinks it's okay to depend on a woman to bail him out! I don't trust that he can manage his money and there is no transparency as to where his money goes. This is the second guy I've dated who is in a financial mess."

I then ask her to tell me about the fertility issues. She says, "We've now had several failed rounds of IVF. If we're unable to have a child, I'm not sure this relationship will survive given our financial issues." I ask what her commitment is to this relationship, and she responds, "When things are going well, I'm an 8 of 10. I know that part of my frustration isn't about him but with life and IFV. I do love him. We laugh a lot together, he supports me, and he helps out. In previous relationships, I've had to downplay my successes in order to protect the man's ego, but I don't have to do that with him, and that means a lot. But when I start thinking about the finances, I'm a 2 of 10!"

"All of that makes sense," I reply. "What's your goal for the couple therapy?"

She responds, "I want to flesh out this whole financial situation. I want to be able to have a voice in couple therapy, and don't want to overly compromise my values. I also want to figure out if this relationship is worth staying in."

I leave this session slightly more concerned than hopeful. Although I'm glad to hear that she's committed and does love him, she has strong feelings about money and dependency that have created feelings of resentment. In my experience, once resentment enters the picture, it's difficult to change. Moreover, her financial concerns aren't simply about needing to have the right framework but rather is a loaded issue with deep historical roots. Her concerns about Marcus helping out his brother aren't surprising in that many middle-class Black couples have the additional burden of providing financial assistance to a family member who is financially struggling (Patillo, 2005).

Marcus's Individual Session

After my standard reminder about limits to confidentiality, Marcus jumps right in. "I'm at a make it or break it point right now, because I feel we have fundamentally different views of what it means to be a family. I'm willing to accept all of her, but she's only open to accepting the good but not the bad, which is counter to how I see family. She looks after her own best interests and not each other's best interests. I feel as though she's ruled by the 'fair–unfair' ethos. She wants to pretend that there is no money, but I can't pretend."

The concerns I had after my session with Beth are only amplified after hearing his perspective. It's clear that they're polarized around this issue, and I'm not sure if they'll be able to recover. I wonder whether he fully understands her history with her father and how much that impacts her perspective. I think that *maybe*, if he could realize that her concerns stem in part from her family history, perhaps that historical context would provide him with more empathy.

I ask him to share his thoughts about their fertility challenges. "I wouldn't have put this much effort into having a kid. I feel that it shouldn't be this hard to have a kid, and it shouldn't be this hard to get along. I think we need to be in a more solid relationship prior to having a kid," he states. I then say, "That's an interesting statement about needing to be in a more solid relationship before having kids. Can you share with me your commitment to this relationship on a scale of 1–10?" He replies, "A 9. When I make a decision, I'm intentional. I also realize that Beth has many wonderful qualities that are hard to find in a partner." I then ask, "What's your confidence on a scale of 1–10 that this relationship will work?" "A 5," he replies. "I think she's a bit selfish, and I don't know if she'll be the 'ride or die' partner I need."

I then ask, "How has your family of origin affected your current relationship?" He shares: "My parents were divorced. I didn't grow up with a lot of money, as my parents both lost their jobs at different points; however, when they were married, they were a team. If one of them lost their job, the other stepped up, and that's what I want with Beth!"

I end with the question "What are your goals for couple therapy?" He states, "I feel undervalued in this relationship, and I want to know if this relationship can work out. I'm willing to work on this relationship, but I can't do this by myself. I also want to know how to better communicate with her around big issues." I thank him for his candor. He then thanks me for meeting and says, "I don't often get a chance to share what I'm thinking and feeling, so I really appreciate this opportunity." That strikes me in a very positive way given that he wasn't overly excited by the prospects of couple therapy.

In preparing for the feedback session, there are many paths I might take. I tend to focus on the areas that have the biggest constraints on the couple's relationship, while also addressing "low hanging fruit" in order to boost the alliance. I also take a strategic approach by identifying which areas I think we need to address first in order to pave the way to address other constraints. With these ideas in mind, I focus the feedback to Beth and Marcus on three primary areas. I want to start by discussing finances through a developmental lens. I want to communicate how the significant financial decisions they've made don't match their stated level of commitment. Next, I want to share the importance of developing a shared vision for the future of their relationship as a way to provide increased clarity and safety for making future relationship decisions. Finally, I want to focus on the fact that neither of them has a good model for how to have a healthy relationship. Because of the prevalence of divorce, lack of marriage, and out-of-wedlock childbirths, many Black people don't grow up in a well-functioning, two-parent household. Thus, I find it helpful to provide Black couples with some basic relationship education identifying the key ingredients and framework necessary for having a healthy relationship.

Feedback Session

I start off by placing their concerns in a developmental context of them oscillating between being a premarital, engaged couple and being an established "married-like" couple working to conceive a child. That developmental frame resonates with them. I continue to use the developmental frame as a way to understand their difficulties. I discuss with them the unintended consequence of commingling their finances while not being married; that is, the degree to which they've merged their finances does not match the level of commitment to their relationship, which has led to some misunderstandings and hard feelings. For instance, Marcus assumed they were working toward a future together forever, so he didn't see a problem with asking for assistance; however, Beth willingly helped, with the understanding that he would pay her back as soon as possible. I empathize with each of them. I also link their feelings to each of their family-of-origin experiences surrounding money. They both agree with my assessment, though Marcus jumps in and states, "I didn't know that Beth was thinking of me as being like her father, because I'm not, but I can understand now why she feels the way she feels." I feel hopeful that his epiphany could be the foundation for decreasing their polarization.

I then discuss the importance of gaining clarity as to where this relationship is headed. I reflect back to them how they are engaged to be married but haven't set a wedding date because she has concerns about his management of finances, yet the two of them are actively going through IVF, which would bond them together. This poses particular challenges, since they both report they don't want to have a child out of wedlock, yet because of Beth's age and family history, they don't have the luxury of figuring this out before trying to conceive a child. I mention to them that they'll have to "build the bike as they're riding it," and the potential risks associated with this approach, while empathizing with them how difficult this is. They both resonate with this feedback, and Beth begins to get tearful. I lean in to ask what her tears are about, and she says, "I love him, and I want this to work and I want a baby, but I'm just struggling with the finances. I vowed to never be with a person who doesn't view money the same way that I do, but I can't imagine a life without him." Marcus leans in and holds her, creating a tender moment.

I conclude by stating that I want to provide them with a framework for how to think about finances and marriage, and to go over core principles for how to have a healthy marriage. I mention that neither of them has a healthy model of marriage, and that this can be one of the greatest gifts they could give a potential child. I normalize how many Black couples don't have a healthy model because of our disproportionately low marriage rate, high divorce rate, and high rate of out-of-wedlock childbirths. I state, "I want to give you this knowledge not only to help your relationship and future family, but to be a beacon of hope for other Black couples." They light up with that frame and say they want to be that exemplar couple. Finally, I state, "I want to help the two of you to improve your communication, and especially improve your ability and confidence to be able to have hard conversations in order to decrease your avoidance of conflict, which, paradoxically, only leads to bigger fights later." That also really resonates with them. I leave the feedback session feeling moderately optimistic that we could make some positive changes, while at the same time realizing the magnitude of some of the constraints this relationship faces.

BEGINNING PHASE OF THERAPY

Given that many Black couples don't have good models for how to have a healthy relationship, it's not uncommon for me to start therapy in a didactic mode, providing couples with a relationship framework (Chambers, 2008). I share this rationale explicitly, as I find that couples tend to be hungry for this information, because they often want their relationships to work but unfortunately don't have a model for how to go about achieving relationship success. Moreover, many Black individuals are skeptical of therapy because they feel it's just venting of problems but never solving them. By providing information and tools, the couple can instantly feel that the therapy can be helpful.

"I need your help," Marcus says to Beth early in the next session. "I want to feel like we're an 'us' and not living separate lives. I want to feel closer to you." Beth responds with appreciation of his willingness to be vulnerable and forthcoming. I also immediately affirm his vulnerability. They both turn to me and express not knowing how to become an "us." This provides me with the opening I was seeking.

"If it's okay with the two of you, I'd like to help you learn how to become an 'us.' There are actually specific relationship mind-sets and skills that can help you become closer."

They both lean in, intently curious and intrigued by the idea of learning. "The inevitable consequence of being raised by a single parent, or by parents with unhealthy relationship dynamics, is that the child has an increased propensity for self-reliance or to embrace an independent mind-set. That independent mind-set does have some benefits, like in educational attainment. However, it may not be as helpful in another context, like a relationship." Their eyes are locked in as I'm speaking. "When we sign up to be in an intimate relationship, we're signing up to play a team sport, not an individual sport, and the rules for success are different. Individual sports embrace an independent mind-set, whereas team sports embrace an interdependent mind-set. By 'interdependent,' I mean no matter what I do, it has an impact on you, and no matter what you do, there's some impact on me, and there's no getting around that. Thus, when we focus on team success, the good news is that we also benefit as individuals, because we're a part of that team. So the key to happiness in a relationship is fundamentally about embracing this interdependent mind-set. Let me stop and check in with how this is resonating with you."

I first check in with Beth, because I'm concerned that she would be the one more resistant to this idea. Beth says, "That makes a ton of sense! However, it also scares me, because I've achieved my success in life by being independent. In fact, I take pride in the fact that I don't have to rely on anyone, but I also see the limits of the independent mind-set in a relationship. Like Marcus said earlier, I'm going to need some help and patience as I work to evolve my mind-set." I lean in and say, "Beth, that's all any of us can ask for! I so appreciate your willingness to be vulnerable in this moment, and your willingness to engage in this process." Marcus immediately jumps in: "This is all that I wanted! I want a teammate to go through life together." This is a tender moment, and I share my hope that this would serve as a positive inflection moment in their relationship.

This couple also expresses a strong allegiance to fairness. Fairness is a concept that has particular salience in the Black community because of the numerous examples of unfairness and injustice, whose etiology dates back to slavery and has continued to present day. Fairness is also a concept that begets rigidity. Again, the central task of any relationship is the management of differences, and successfully managing differences requires flexibility. Fairness is also a concept that is inextricably linked to trust; that is, once there's been an instance of unfairness, there's a risk that a trust issue may ensue. With a similar etiology to fairness, trust has followed a similar trajectory in that many Black individuals struggle with trust (Chambers & Kravitz, 2011). Most importantly, once trust has been broken, it can be hard to forgive.

It became clear to me during the assessment that both Beth and Marcus struggle with fairness and trust, and it seems as though they haven't been able to forgive. In the next session, we focus on distilling those concepts, as well as the historical significance of those concepts to the Black experience. Specifically, I discuss the unique history of mistrust and unfairness between Blacks and numerous institutions in our society, and I use that to contextualize and normalize some of the challenges we have with fairness, and especially forgiveness, in our relationships. The interaction between the macro challenges with unfairness combined with one's personal history of betrayal can be a powerful constraint for forgiveness among Black couples. When I provide a framework for forgiveness, Beth becomes tearful: "I've never forgiven anyone! It's too painful to risk getting hurt again. I've never even forgiven my father." Marcus goes over to console her, then becomes tearful and shares, "I don't think I've ever forgiven my father for not being there for me the way I needed him to be." I offer softly, "Both of you are in the same boat of holding onto past hurts and resentments. I wonder if the two of you can use this relationship as an opportunity for healing by taking care of each other's wounds and providing each other with a context where it's safe to forgive and to be vulnerable?" They not only agree to this but express excitement by the prospects of this new way of relating.

In the next session, they announce excitedly, "Doc, the wedding is back on!"

"Oh my gosh!" I reply. "That's terrific news—can you tell me about how you came to that decision?"

Marcus says, "We spoke and the last couple of sessions really resonated with us and helped us to realize how much we love each other and can't see a life without each other!"

Although I'm always a bit skeptical when change happens so quickly, it was a nice reminder of the importance of having the right framework and the benefit of contextualizing their relational pain in the historical context of Black pain and triumph. Because the couple was doing better, we agreed to meet monthly. They continued to do well. The relationship paradigm shift seemed to stick. I also taught them communication skills centered on how to have difficult conversations given their propensity to avoid talking about hard issues. Everything seemed to be going well, until it wasn't!

INTERMEDIATE PHASE OF THERAPY

"We just found out that Marcus is being sued because of one of his brother's unpaid bills! This is why I can't trust him with finances or his ability to take care of business," Beth says, exasperated. "I told him that it's his debt, and I need him to take care of it!"

Marcus jumps in, "You see me in this situation, and you have the means to help me out and you don't. That's just selfish and wrong!"

Beth continues, "Plus you had the nerve to bring a contractor over to the house. Why would you do that when you don't have any money and I'm not working, and your brother still has this debt, and you're being sued? That makes no sense!" She says, "I often pray to make my ego smaller because I want to be with him, and I don't want to break up."

They're so angry and triggered that, despite my multiple attempts to interrupt, they can't stop themselves from continuing to argue. I sense that part of their inertia is because they don't often talk about hard topics, so once the issue is brought up, they end up "vomiting" all of their feelings, frustrations, and perspectives. I'm aware of feeling ineffective to be able to turn this session into a productive one. To be honest, this is the dynamic I expected after the initial assessment, because the issues of finances and each of their family-of-origin experiences result in their being polarized. Money can be challenging for all couples, but trust and money can be especially layered in Black families. It's not uncommon, for example, to hear intergenerational narratives of "make sure you have your own money that you keep separate from your spouse." It's well-intentioned advice that can have unintended, paradoxical consequences of further complicating the relationship. I eventually end the session by suggesting we meet next week given how triggered they each are. I also encourage them to recall the progress they've made over the previous months in an attempt to help them feel more hopeful and less polarized.

Although they come into the next session with a noticeably lighter affect, it's clear they are still struggling. With a look of hesitancy, Beth states, "I need to know that Marcus is working as hard as he can. I feel like I'm suffering, yet I'll be forced to work a job that's stressful because I can't depend on him to earn more money. It's bigger than just money. I need him to help out around the house and exercise, as well as to show some hustle with making more money and paying off debt."

I reply, "That must make it hard for you to be in this relationship because you love him, but you need to know you have a partner, and right now it doesn't feel like you have that partner." She emphatically agrees with my reflection. I go on to ask, "Does this also make you anxious and worried about whether or not you can trust him and depend on him?" She again agrees. I ask Marcus how he feels about Beth's comments.

He replies, "We have no conversations about how much money to contribute to anything. We don't talk."

I state, "That must be frustrating to also feel like you don't have a partner. That you wish you had a partner where you could work together and talk about these issues and problem-solve together." He emphatically agrees. I then turn to them both and state, "It's interesting that both of you are in the same boat of not feeling like you have the partner that you desperately want and need." That frame engendered some warmth in the room as they seemed to become less polarized.

I have a few options regarding where to go next. I could discuss more about how they're a team as a way to amplify the depolarization. I could try helping them to restate their concerns from a place of empathy in order to help them have a more connected conversation. However, I decide to go in a different direction. Early on, we briefly talked about finances, and once they started to get better, we never revisited it. I remember how well they did in the first few sessions when I provided them with information and a relationship framework, and thought it would be good for me to provide them with a financial framework for understanding money and marriage. Moreover, that framework is consistent with the interdependent mind-set we discussed in the beginning phase of therapy.

With them in a more reflective rather than reactive state, I broached the idea of sharing a framework for thinking about money in the context of marriage and asked if they would be interested. They both look intrigued and nodded, so I continue. "First, money is a top reason couples get divorced, and that's true for both rich and poor couples. That's because it isn't about the amount of money one has, but rather the psychological variables that money represents. Money represents issues of power, anxiety, fairness, trust, and dependency. It also represents a sense of an 'us,' or a sense of separateness. Although the mismanagement of money is a huge risk factor for divorce, money can also be a huge protective factor; that is, if you set your money up correctly, it helps fortify your connection and operationalize the concept of interdependence. One definition of intimacy is the co-creation of a shared vision. When a couple's behaviors and decision making are aligned in order to actualize a shared vision, there's no greater feeling of teamwork than that. And just about all visions have a price tag associated with them, so if we can create a vision and then actualize it, then it will help you feel more connected." They're now leaning in, fully engaged.

"Now, there are two principles that are critical for money and marriage to work well. The first is this notion of *our money*; that is, it doesn't matter who makes more or who makes less, we have one pot of money that has to take care of everyone in the family. Of course, there are important nuances to factor in when operationalizing the notion of 'our money,' such as family inheritance or second marriages, but the idea is to conceptually approach finances as a team. The second principle is *transparency*. Some of the worst cases of infidelity I've ever treated were financial, not sexual. For example, one person has a secret stash of money that their partner doesn't know about until years later, or a partner has a huge amount of debt about which their partner doesn't know. If you operationalize the concepts of *our money* and *transparency*, then it's hard to go wrong. Deviating from either of these principles increases the risk of having marital problems. Let me pause there and hear each of your reactions to what I've just shared."

I'm anticipating that Beth is going to struggle with what I put out there. Beth says, "I *really* like the idea of transparency! I have no idea what he's doing with his money, and I think we need transparency. The concept of 'our money' is a lot harder for me. It makes a ton of sense and I actually agree with it in theory, but I'm not sure if I can get there given my past." I thank her for her candor. Marcus responds as I expected, which is that he wholeheartedly resonates with what I shared. This takes us to the end of our session, and I encourage them to reflect on this further and share their perspectives next session.

As Marcus enters our next session, he says, "Doc, we tried to talk after our last session and the conversation ended badly. I still struggle with how to communicate with her. We also aren't aligned on decisions we made in the past. We can't get on the same page about the facts." Beth jumps in and says, "I agree, and that's because you're living in some alternate universe." I can sense where this is going, and I want to make sure this session doesn't devolve like the one a few sessions earlier. I jump in and state, "Look, let's not relitigate the past. It's clear that what happened in the past means there's an opportunity to have better alignment moving forward. The two of you have difficulty communicating about hard topics, and when you do talk, the conversation lacks details. I believe this moment presents an opportunity to learn to discuss the details and to make a plan before making a final decision versus making a decision and then trying to retrofit the plan." That seems to resonate with them, and it slows down the frenetic energy that's building up.

"It sounds like the two of you struggled communicating after last session, so let's review some of the communication skills." I want to take more control in this session to keep them on a less reactive path. "Remember there are three keys to having a soft start-up to a difficult conversation. First, remind each other that you're on the same team, and that you're communicating with your teammate, not your opponent. Second, assume good intent, and finally, seek opportunities to call yourself out rather than try and call your partner out." They both sheepishly nod as if to indicate that they're a bit embarrassed that they aren't using those skills. I then help them to implement these communication strategies while having this difficult conversation about money.

Their differing view about debt is at the center of a lot of their disagreements. Marcus states, "My goal isn't to have zero debt. I'm focused on getting rid of bad debt, but I don't see all debt as bad."

Beth jumps in and says, "Well, I think all debt *is* bad! I want to pay off this house as soon as possible because I don't want a mortgage!"

As they're starting to escalate, I intervene and state, "Look, what we're talking about is debt tolerance. You'll find millions of individuals who view debt like you, Marcus, you'll also find millions of people who view debt like you, Beth, as well as millions of people whose views differ from both of you. When it comes to debt tolerance, there isn't a right or wrong; rather, the two of you see this differently. Remember, the central task of any close relationship is the management of differences. How much debt one has before they become anxious is a threshold issue that often stems back to what messages about debt they received growing up." This seems to resonate with them as I try again to help them become less polarized.

I then review the nuts and bolts of how to create a budget, and I emphasize that "a budget is a reflection of our values in terms of where and how we choose to spend money. Thus, the opportunity that budgeting presents is to help a couple clarify their values and to have discussions focused on co-creating a shared vision. I recommend that the two of you start creating the budget and to expect that there will be differences and to use the communication skills to help navigate those conversations. I also want the two of you to start the habit of meeting at least weekly to review the budget as a way to prevent avoidance." They both verbally agree with this approach, though Beth has a puzzled look on her face. I ask her, "Are you okay? How is this sitting with you?" She softly says, "I'm just digesting all of this, but it all makes good sense." I turn to Marcus and he says, "I'm realizing that I need to be more flexible and start making some changes in order to help this relationship get on the right track."

As we finish the session, I wonder if Beth is struggling with this, as my formulation is so different from the mental model she has about finances. And sure enough, later that evening, I receive an email from Beth stating, "Dr. Chambers, I'm really struggling, and I'd like to set up an individual appointment to see you as soon as possible." I respond, "I'm happy to see you and I have an opening tomorrow if that works for you. However, please let Marcus know that you're coming to see me and remember my policy of not being the keeper of secrets."

Beth enters the session visibly shaken. She starts off, saying, "I think I just need to vent for a bit and then hear your perspective. I'm frustrated. I keep finding men with money problems, and I never wanted to be in this situation. I also have some gender role expectations as I wanted to be with a man who is ambitious and wants to be a provider. I know that isn't the most feminist thing to say, but it's how I feel. I never wanted to be the primary breadwinner and I don't want a lifestyle that depends on my income. I need to see Marcus make some sacrifices and not be so complacent. I know I'm being judgmental, but I also have to be honest with myself. The way he's operating with money is just exacerbating my anxiety. In fact, I'm hoping that you can provide me with some tips for managing my anxiety."

As she shares her perspective, I think to myself about how familiar this pattern is among many Black couples. A disproportionate number of Black women are more educated than men and end up with higher paying jobs. Thus, many of the women end up falling into the provider role by default, but then end up resenting that role. This is consistent with decades of research demonstrating the mate availability issue among Black men compared to women. This well-documented finding of there being a dearth of marriageable Black men is well known in the Black community. Thus, this can further complicate decisions of whether a Black woman, for example, should accept her partner's financial struggles, because it may be unlikely for her to find a Black man who is able to match or exceed her role as the provider.

The paradox of gender role expectations with a feminist mentality is also one that I've encountered. I validate Beth's concerns and discuss them through a sociological lens of the Black experience. I try to do so while also expressing compassion and empathy. I let her know that this isn't uncommon. I then try to help her focus on what Marcus does bring to their relationship rather than focusing on what he doesn't. That seems to resonate with her, as I have her list and verbalize all of the positives he brings. I then discuss her anxiety and let her know that "anxiety disorders are essentially about perceiving danger when in fact there is no danger. It's like having a lot of false alarm bells going off." She immediately says, "*Yes*! That makes so much sense!" Her affect shifts and she leaves the session expressing more hope. I respond by saying, "I'm glad you find this helpful, and I'll be cheering the two of you on to have a great couple of weeks until our next session."

I reflect on the session, which feels quite positive, and I'm hoping that it will become a true inflection point. Sure enough, they come back in 2 weeks and both report that things are going very well! They took to heart my suggestions and have started to use money to build trust and to build a vision. Beth reports, "I'm cautiously optimistic as he's made some real progress, as he's exercising and making a plan for paying off the debt." Marcus adds, "The weekly budget meetings seem to be helping us stay on track, and I feel like we're a team, which is all I wanted." Beth adds, "I'm even starting to be less judgmental of him and accepting of who he is." They stay in this positive place for the next couple of sessions. I'm feeling hopeful that perhaps this time the positive change will stick. We end up taking about a 6-week break because Beth has an upcoming IVF procedure and wants to focus her energy on that.

CONCLUDING PHASE OF THERAPY

As the next session starts, Marcus appears dejected and Beth actually has a look of despair. What I feared had in fact occurred. "The egg transfer didn't work," she states, choking back tears. "My doctor and I agreed that this would be our last attempt, and now I need to try and reimagine my life. I need purpose." I processed her feelings, offered empathic reflections, expressed sympathy—all the things a therapist is supposed to do—yet I feel helpless and sad for both of them, especially for Beth. Her life revolves around the vision of being a mother. I ask Beth, "Are you interested in exploring adoption or surrogacy?" She says, "No, I'm really not interested in alternatives." I ask Marcus how he's feeling, and he states, "I'm also disappointed that this last round of IVF didn't work. We've put a lot of time, money, energy, and hope into this process, and so for this to come to an end without the outcome we were looking for is a hard pill to swallow."

Over the next few months, our sessions alternate between a return to focusing on finances and the evolving struggle of grieving and acceptance. When the focus is on finances, the therapy returns to old refrains of Beth needing a financial partner and struggling to accept Marcus's debt, while he expresses concern that Beth's desire to marry him is dependent on his being the financial partner she feels he should be. When the focus is on accepting a life without children, Beth is the center of those conversations as she expresses not knowing what marriage means without kids, struggling to figure out the purpose of life without kids, and still struggling with anger. Interestingly but not altogether surprising, as she begins to accept life without kids, she becomes increasingly intolerant of Marcus's approach to work and finances.

They come into session the following week and report that they attempted to talk after our last session, but it didn't go well. They disclose that things "got really bad," to the point that Marcus told Beth, "If you can't accept me, then maybe we should just break up!" The next day, Marcus apologized. I ask Marcus if he can understand why she's so triggered by the finances. In that moment, I want Marcus to see Beth not as someone who is being obstinate for the sake of being obstinate, but rather to really try to understand. I then have Beth share again her childhood experiences of her dad and money as a way to try and help Marcus contextualize her perspective. With tears in her eyes, she shares heartfelt moments of childhood anguish and confusion over a father who would steal money from her. She states, "How could my protector be the perpetrator? And if my dad can take advantage of me, then how am I supposed to trust any man?"

Marcus is listening intently. I ask Marcus, "What are you feeling in this moment, listening to Beth?" Marcus says, "I know I've heard this before, but for some reason I feel like I just got knocked over with a ton of bricks! I'm not sure why I never realized before just how deep-seated her issues with money and trust are, but they're huge issues! I don't want her to feel this way, and I want her to know that she can trust me. So I'm going to get another job that pays more, because I want her to know that I care more about her well-being than this job I currently have." Beth's eyes well up with tears—reflecting a look of disbelief combined with skeptical hope. Marcus says, "I don't want to prematurely give up on this relationship, because there's so much good in this relationship." This moment leads to a tender sequence, which I amplify! I leave the session moderately hopeful that perhaps this moment of tenderness could result in a meaningful moment that begets connection and hope.

Creating hope is an essential element of therapy, but in some instances it can deepen disappointment for all participants when best efforts still fall short. The next time we meet—a year and 3 months after beginning therapy—Beth announces that this would be the couple's final session, because she has decided to end their relationship. If it's possible to be both stunned and not surprised at the same time, that would best capture my reaction! The last session had left me hopeful that they were possibly on a better trajectory toward healing, whereas from the very beginning, I knew they had many strong constraints facing their relationship. She goes on to say, "I realize that I'm making compromises not consistent with my values."

Marcus jumps in. "She's my family. We built this house together. I don't know what I can do, but I love her and always will! It's tragic that this can't work. I didn't see this coming. I thought we were sticking to the plan. I would've done anything to save this relationship." His sentiments fall on deaf ears as Beth responds, "I'm pissed off that I've given so much money and time. I don't have any more to give! It's clear that he doesn't get how much I've done for him." Marcus continues to express his sadness and despair. "I feel homeless and vulnerable. She promised me when we were looking for a house that we would be together forever. Now she's kicking me out, and I would never do that to her." Both of them have tears in their eyes.

I also feel some of that anguish, as I find some of the hardest sessions to witness are when one person decides to call it quits and the other person is feeling despair and devastation, and is desperate to do anything to save the relationship. I give them space to process their feelings and to communicate what they need to share. Because this is their last session, I broach the logistics of their breakup. The session continues to ebb and flow through the familiar dialectic of anger and sadness. At the end of the session, they both report that our work together has been helpful to them and that they appreciate my efforts to guide them through this relationship maze. I encourage them to consider brief individual therapy as a way to reflect on their own contributions toward why this relationship didn't work, to enable them not to carry that baggage into other relationships. Toward that end, I also offer a one-time individual session with each of them, if they would like. Finally, I thank them for the privilege of letting me join them in their journey, and I share that although this wasn't the ending either of them wanted, I hope that with time they find clarity and peace with this tumultuous chapter of their lives. Privately, I recognize my own mixed feelings of sadness and disappointment on their behalf, and my regret that they hadn't come to see me a few years earlier, when our efforts to improve communication and manage differences might have had more enduring impact.

FURTHER REFLECTIONS AND IMPLICATIONS

I'll remember Beth and Marcus for a long time to come. The most challenging aspect of this couple was the fact that as they were trying to launch into marriage, they were held back by so many constraints stemming in part from difficulties in shared decision making, as well as lingering unresolved issues from their respective family histories. There was a heaviness associated with this couple that you usually don't see with premarital couples, in that they had made major financial and life decisions (buying a house together, loaning tens of thousands of dollars, and going through IVF without the firm commitment of marriage) that one usually associates with more established married couples.

Looking back, I wonder if I gave homework assignments without enough scaffolding. There was a pattern of my giving an assignment or encouraging them to talk and then the next session they would be struggling. On the other hand, I wonder if I should have done more along these lines. Given their propensity to avoid, perhaps if I'd given more homework the issues and problem sequences would have presented themselves earlier and more intensely, providing the opportunity to intervene to construct solution sequences. Although I shared with them the benefits of meeting weekly and then titrating sessions, they were resistant and—given his ambivalence about therapy—I was concerned that if I pushed harder I could jeopardize the therapeutic alliance, especially with Marcus. I also keep thinking about the second to last session, when Marcus finally was able to connect and understand Beth's emotions around finances. What would have happened if he had come to that understanding earlier, and was there anything I could have done to accelerate that? Perhaps they just had to follow the natural iterative arc that many couples have to go through when discussing difficult, polarizing issues. Unfortunately, for Marcus and Beth, that last iteration came too late.

I also reflect on the impact of the failed IVF. We know that many couple relationships don't survive the death of a child for many complicated reasons. For Beth, the failure of IVF was analogous to losing a child. She felt lost, directionless, purposeless, angry, and devastated. Beth seemed unable to overcome this existential crisis, and she seemed to lose her motivation to continue to work on this relationship.

This couple had many interwoven layers that provided a rich texture for understanding them. First and foremost, this was an upper-middle-class, Black couple. Through one lens, they fit the prototype of many Black couples, in that they struggled with issues of gender disparities; were children of divorce who lacked a model for how to have a healthy romantic relationship and how to effectively manage differences; lacked clarity around gender roles and conflict around leadership, power, and empathy; had heavy work stress that included racial pressures to succeed in a White-dominated world; had issues with cohabitation, which we know for a disproportionate number of Black couples doesn't serve as a precursor to marriage as it does for a higher proportion of White couples; and finally, were subject to the historical challenges for Blacks around trust, vulnerability, and forgiveness. Beth and Marcus struggled with all of these issues to varying degrees. Yet, despite all this, Beth and Marcus also demonstrated many aspects of resilience through their commitment to each other over the years and their willingness to engage in couple therapy for 15 months.

In addition to those challenges that are amplified for Black couples, Beth and Marcus also were burdened with problems that can plague many couples, most notably, money and infertility. Either of these issues on its own would be enough to cause relationship problems, but the combination of these issues layered upon the unique, race-linked challenges for many Blacks only exacerbated the intensity of the difficulties Beth and Marcus faced.

I felt a special connection to both Beth and Marcus. I admired Marcus's persistent hope that things could get better, and I especially appreciated experiencing another Black man wired toward relationships. The stereotype of the Black man doesn't include a sensitive, relationally driven, heterosexual man—and I was drawn to that in Marcus. I also connected with Beth through her deep values around education and achievement. I resonated with the stress she described as an executive in a major firm, and the many layers of complexity that come with being a member of the ethnic/racial minority community in a role of power.

I believe these diverse aspects of my own identity also helped each of them to connect with me. I'm often asked by colleagues or trainees how they, as highly educated White couple therapists, can work effectively with a Black couple? Although the answer to that question often starts with encouraging them to learn about the sociopolitical and historical context of Blacks, I actually believe the answer lies in cultivating critical consciousness (Kelly, Jeremie-Brink, Chambers, & Smith-Bynum, 2020). Critical consciousness requires both awareness and sensitivity. It's more than awareness, because awareness alone is a cognitive process—one can have awareness and all the information in the world but lack sensitivity. When there's also sensitivity, there's the realization that what you say may be experienced in a negative way. Thus, the goal is to have both awareness and sensitivity. Finally, it's important to embrace cultural humility, whereby we adopt "not knowing" as an ethical stance that empowers connection. Cultural humility helps us to facilitate and engage in authentic connections that beget curious conversations between you and the couple rather than presumptive or judgmental conversations. People of color are highly attuned to being judged, and so a White therapist who enters the therapy space with the ability to authentically communicate curiosity is in a better position to develop a strong therapeutic alliance. Finally, it's important for White therapists not to overassume or underassume the impact of race—as both are problematic.

I was grateful for the opportunity to have that final session with Beth and Marcus rather than their simply canceling or not showing—leaving me to wonder what happened or how they're doing. I believe that their choice to come in for a final session after deciding to end their relationship was testament to our alliance, and for that I was very appreciative.

When working with Black couples, sometimes race is in the figure and sometimes it's in the background, but race is never absent. For Beth and Marcus, the issues of race oscillated between being the figure and being the ground. But ever-present was their humanity and their genuine desire for connection. Ultimately, Marcus and Beth's relationship wasn't healed. But I hope that our work together positioned both partners to create healthier new relationships as they moved forward separately.

REFERENCES

Breunlin, D. C., Russell, W. P., Chambers, A. L., & Solomon, A. H. (2023). Integrative systemic therapy for couples. In J. L. Lebow & D. K. Snyder (Eds.), *Clinical handbook of couple therapy* (6th ed., pp. 318–338). New York: Guilford Press.

Chambers, A. L. (2008). Premarital counseling with middle-class African Americans: The forgotten group. In M. Rastogi & V. Thomas (Eds.), *Multicultural couple therapy* (pp. 217–234). Thousand Oaks, CA: Sage.

Chambers, A. L. (2012). A systemically infused, integrative model for conceptualizing couples' problems: The four-session evaluation. *Couple and Family Psychology: Research and Practice, 1,* 31–47.

Chambers, A. L. (2019). African American couples in the 21st century: Using Integrative Systemic Therapy (IST) to translate science into practice. *Family Process, 58,* 595–609.

Chambers, A. L., & Kravitz, A. M. (2011). Understanding the disproportionately low marriage rate among African Americans: An amalgam of sociological and psychological constraints. *Family Relations, 60,* 648–660.

Kelly, S., Jeremie-Brink, G., Chambers, A. L., & Smith-Bynum, M. A. (2020). The Black Lives Matter Movement: A call to action for couple and family therapists. *Family Process, 59,* 1374–1388.

Lebow, J. L. (2014). *Couple and family therapy: An integrative map of the territory.* Washington, DC: APA Books.

Lebow, J., Chambers, A. L., Christensen, A., & Johnson, S. (2012). Research on the treatment of couple distress. *Journal of Marital and Family Therapy, 38,* 145–168.

Pattillo, M. (2005). Black middle-class neighborhoods. *Annual Review of Sociology, 31,* 305–329.

Pinsof, W. M., Breunlin, D. C., Russell, W. P., Lebow, J. L., Rampage, C., & Chambers, A. L. (2018). *Integrative Systemic Therapy: Metaframeworks for problem solving with individuals, couples, and families.* Washington, DC: APA Books.

CHAPTER 10

Addressing Gender, Class, and Racism in a Mexican Transnational Couple

CELIA JAES FALICOV

> *Editors' Comments*
>
> How should a clinician adapt couple therapy to a specific population? In this highly informative chapter, Celia Falicov applies her multidimensional ecological comparative approach (MECA) to a traditional Latinx couple whose lives now transect their Mexican cultural and sociopolitical heritage with the evolving sociocultural perspectives of their adult children who've immigrated to the United States. Although her chapter focuses primarily on ecological dynamics impacting therapy with a Latinx couple, Falicov's innovative conceptual model and related assessment paradigm offer a structured process for incorporating important distinctive aspects of any specific cultural and sociopolitical context to couple therapy.
>
> Throughout her narrative, Falicov shares her internal dialogue about choice points in the therapy involving both formulation and intervention drawn from broad methods in couple therapy and how those specific methods might play out in a traditional Latinx context. This case study also speaks to the sometimes unacknowledged or unstated legacies of color and class discrimination that often are experienced by Latinx and other marginalized groups.
>
> Falicov's case study reflects the work of a skilled couple therapist that builds on partners' complex identities rather than relying on simplistic stereotypes about Latino/as. She hypothesizes and formulates and creates marvelous ways to build a strong therapeutic connection with the couple and balance her alliances with both partners. She draws from a lifetime of experience in how to speak with Latinx couples who not only share in common with her some important aspects of life circumstances but also have much different lives and belief systems. She offers the reader many specific guideposts for how to address gender, class, and race and their intersectionalities.
>
> The chapter describes how to engage and help a couple with issues of possessive love and severe jealousy in the context of couples who view jealousy as a sign of

> love—a view based on their cultural, sociopolitical, and personal locations. The chapter also shows how to skillfully explore the appearance of one instance of intimate partner violence prompted by jealousy that should not be ignored in therapy. Falicov wonderfully shows us how to join with, rather than threaten, the couple system and how, as a welcomed visitor in the couple's world, to reframe problems in ways that solutions become accessible.

I became a family therapist long before I started seeing couples. Perhaps this preference was anchored in my social location during my formative years. I lived my childhood and adolescence in a Jewish enclave of Buenos Aires, Argentina, in daily connection with three generations of my extended family. My parents, grandparents, uncles, and aunts were immigrants from Eastern Europe. I was the first person born in Argentina in my nuclear family, so my interest in the cultures and contexts of immigrant families started early in my life. Concerns about identity, language, and culture change were intensified when, as young adults, my husband and I became Spanish-speaking immigrants to the United States. A few years after this migration, as a doctoral student in human development at the University of Chicago, I began to think about the life cycle transitions of couples and families. These academic and personal interests in culture, social context and life cycle transitions naturally led to a clinical practice with Spanish-speaking immigrants in the United States.

Systems-oriented therapy brings together many of the elements I learned to value personally and professionally. It's eminently contextual in that it always looks at individuals and families in their social context; it is developmental insofar as it always evaluates family stresses in the light of life cycle transitions and other temporal events; and it is culturally relative, since its concepts and interventions always consider that behaviors and their meanings shift according to the culture and social context of the couple and family.

Over many years of work with Latinx couples and families, I became aware of the enormous cultural diversity and the varied sociopolitical contexts across Latin American countries and within Latinx communities. Attempting to construct therapeutic strategies appropriate for this diversity of culture and context, I developed a clinical framework that could incorporate a plurality of sociocultural variables rather than only ethnic-focused content generalizations. My other motivation was to acknowledge that cross-cultural work, even among therapists and clients who share language and some cultural features, is fraught with risks of misunderstanding or preconceptions in meaning making. My hope was to develop a rich conception of culture and contexts, free from preconceived static stereotypes yet allowing for cultural consistencies as well as contradictions, uncertainties, and hybrid sociocultural views to emerge from the clients themselves.

With these thoughts in mind, I proposed a multidimensional ecological comparative approach (MECA; Falicov, 2014, 2017a). It encompasses four universal domains in which cultural diversity and sociopolitical inequality may appear. Two are migration (and other uprootings) and ecological context capturing sociopolitical dimensions such as social inequality and discrimination. The two others are family organization and family life cycle addressing diversity of values and belief systems. Although MECA offers guidelines for inquiring about these four domains, the questions are content free—facilitating therapists' "knowing with" clients as the experts on their cultures and contexts rather than "knowing about" clients' cultures a priori as some cultural "competence" approaches encourage. MECA also offers interventions related to issues that arise from cultural diversity (e.g., questioning mainstream attachment theory) or from sociopolitical inequality (e.g., empowerment and resistance to oppression).

The MECA framework also aided my own cultural and sociopolitical self-reflexivity. Indeed, the therapeutic encounter is not culturally neutral, even when a therapist shares some similarities with a client's language or recent immigrant experience. Practitioners bring into their conceptualizations their cultural ideas derived from mainstream psychological theory, their inevitable hierarchical position, and their own sociocultural upbringing or their personal experiences and preferences. MECA provides a way for therapists to exercise "cultural humility" by comparing their own cultural values and social contexts in the same four domains of their clients, thus gaining awareness of cultural overlaps or differences and recognition of the power differentials that may unwittingly promote social injustice in treatment. My book *Latino Families in Therapy* (Falicov, 2014) provides concepts, case examples, and templates to incorporate issues of culture and context when working with Latinx immigrants, with variations according to country of origin, and examines the culture and the sociopolitical position the therapist brings to each case. The use of MECA with Latinx couples is also discussed in Falicov (2017b).

In this chapter, I illustrate the use of MECA in my work with Piedad and Francisco, a middle-aged transnational couple from Mexico presenting with possessive jealousy of Francisco toward his wife. Despite my interest in including culture and context in clinical practice, I don't believe that culture should be approached as a reductionistic explanation or a justification for the behaviors observed. We should never lose track of the universals that unite us, nor the particulars or unique features of each person, couple, or family system, as well as the sociocultural contexts of the communities from which our clients come. MECA is a framework for integrating culture and context in systemic practices for any cultural group, including dominant ones, and can be used to question or modify mainstream approaches to practice that, of course, are also the products of specific cultures and contexts.

As I contemplate this case, I consider that intimate jealousy as a threat or fear of loss or exclusivity in a valued romantic relationship is nearly universal and generally regarded as needing containment when intensely obsessive and persecutory. However, cultural beliefs and meanings attributed to jealousy vary. In some cultures, jealousy is seen as a proof of true love and protection of a monogamous relationship. In others, it is considered an oppressive entitlement, often gendered. Yet in still other cultural settings, jealousy may be seen as both loving and oppressive. If these cultural meanings are ignored or are not deconstructed in therapy, jealousy could be incorrectly regarded as only individual or couple pathology. Nevertheless, the individual histories of each partner need to be considered as they add subjective meanings that complicate the experience of jealousy. Consistent with a relational lens, I assume that jealousy in a couple is part of an interactional pattern and, if not caused by the interactional communication itself, is at least maintained by an interactional history or repetitive pattern over time. It is universal and influenced by cultural understandings of interactions in romantic relationships that become visible when working with the particulars of a couple.

INITIAL ASSESSMENT AND CASE FORMULATION

The request for couple therapy for Piedad (age 56) and Francisco (age 63) came from Lucía, their 27-year-old daughter. She called to ask (in English) if I would see her Spanish-speaking parents. They had never been in therapy but had a history of long-standing conflicts triggered by her father's jealous possessiveness of her mother. I asked if she was acting on her own by making the phone call or if she had discussed this idea with her parents. She replied that she was one of six children, four now living in California and two others in the small town in Mexico where the parents were born and lived for several decades. The siblings in both countries were all in agreement that the parents needed couple therapy. Their parents had been a little more reluctant, particularly Francisco, but had agreed with Lucía's making an appointment with a Spanish-speaking therapist.

The fact that it was their daughter calling for an appointment confronted me with my first therapeutic choice. Should I include the daughter in the first session, as she was the referring person, and might this facilitate the encounter with the parents? Many thoughts came to my mind. Concerns expressed by offspring usually provide a powerful motivation for parental change in most cultures, but perhaps even more intensely among collectivistic Latinx, where it can be an acceptable cultural practice for a family member to make the first inquiry. On the other hand, including Lucía, an acculturated person who might articulate her parents' marital issues from her or her siblings' perspective, could deprive me of the initial information I might obtain from hearing directly from her parents and from observing their interaction. I remembered an old dictum from Carl Whitaker: "Clients are in charge of the initiative; therapists are in charge of the structure." Because I thought it would be advantageous to have the couple take the initiative, I told Lucía that it would be best if she gave them my phone number, so that we could find a mutually acceptable time for a session. I kept it in my mind that Lucía and perhaps her siblings might be a therapeutic resource in the future. I've learned that when children express emotional concern for parental conflict, convening them either as an actual or as an imaginary presence can be a powerful source of parental motivation and change.

Two days later, Piedad called, and we arranged a time for the first session. Following a conventional guess on my part, I asked if her husband was going to be the driver and, if so, would it be okay with her to put him on the phone, so I could give him the address and instructions. His coming to the phone gave me an opportunity to introduce myself. With this gesture, I had now made a kind, joining move of acknowledging each of them and telling them it would be a pleasure to meet them. This rather formal personal approach continued in our initial in-person introductions. In the literature about Latinx values, this preferred style of relating with courtesy and politeness that conveys interest in connection is labeled *personalismo*.

Francisco had piercing black eyes, black hair and a large moustache, blue jeans, cowboy shirt, pointy boots, and a belt with a big buckle. He looked like the stereotype of the Mexican *charro,* or cowboy. Piedad, a good-looking woman, was smartly but simply dressed, hair cut short, no makeup. Her skin was lighter than Francisco's, and she was also physically larger than he. I presumed that given their generation and their native small-town location, not using their first names right away might command greater seriousness to our encounter. When I shook hands with each, I was *la Doctora Falicov* and they were *el*

Señor y la Señora Torres. In time, I asked their permission and granted mine to use our first names. But we all continued throughout to use the formal *Usted* (you) in Spanish instead of the informal *Tú*.

How one approaches initial greetings with Latinx clients is important. With my younger clients who come from large cities in Latin America or Spain, I ask how they would like me to address them. Usually, they'll tell me to use their first names and the familiar *Tú* or *vos* in Spanish, depending on the country of origin. I'll then respond that they can call me Celia and *tutearme* (the verb for using the more informal *Tú* or *vos*). I make it clear that it's their choice. It is important to ask, as there are some countries where the formal *Usted* is used between parents and children. Use of first or last names, or formal and informal ways of addressing others, is a sociocultural narrative, emblematic of the nature of the relationship. It's at this introductory phase that first cultural negotiations begin to take place and provide an avenue to express that culture is present and informs our interactions.

I told Piedad and Francisco that I would like to get to know them and their families first, before we focus on the problems that bring them to talk with me, and that I would do this by asking them some questions about their lives. I frequently use MECA questions to know crucial elements of their family and community life, to initiate a therapeutic alliance, and to delay an early focus on potentially explosive presenting issues. This information, once obtained, also allows me to locate myself in terms of personal, cultural, and sociopolitical similarities and differences. Probably I had already begun to fill out the four domains in the MECA template when talking to their daughter over the phone. I learned that four of their six children, two young women and two young men, migrated to the United States in their late teens and early 20s to study and to work, with the aid of uncles who had migrated from Mexico earlier and were settled in California. Just as their daughter Lucía had already mentioned in the initial phone conversation, two of her brothers had remained in Mexico but one of them had married recently and moved to another city to be close to his wife's family. I asked Piedad and Francisco about their emotions connected with these separations and reunifications with offspring across countries, a topic I regularly address with immigrant families. They shared that it had been difficult for several years living with the family fragmentation of what I've called "living with two hearts, one here, one there," a metaphor I shared when they told me about their family separations. Most clients feel understood and cherish this image, often carrying it with them. So did Piedad and Francisco. I also asked if their children's migration reflected family values toward education or better economic opportunities or if they had other reasons. These inquiries about personal or cultural values and strengths are always included during MECA explorations.

The couple's health and work situation had begun to change recently. Francisco had developed intense back pain and had been delegating his small farming business, the *milpa*, to the oldest son, who had remained in their original rural town in Mexico. Work, income, and status are part of ecological context that have implications for family survival, self-esteem, and networking. But this information also related to life cycle transitions, because the mature judgment of this son was trusted, which meant that Francisco and Piedad could now come more often to California to visit their adult children and their growing families. Their visits had lasted 3–4 months, but they considered expanding their next visit to 6 months and eventually staying permanently, since more of their children and grandchildren were in San Diego. They were entering a retirement stage with its constraints in work and health, while simultaneously facing the adaptations of becoming prospective immigrants.

I explored their lived environments and learned that the couple had been stable contributors to their community—Francisco through his many work acquaintances and his domino games in their hometown central plaza, and Piedad with her involvement in the local Catholic church and charity work. When asked about the nature of these social networks, Piedad in a rather jocular tone used a sharp metaphor to describe how she viewed her husband. She said that in their community, Francisco was "the light of the street," but then she added "and the darkness of the home." In Spanish, *luz de la calle, oscuridad de la casa* shocked me a little. It told me that he cared to be a public charmer, to present his best side to the community—but to her, he showed the opposite, an ominous dark presence in their privacy. This opened a door to their problems, so I nodded but didn't explore its meaning further. Perhaps I wanted to continue with my MECA-guided assessment and not yet delve into negative details of the presenting problem. Or perhaps the image offered by Piedad worried me and I needed time to think how to approach it. I often store such thoughts until they're better formed or fit the moment better, so I continued to ask about community supports for her and for him, such as the presence of *comadres* and *compadres*— close friends of a woman or a man, or godmothers and godfathers of their children, as these are common relationship roles in Mexico. In this context, I asked if they belonged to a faith community. Piedad said she was a churchgoer and that this activity provided comfort and support. She added that their life would be better if Francisco was not so reluctant to accompany her to church.

I next asked about their family organization. They both had grown up in traditional patriarchal ideologies, where men worked hard to support large families and women were devoted mothers and wives. The couple described their families of origin as very different: Piedad's father had a small furniture store in the center of the town, and she was one of five children, whereas Francisco's father was a farm worker who managed to support his wife and their 14 children. Piedad said that her two daughters, now living and working in San Diego, had shown her more modern types of marriage. Francisco nodded in agreement and called the daughters *recias,* meaning "strong," and in this context not to be argued with or shy. Piedad said she wasn't critical of Francisco, as he was a good provider, a good companion and father, and a loving man. They were both aware of their traditionalism and said that it worked for them because couple complementarities are expected in traditional marriages. I commented that Piedad was describing strengths and compatibilities in their marriage. Piedad agreed and added that she knew that they had come to therapy to talk about problems she had with Francisco's behavior, but she also didn't want to give me a wrong impression about him, as he was also those other good things. I congratulated her for her equanimity in talking about Francisco's qualities. This prompted Francisco to tell me that Piedad was beautiful and elegant, a loving mother, devoted wife, neat to a fault, a good cook, always calm and correct, *esta güerita mía* ("this blondie of mine"). I'm familiar with the term *güera* and *güerita* and nodded, indicating that I understood the Mexican slang that describes a blond and light-skinned person. These comments made me wonder internally about the impact of skin color in their relationship.

When I then continued to inquire about their family life cycle, what stood out was that Piedad said that they had both been raised in a very strict way. She related that when their sons were young, she didn't tolerate it if Francisco wanted to belt them, as he had been harshly disciplined by his own father. Francisco understood her reasons and stopped, leaving much of the discipline to Piedad. He believes that giving up his punitive approach has made the children love both of them.

I decided to broach what I think of as the inevitable triangle of therapy. I wondered whether my being a woman could have empowered Piedad to reveal more than her husband. Being outnumbered by two women might threaten Francisco, who was anticipating being blamed for his behavior with Piedad. So I asked each of them how they felt about seeing a woman. Piedad answered that she was confident that I would understand her. Francisco said he knew that things were changing and not all doctors are men, but the most important thing is that I came highly recommended to his daughters as an educated person. He then used a *dicho* and said, "*A buen entendedor, pocas palabras bastan*" ("for the good listener, a few words suffice"). *Dichos* (proverbs and sayings) are an important type of brief communication in Latin America that usually embeds complex ideas with a few words. They can be serious, sarcastic, fun, or light colloquial messages.

Next, I shared that I am a secular Jew, but that having grown up in a Catholic country, I know a fair amount about Catholicism. I wanted to make sure they felt comfortable with me. They replied that in their small town, they never met a Jew, but they weren't prejudiced and what mattered is that "you're an educated person." I didn't approach the issue of race and colorism, as in my mind it would have been premature. There was a gradation of color in the room, with Francisco being rather dark, Piedad much lighter, and myself still perhaps a bit lighter. I'm aware of the complex, and often simultaneously open and denied, hierarchies of color in Mexico. I didn't know at this point the relevance of racial issues for this couple and for their presenting problem, though Francisco had already mentioned Piedad's fair skin as part of her beauty. I've written elsewhere about the importance of listening with a wider ear for "openings" that allow for conversations about race, gender, and class. I waited for these openings to come from either one of them again later, so that I could explore them with curiosity and respect.

At the end of the first session, I thanked them for telling me so much about their lives and how impressed I was by their remarkable dedication to their family. I added that I'd think about them and in the following session we could concentrate on the issues that causes their current suffering. Interestingly, Piedad said that the questions I asked were like "a mirror" to their lives. This felt like an invitation to join with their family values further, so I said that I would enjoy seeing a photo of their children and grandchildren at some point.

After they left, I reflected on the MECA domains that may be tied to possible areas of vulnerability and to the presenting problem. I believed that ecological context influences such as Francisco's concern with his social reference group and the recent family life cycle changes of health and work may have exacerbated a tendency toward jealousy. The prospects of immigration may not be an issue yet, except for the more intense witnessing and intervention about the couple's interactions by the adult daughters acculturated in the United States. The family organization dimensions of patriarchy and traditional gender roles were likely contributors to the domineering aspects of jealousy.

The MECA framework I use furnished the opportunity to know the couple more broadly than their presenting problem and provided elements of cultural and personal identities that I could return to in my future conversations with them. After this first session, I reflected on what I heard but chose not to focus on. What had been told indirectly? What did it mean that Francisco was so concerned with being liked or approved of socially, while he behaved differently in private? What did Piedad think that Francisco would gain by going to church? Why did she have to help him control his violent parenting, so that he wouldn't inflict his childhood hurts on their children? What were the cultural changes around gender roles they were learning from the daughters? How could any of what I learned in the first session be related to the presenting symptom or concern? I also became aware that many of the more revealing comments came from Piedad, whereas Francisco's comments were more conventional or superficial, despite my attempts to engage him. Perhaps he was being the "light of the street" with me too, evading his or their darkness. I usually keep in my mind these unexplored complexities as topics to address more thoroughly in future sessions. When I see a couple, they become part of my thoughts and my caring outside the session.

BEGINNING PHASE OF THERAPY

I learned in the second session that the incident that precipitated the referral to couple therapy had occurred following a family gathering in San Diego, with many nuclear and extended family members present. During this party, a 32-year-old male nephew, in a wheelchair due to a chronic disability, approached Piedad from behind and put his hands on her arm, saying, *"Mi Tía linda, mi Tía buena"* ("my pretty aunt, my good aunt"). Piedad turned around, reached for his hand, and smiled at him saying, *"Este muchacho tan cariñoso"* ("You are such an affectionate lad").

She didn't realize that her husband was watching them like a hawk. His fury mounting, he intervened by moving her away from the nephew and insisting they go home. The minute they got home, he had an intense fit of jealousy, accusing her of carrying on an affair with the nephew and pushing her physically when she denied it, defending herself from this absurdity. Piedad's concern for her safety and reputation prompted her opening up to her daughters. I asked whether there had been previous incidents of jealous outbursts or whether this was the first one. Piedad answered that these occurred from time to time in their hometown in Mexico, but recently there had been a few years of peaceful coexistence without these incidents.

I asked Piedad what made her turn for help to her daughters and even her sons. She said that despite jealous questionings over the years, Francisco had never gotten violent toward her. Francisco had mentioned two recent changes: his back injury and his delegating his farming small company to their oldest son. I wondered whether these issues intersected with his masculine identity in ways that diminished it, in his own self-evaluation or in his community interactions. I kept in mind that these changes could have contributed to lower self-esteem and his clinging to the love of his wife as the most affirming aspect of his masculine worth, but I chose not to advance this simple hypothesis, as it could justify or excuse the increase and severity of Francisco's jealous outbursts prematurely. I must add though, that with some frequency, though not always, I return in my work with couples to my "first thoughts as best thoughts," like Buddhists say.

Instead, I asked them to describe other incidents of jealousy that happened in the past. While the occurrence of jealousy wasn't predictable, the pattern that emerged was repetitive. It always involved a social situation in which Francisco felt that Piedad's attention was directed to or taken by another man. Francisco then questioned her, insinuating that she showed interest and even fascination in the other man. Until the recent incident, her response during these episodes was equally repetitive. She always calmed him down, appeasing and reassuring him of her love and devotion to him only. But this last time, she felt he'd gone too far. It was outrageous that he suspected a disabled young person in a wheelchair and proceeded to humiliate her publicly by "making a scene."

Once I have clarity about what's being described, I regularly ask about the couple's own guesses or theories about why a problem exists. Once I know their theories, I might add a collaborative comment as my guess about a connection between the presenting problem and other issues in their lives. Francisco's guess was that he becomes so jealous because his love for Piedad is so intense, he can't tolerate the idea of a potential rival. He considered his feelings normal, particularly because Piedad is so beautiful, so refined, so elegant, and such a great person. He thought that many men would be attracted to her. Piedad interrupted him, "That's what your explanation always is—that your love is so deep, and I always believed you, that your jealousy is a proof of how much you love me. But this is what we've been doing all these years and now I think something is too much, something is wrong."

The thought crossed my mind that this interpretation of jealousy might have cultural roots but did not want to invoke this idea as most couples come to therapy when the need for change has become evident and one or both partners question a pattern. Now Piedad could pronounce, "Something is wrong and has to change." She had always assumed a complementary position in relation to Francisco's jealousy by mildly protesting his accusations while placating and reassuring him about the purity and loyalty of her love toward him. She had never gotten angry at the injustice or demanded that he stop oppressing her. For Piedad, who had been raised in a patriarchal setting aspiring toward middle class, being virtuous and "put together" was expected of her; arguing, confrontation or anger, whether justified or not, in her mind wasn't what a good woman is "supposed" to be. Nevertheless, several exceptions demonstrated her agency—right now, it was her interruption of Francisco's regular argument that his jealousy was proof of his intense love. She had also reached out to her children recently, a move that led the couple to therapy. She had also expressed her opinion that he would benefit from churchgoing, and early on, she stopped his abusive behavior with the children. My tentative hypothesis was that perhaps Piedad needed to adopt a more symmetrical power position in relation to Francisco's jealous outbursts, by setting boundaries and telling him that his behavior wasn't acceptable to her. This would be a change from her rushing to a complementary, appeasing position. But expressing anger at injustice toward her was not spontaneously part of her repertoire. It may have been possible for me to ask what would happen if she became angry with him, but it seemed risky to do so, as it might appear I was siding with her against his wrongdoing and, if so, the nascent therapeutic alliance with him might be endangered. And there was another risk: "Assertiveness training" has been identified as a potential for greater conflict and even violence, besides not being a culturally syntonic way of relating among traditional Latinx couples. In truth, I hadn't yet discarded the possibility that jealousy might have developed into more incidents of violence, but disclosure of violence may be hidden in the beginning stages of therapy or minimized throughout, as it is socially reprehensible in any culture and social location.

The meanings, reasons, and consequences of jealousy are multiple, and I still didn't know enough to venture any intervention, so I returned to my question about their guesses as to why this repetitive, jealous pattern had installed itself in their relationship. Piedad offered a historical explanation for Francisco's surveillance of her. He was the youngest boy in a very large family of 14 siblings, many of whom were girls. He was told by his parents to watch them always at dances, in the street, and at school for potential misbehavior and, particularly, for being seductive or simply being courted by tempting men, young and old. Francisco was always praised for bringing back information about the sisters to the parents. Piedad believed that he got used to making things up that would raise doubts about the sisters' behaviors, presumably because he gained parental favors and self-importance with such lies. Piedad now worried that he might have been making up stories about her, too. She thought that sometimes he inquired about her activities from others in their circle, another reason why she'd felt that his jealousy has gone too far. He denied her accusation that his *sospechas* ("suspicions") served to spread problematic rumors about her; he added that it was he who was much more deeply damaged by how their community may judge him, if other men showed interest in her and she didn't outright reject them. The therapy hour became rather heated, with each claiming that the other's behavior was damaging to their reputation. I empathized with both of their concerns, as it sounded like issues of public honor are culturally very important for their well-being and community standing. However, I ventured that if we could return to focus on what was happening between the two of them, they might become better able to help each other with these concerns about social standing.

There was a reason for my moving back to the relational aspects between them. I wasn't surprised by their concerns about the opinions of others in their communities, particularly commentaries about the sexual morality of women. Piedad had already described Francisco as *luz de la calle, oscuridad de su casa* ("light of the street, darkness of the home"). She was referring to the fact that in social circumstances, Francisco was charming and seductive, a loquacious and dashingly dressed *bon vivant*, indeed, the light of the street. He illuminated what he touched by helping everybody, never saying "no" to favors asked. He paid for all the drinks. He hired groups of mariachis to throw parties and spent considerable money in social situations. With Piedad, too, he could be extremely affectionate, generous, and passionately romantic. He would even arrange to deliver a musical message of love to her, a *serenata*, an old custom more common in Mexico than elsewhere in Latin America.

But there was the other side, the oppressive darkness of jealousy only revealed behind doors. The triggers for displaying his overbearing possessiveness and control were small and trivial social situations, but when they occurred, Francisco spent time monitoring Piedad's activities, questioning relationships with other men, becoming suspicious and accusatory. In urban areas, and even more so in small rural enclaves, Latinos are often surrounded by an intensely involved network of family, friends, and acquaintances that scrutinize, tease, banter, or give advice. I've expanded elsewhere on a phenomenon I call "in the cultural gaze of others" to describe an experience of feeling exposed by the scrutiny of others in community settings (Falicov, 2010). Men and women may experience a profound sense of shame and humiliation when found wanting or at fault in their traditional cultural gender expectations by the witnessing group.

Piedad also had not told anybody about the jealousy issues, preserving the image of the perfect marriage. I thought this concern about their community's opinion would be hard to change, since their group identity was inextricably tied to their personal well-being. Even with their recent transnational lifestyle, the extended family and social network in the United States may function similarly as in the country of origin. I didn't feel it was a therapeutic option to work with them on not caring about *el que dirán* ("what they will say"). The family and its social network may be a constitutive part of Latinx identity for many. So I asked Piedad if it would be acceptable for her and their children if Francisco remained the "light of the street" if he stopped being the "darkness of the home." She wholeheartedly agreed. I decided then to direct our attention to a topic that Piedad and Francisco had brought up as part of their couple belief system: equating jealousy with love.

Both jealousy and love seemed inextricably connected in their minds, but I thought that separating them could potentially expand the alternatives for change. In addition, whenever the experience of violence is mentioned, I feel the responsibility to explore it further, since, as I mentioned, social desirability may impede total transparency. I decided to share the following story to open conversations relevant to equating love with jealousy, and even violence. There is some practice-based evidence that telling stories is especially both a convivial and an insight-oriented strategy when working with Latinx clients. The story that popped in my head was about a client, a beautiful Guatemalan woman who limped. Her husband had shot her in the leg several years before when she was in front of the mirror putting on makeup to go out with him on their anniversary. She believed him when he said that he couldn't stand how beautiful she looked and wanted no other man to ever have her, that nobody could ever love her the way he did. Ten years later and with a leg disability, she has become fully aware of this abominable injustice. This was not the first instance of jealousy and brutality on his part, but she, who had suffered much parental deprivation and abandonment in her childhood, always told herself that nobody had loved her as he did in such an intense way. She could now see that he assumed that she was his property and believed he had the right to control her, at the cost of hurting her, with her implicit approval.

While Francisco and Piedad agreed with me that this was an extreme example, it somehow stirred their emotions as it had mine, and opened an avenue to speak about the effects of love as entitlement to hurt, to love as a wish to own the other person and make them behave according to one's wishes. I asked if there were meanings of love for them other than jealousy. What were they, and could we list them? Parental love, filial love, fraternal love, romantic love, erotic love, domestic love, companionship love. In these stimulating conversations about difficult definitions, Francisco initially appeared more confused than Piedad, but both were equally engaged. Gradually, a narrative of their love relationship emerged about how their love began, their early marriage, how love changed when they became parents and again when their children left, what parts of love fit or did not fit with traditional gender expectations and whether there were early conversations about jealousy.

Talking about different conceptions of love in marriage provided a safer avenue to frame their issues than calling Francisco's behavior an abuse of his power, or Piedad's acceptance as incorrect submission to his domination. More poetic, more traditional and less politically flavored, the discussion of gender and love felt culturally consonant for both partners, while they recognized that their children's marriages were culturally egalitarian.

Since Piedad had offered a historical hypothesis for Francisco's need to control the behavior of women, I asked them if there was anything in Piedad's past that might contribute to her belief that jealousy and surveillance of women is a form of love. She said that she'd been thinking recently that her father wasn't an emotionally expressive man and even her mother was rather cold, but they both were concerned and protective of her and her sister's behavior toward boys and men. So perhaps when Francisco was so jealous, she felt that he was expressing love toward her. She also realized that her parents' marriage had been cold, with her mother expecting affection from her husband but not demonstrating any herself. Piedad wondered if she was like her mother, because she wasn't very expressive or appreciative toward Francisco; perhaps she feared that if she demonstrated affection or even attraction, Francisco would consider her an "easy" woman, a common oppression of women's sexual expression in patriarchal systems. I then asked Francisco if he could tell Piedad how he would react if she told him how much she loved him, not as a reassurance of love provoked by his jealousy, but as her genuine initiative. Would he judge her in the ways she feared? He said "no"—that his own mother was affectionate toward his father, and he saw his own daughters being demonstrative with their husbands. He reflected that he had accepted that Piedad's relative coolness was due to her growing up in a different social class environment and having a smaller family in which people were more rational than emotional. "It wouldn't be natural for her," he said.

I left them to think about this issue, wondering aloud if it would be out of character for her to be more demonstrative? And on his side, would he believe that he was deserving of her love if she demonstrated it more? Since by now I had heard some openings to race and class differences, I ventured raising consciousness of the influence of skin color and social class with a somewhat ambiguous phrasing. Would their class and color differences have anything to do with how they relate to each other or with their expectations of each other? In my mind, I thought that relationally, jealous domination was tied to the patriarchal privilege of gender he had, whereas she may unwittingly represent the privilege assigned to color and class in colonized societies.

INTERMEDIATE PHASE OF THERAPY

They both came to the next session with thoughts stimulated by the discussion about different forms of love. Piedad said that our discussion was lacking a type of love that she called *amor con respeto*—"love with respect." *Respeto* is a core value in Latinx relationships. It refers to interpersonal obligations of mutual deference and good treatment with all people, even with those lower in the hierarchy, such as children or employees. Some authors believe that respect in English-speaking countries relates to merits deserved or gained through behavior and accomplishments rather than being deserved simply by being a human being, as it is in Latin American cultures.

I'm never sure what exactly is meant by "respect," as it's one of those ubiquitous abstract concepts that can vary culturally and personally, so I ask and don't assume its meaning. Privately, I wondered whether Piedad couldn't respect Francisco because of his absurd jealous scenes or whether she was the one who felt disrespected by his suspiciousness, so I asked her if she could tell me a little more about what she meant by "love with respect." She answered that she thought there was a difference between fear and respect; that she wanted to love Francisco without fear. By making his *sospechas* ("suspicions") public the way he did at the party, she feared that he had demeaned her in the eyes of the family and the community. And after he pushed her when she rightly defended herself, she couldn't trust that he understood how his behavior was affecting her—what effects it could have on her own self-respect, on her well-being and that of their children. His jealousy no longer felt loving and respectful, and that could make it difficult for her to reciprocate love and respect. She added that Francisco was very romantic and used to say the following in Spanish: "I hope you don't doubt my love. I no longer must conquer the sky. Since I've already gotten my little star, you're the most important thing in my life. For me, you are and will ever be everything, my moon, my star." She said, "At that time, I felt that it was love, but if he said the same thing today, I couldn't believe him."

Francisco understood that Piedad was wavering in her trust of him and that perhaps, by disentangling love from jealousy, she was asking him for a different form of love. He seemed to take her position seriously and instead of asserting his entitlement to jealousy as he had before, he now said he wished he could stop it. But it wasn't easy. When he was seized by doubt, his feelings of threat were so intense that he feared a heart attack. He described his heart racing, his eyesight becoming blurred, his blood pressure mounting, his anxiety so intense that it felt like panic. I wondered aloud if they were both seized by a tyranny of jealousy (*la tiranía de los celos*), by which I meant that they were both oppressed. They agreed that jealousy was a heavy burden for them and for their children, too. Piedad was very relieved by Francisco's acknowledgment that he had to do something about his jealousy problem, though he wasn't truly apologetic or accountable for the injustice she suffered. But one could for the first time envision his vulnerability. Piedad brought back the idea that church might have a calming effect on him, as it does for her. Francisco appeared reluctant or dismissive of this idea, but I supported him by saying how remarkable it was that he did want to do something about his "jealousy problem." But what could help? Did he have any ideas about how to cope with the intense effects of his suspicions? He ventured that deep breaths and leaving the scene might do something. I supported these ideas. (I responded by telling a little story from my professional past. I had a Norwegian professor who told us that in his country, when a husband was upset or angry, he left to walk in the woods, sometimes for many hours or days. When he came back, he had resolved his feelings on his own.) I added that, as a young psychologist, I thought everything had to be talked out. But now, I think that not everything in marriage can be clarified by talking or by confrontation. Sometimes one must just let go. I was honest, but I did this purposefully, as I thought Francisco depended too much on Piedad's reassurances, a dependency that probably perpetuated her oppression. Indeed, I saw Piedad wincing (with annoyance?) whenever she talked about how he turned to her (pestering?) with questionings. Perhaps she wanted him to go to church to relieve these pressures on her. I thought it could be useful for him individually and relationally to rely more on his own soothing capacity.

In this intermediate phase, I wanted to return to the possible effects of race or skin color or social class on their relationship. Since they had not responded to my previous question on the topic, I felt I must state my viewpoint rather than assume they would understand why I ask. Most people think that therapy is about inner lives and an interpersonal dynamic independent from sociopolitical contexts, so I locate myself with some version of the following: "You may wonder why I asked the question about race, skin color, and class. It's because, as a psychologist, I think there's an unjustified and unfair prejudice in most societies about skin color—darker people suffer more obstacles and must deal with more racism than White people. This situation causes stress and suffering even if people don't talk about it. I wonder if you agree with that and, if so, how have those stressors affected the two of you?"

Perhaps Francisco didn't feel safe to bring the effects of colorism and racism into his awareness or in this therapy setting, with his wife and a White therapist. Or perhaps he was exercising cultural resistance when he answered that he was proud of his brown color, his *sangre de indio*, his "Indian blood," the blood of noble men, just like his father and brothers. He said his worry about being discriminated against centered on his occupation and socioeconomic class relative to Piedad's family. He was a farmer and so was his father. Growing up, they lived on the farm and his mother washed the clothes of her 14 children in a big old sink outdoors, whereas Piedad's family had a business and lived in a house in town and the mother had help. He always thought that Piedad's family thought they had Spanish blood (associated with whiteness in Mexico) and felt that she had married down; he never felt comfortable around them. Piedad had heard before how Francisco felt about her family's acceptance of her marriage to him, but she minimized his feelings, saying that he was exaggerating. It was hard for me to know if she couldn't validate Francisco's experience of color and class to protect him from the pain of rejection by his in-laws—or whether she was protecting her family of origin by not revealing their color and class allocations of inequality among family members, a rather common favoritism toward family members of lighter skin.

Piedad had never validated Francisco's perceptions of discrimination. I asked her if she were to think further about this issue of class difference and its effects on them, what kinds of things would come to her mind? She said that she was 20 years old when she met Francisco and she was mesmerized by him—he was tall, good looking, and confident. He worked hard with his father on the farm and was likely to become a good provider, as he certainly did become. "I didn't think my parents would object but, yes, they may have had reservations about our marriage early on." She was quick to insist that now everybody in her family knows that Francisco *nos cuida a todos nosotros*. Translated literally, this would be "He takes care of all of us," but this may not say it all. In Spanish, it could mean "He nurtures us, he protects us, he supports us materially." Indeed, Francisco's caring showed remarkable family dedication. Piedad's statement that there were early objections to her marriage to him validated his feelings of discrimination. The addition of current family views about Francisco's contributions to family well-being was, of course, a more empowering relational narrative than the rejection he feared from his in-laws. It was likely that Francisco had always felt insecure about his class status, his education and manners, his poorer background relative to Piedad. He must have always felt threatened, perhaps by the unlikely possibility that she would leave him for a higher-status candidate, but even more so, if he became physically impaired and less able to "take care" of all of them. His control of her via jealousy might have always been an expression of his insecurity while also exerting his *hombría*, his "masculine power." Piedad, on the other hand, appeared to have fallen in love with him when young in part because his adoring passion fulfilled a scarcity of nurturance from her parents. As a privileged person, she may have been less sensitive to the sufferings of socioeconomic inequality.

CONCLUDING PHASE OF THERAPY

We were approaching the time when the couple had to return to Mexico. Their tensions with each other appeared to have decreased, and they reported having spent time walking and talking about the topics we had covered in the session. Piedad mentioned that while they didn't want to lose the romantic aspects of love, they were still talking about whether jealousy was a demonstration of love or a distortion of love. I mentioned to Francisco that, in the previous session, Piedad clearly showed more appreciation for many other qualities in him than for the purported jealousy as love. Could he name what was meaningful to her about him? What was good for her? What did she appreciate? Could he think of qualities that she valued as caring for her and the family? Interestingly, he couldn't come up with any self-descriptions, positive or negative. He felt that therapy conversations pushed him to move from action to thought, that he had to think and talk more than he ever did; he had never been prudent or analytic, but perhaps he needed to be. He finally said, "True, I'm a very hard worker, but without my back I can't work, and I don't know if we can live with dignity if we depend on my son's work." Francisco and Piedad had never talked about the impact of his back injury and his retirement on his self-esteem and on their relationship.

Even before I had time to invite them to a fuller discussion of these topics, Francisco added, "Now even the children are against me, naturally preferring their mother. They're even hinting that they might keep her here and won't let her go back with me." I had no idea about this, so I said, "Really? Did you know about this, Piedad?"

She hesitated and replied, "Yes, Lucía and Adela [the other daughter] asked a friend who had a therapist friend, and from her they got the idea that it would be better for me to stay here in San Diego. I told them I wasn't doing that, that I was going home with Francisco. But I didn't know that Lucía had told her father about this idea." At first, I wondered if Francisco had come to therapy motivated by the daughters' threat—but I quickly realized it didn't matter how he came to therapy. So, I turned to ask Piedad how she felt when the daughters suggested she stay with them. She answered, "My home is with Francisco, and I want to be with him in peace." I asked Francisco if Piedad's answer affirmed her commitment to him—indeed, he hadn't known that she refused their daughters' plan and wanted instead to come to therapy with him.

We talked about how their relationship will continue in their hometown with Francisco being home more. Could they work together to anticipate situations that might lead to jealousy? How can love be expressed in other ways? What do men who work less than before do in their town? Could he remain as a consultant to the son in the business?

A typical question I ask at the end of therapy is how they would handle a relapse—a reappearance of the symptom or pattern that was disturbing to them. Francisco said half-jokingly, "Ah, do you [looking at me] want me to be a *mandilón* [a Mexican slang word for a henpecked, submissive, or compliant man, fearful of the wife] all the time?"

I answered, "No, I know that you're a strong and dignified man who is deeply valued by your wife and children, so why let yourself be oppressed by the tyranny of jealousy, which may rear its ugly head at times, for example, when you fear being criticized by other men?" Piedad said she worried that Francisco might get the wrong interpretation about something she did innocently. But it would help her to think about what we talked about in therapy, that he doesn't own her, and that she wants to be loved with respect and love him with respect. They both asked, "How about we call you if we have another flare-up?"

I replied, "Yes, you can do that, but let's think about whether there's something the two of you can do that will be sort of like therapy." We came up with the idea that every Sunday evening, they would sit down and review the week, and if there was anything that happened that provoked his insecurity or his jealousy, he would talk with Piedad about it. And if there were any times during the week when she needed more respect and space from him, she would say it.

Francisco and Piedad stayed married. They both agreed that they loved each other better this way, albeit with less dramatic passion. They planned to spend more time together in their hometown and for Francisco to remain involved in the business without doing any heavy work, but advising the son and seeing that things were done the way they were when he was the sole proprietor. Their children appeared to feel comfortable with the progress their parents made and the safety of their mother. They happily agreed to their parents' return to their hometown and making plans to gradually increase their visits to San Diego.

FURTHER REFLECTIONS AND IMPLICATIONS

It took me a while to feel comfortable working with this couple. Despite similarities in language and a rather close understanding of culture between us, I felt some initial tension. Several factors may have contributed to this. Therapy wasn't a known place for them, so we needed to find the right tempo to develop trust and ease. They accepted therapy to appease their adult children, and only at the end did I find out there was a threat of separation for this couple instigated by their daughters. Because of the couple's generation and their social and geographical location, there was a clear configuration of patriarchy. Capozzi (2022), in a useful typology of men and patriarchy, writes about stereotypical masculinity in referring to men who embrace gender normative masculinity views with no awareness of the personal privilege and power inequality those views endorse. In these cases, she claims therapy is unlikely to penetrate this ideology. In fact, in my experience, some of those men may even claim that it is women who exert power over men. Some women in these rigidly patriarchal arrangements may also consider the power imbalance as "the natural order of things."

For myself and perhaps other clinicians, particularly women, entering clinical situations of possessive jealousy in patriarchal contexts may be fraught with negative emotions and even judgments. I was aware that I needed to choose my words carefully to ensure their cultural safety in help seeking rather than defensiveness or distance. I considered what would be helpful versus unhelpful paths. If I had said to Francisco that his drive to dominate and control Piedad is based on *machismo*, I might run the risk of justifying his behavior as culturally dictated and therefore common or even acceptable, including in the eyes of both partners. On the other hand, if I had expressed even subtly my disapproval of patriarchal entitlements, I could be seen as critical of Francisco at a time when he is already being accused by his own children and his wife. (See my 2010 discussion of machismo as a denigrating attribution of dominant cultures toward Mexicans and the need to consider greater complexity about Latinx masculinities, a complexity that allows for transformative uses of culture in clinical practice).

In my work with Latinx couples in traditional patriarchal arrangements, I often talk about gender and love before addressing gender and power. I do so, fully cognizant that gender power differentials organize multiple aspects of marriage, and even more so in traditional hierarchies. However, using a language of love rather than one of power shifts the focus to emotions, a topic at the heart of Latinx values. Talking about love decreases the distance and polarization associated with conversations about power. Romesin and Verden-Zöller (2009) encourage a legitimization of conversations about collaboration, help, sharing, and security as a counterpart to the language of domination, authority, and power valued in patriarchal societies. Some therapists, confronted with rigid, traditional gender dynamics, equate the woman's agency with leaving and her staying as victimization, as we saw in the advice given by a therapist to Piedad's daughters. This is a simplistic traditional approach. Instead, I favor third-wave intersectional feminism grounded in anti-oppressive, nonviolent, and socially just practices, and therefore question reductive essentialist arguments that suggest patriarchy is the only cause behind jealousy as a form of gender violence. This position embraces a variety of explanations and treatment options (George & Stith, 2014). It's important for clinicians to honor complex forms of agency when women demonstrate it in gendered relationships, as is the case in many immigrant groups. In Piedad's case, I could support and amplify those actions that showed her ability to be an agent of change in her own life while attempting to preserve couple and family unity. I must confess that I chuckled when I heard about the daughters' offering Piedad shelter from persecutory jealousy in their homes. I have three grown daughters, and I know they've empowered me to stand up to gender injustices while acknowledging our diverse gendered upbringings. Cultures, of course, are generational and fluid, not fixed.

I considered whether a narrative of externalization of jealousy might be a helpful way for Francisco to resist his bouts of jealousy. But I worried a little over two possible effects that might have on this couple with their mutual adherence to patriarchy. First, it might imply that Francisco's behavior toward Piedad was individual and not relational, although sociopolitically based. And second, that externalization might give the erroneous impression that Francisco was less responsible and accountable for his behavior. I decided to label jealousy as a tyranny that oppressed the couple without discussing the patriarchal or colonized ideology that supported it.

Piedad had eased the way to bring up exceptions to negative uses of power of domination and adulation. She described Francisco as an excellent father, who had raised his daughters without imposing his authority excessively; he had listened to her when she objected to physically disciplining their boys, and he was compassionate and loving to other people in his community. In retrospect, I wonder if I could have suggested meditation groups as a calming space for the stresses caused by jealousy or for Francisco alone, since Piedad had the church as a calming space. For more than a decade, mindfulness groups have gained popularity among Latin American immigrants, men, and women, and it is the type of intervention that would have gained the approval of their children. If they return to San Diego and to therapy in the future, I may encourage Francisco to attend a men's group called *El Hombre Noble* ("The Noble Man") that takes place in Los Angeles, but virtually as well. These groups focus on creating awareness about the contradictory identity expectations Latino men internalize, and how to discover in oneself healthy cultural values and honorable roots inherent in precolonial Latino masculinity, in contrast to what the group leader, Jerry Tello (2019), dubs as "toxic masculinity."

Information from my MECA-guided assessment provided a helpful lens on other sociopolitical inequalities. In addition to the gender inequality in a patriarchal setting, the intersecting oppressions and lived experiences of Francisco and Piedad were quite different. While they shared language and nationality, there was cultural diversity and even more so, social inequality in their histories. We could speak of their marriage as being akin to an intermarriage in which Francisco lived with fears of feeling diminished in Piedad's extended family's higher social circles and, even at a deeper level, a dread of losing her to a more attractive suitor. Once a more empathic framework evolved, it was possible for me to understand Francisco's distressed emotions without endorsing his oppressive actions toward his wife. I also viewed that Piedad's acceptance of his behavior was based in part on her own need to fulfill love absences in her growing up. One could view these mutual vulnerabilities as anchoring their interactional perceptions of jealousy as love, a perception that needed their reflectivity (Scheinkman & Werneck, 2010).

There is abundant evidence that Mexicans and other people of color in Latin America suffer external and internalized racism. Mexican men often make a point of introducing themselves as having a father or grandfather who was Spanish or even Italian or French, tacitly implying racial superiority—as though just being Mexican may indicate being indigenous and therefore of less status than someone from a White European background. In the 1960s, the Chicano movement labeled this wish to be White as "colonized mentality" and more recently has been seen as "internalized colorism" (Adames & Chavez-Dueñas, 2017). Had I continued to work with this couple, I might have been able to broach again the issue of how skin color and racism was a significant dynamic in their interactions. At the end of the therapy, when they brought me a family photo, I referred to color indirectly saying that they had beautiful children and that some of them looked like Piedad and others like Francisco. I felt it had been productive earlier in the therapy when bringing up skin color allowed Francisco to speak about the impact of social class inequality on his self-esteem when he sensed that Piedad's family of origin had reservations about approving the marriage.

One issue remained slightly worrisome in my posttherapy thoughts. I believe that Francisco understood that his jealousy was destroying the possibility of a continuing relationship with his wife and children, particularly his daughters, but how repentant was he? Unfortunately, at no point did he show empathy for Piedad or the suffering she had endured. Perhaps the relationship with her was the only place he thought he could still display his dominance by not admitting wrongdoing. Could he erupt into jealousy or violence as he progressively lost more social power through limitations of health and socioeconomic status? If I were to have an opportunity to work with them again or for a longer time, I would have had one or more individual meetings focused on information and prevention with each one, as I usually do when there is any hint of danger of oppression or of violence.

Couples' presentations of jealousy and possessive love come to our attention typically framed in the context of individual or relationship characteristics. However, it is likely that jealousy, with its interpersonal intrusive demand and despair, is a symptom of a much larger malaise that includes inequalities of gender, race, and class that require future collective sociopolitical and cultural change. In our work as couple therapists, we must acquire tools, such as MECA, to understand how sociocultural diversity and inequities are intertwined with individual and relational distress. Acknowledging our own intersectional locations can help us become sensitive to power and ethics with cultural humility. Only then we can help make visible and learn to dialogue about these issues both in the intimacy of the private hour, and in the public institutional domains where issues of gender, race, and class inequality contribute to the perpetuation of individual, family, and societal suffering. At all levels, activism lies in transforming relationships of domination to partnership systems.

REFERENCES

Adames, H. Y., & Chavez-Duenas, N. Y. (2017). *Cultural foundations and interventions in Latino/a mental health: History, theory and within-group differences.* New York: Routledge.

Capozzi, F. (2022). A multi-level guide to work with male clients in couple and family therapy from a gender-critical perspective. *Journal of Feminist Family Therapy, 34,* 178–195.

Falicov, C. J. (2010). Changing constructions of machismo for Latino men in therapy: "The devil never sleeps." *Family Process, 49,* 309–329.

Falicov, C. J. (2014). *Latino families in therapy* (2nd ed.). New York: Guilford Press.

Falicov, C. J. (2017a). Multidimensional ecosystemic comparative approach (MECA). In J. L. Lebow, A. L. Chambers, & D. C. Breunlin (Eds.), *Encyclopedia of couple and family therapy* (pp. 1–5). New York: Springer.

Falicov, C. J. (2017b). Latino/Latinas in couple and family therapy. In J. L. Lebow, A. L. Chambers, & D. C. Breunlin (Eds.), *Encyclopedia of couple and family therapy* (pp. 1–7). New York: Springer.

George, J., & Stith, S. M. (2014). An updated feminist view of intimate partner violence. *Family Process, 53,* 179–193.

Romesin, H. M., & Verden-Zöller, G. (2009). *The origin of humanness in the biology of love.* Exeter, UK: Imprint Academic.

Scheinkman, M., & Werneck, D. (2010) Disarming jealousy in couples relationships: A multidimensional approach. *Family Process, 49,* 486–502.

Tello, J. (2019). *Recovering your sacredness.* Hacienda Heights, CA: Sueños Publications.

CHAPTER 11

Therapy with Intercultural and Interfaith Couples

REENEE SINGH

> *Editors' Comments*
>
> Reenee Singh offers in this chapter a wonderful example of how to work with multicultural couples. As she points out in her introduction, today's couples are increasingly multicultural. While life of a couple in prior generations largely consisted of pair bonding within cultural enclaves, the 21st century has made such considerations about partner selection fairly low in importance, leaving many couples with the challenge of figuring out how to navigate such differences.
>
> Singh provides a superb road map to such exploration. She offers specific tools to facilitate this process—the cultural genogram and the culturegram—that help articulate the cultural underpinnings of individual and family experience. She shows us how to bring a focus on culture into couple therapy, and how to place it in the context of the overall therapeutic process. She writes not only from the position of a therapist and trainer who has spent a lifetime working with intercultural couples but also from the lived experience of intercultural life. She shares the benefits of both her professional and personal experiences in her work with Ali and Rachel.
>
> Singh also emphasizes that intercultural therapy is not only about culture but it also needs to be grounded in a deep understanding of culture and the therapist's interface with the cultures represented in the couple. This combines with the understanding of other key aspects of couples' lives, such as the intersection of race, country of origin, gender, social class, and faith traditions and the like, as well as across different life experiences. And while Singh offers a compelling example of intercultural facets in a man of Pakistani origin and Muslim faith and a White English woman, it is important to keep in focus that the same understanding of culture is also important in couples who may be less different in cultural origin; that is, whatever differences there are in culture still often make a substantial difference to couples, and may be even more important to their extended families. From this perspective, Singh's narrative of intercultural couple therapy has broad application when "culture" is extended as well to the specific cultures of gender, generational cohort, or other aspects of intersectionality, such as urban versus

> rural upbringing, liberal versus conservative affiliations, and myriad other facets of social as well as psychological location.
>
> Finally, Singh's chapter can also be approached as a fine example of the sorts of issues that can emerge at the birth of a first child, a time when a new set of issues comes to the fore for most couples.

I watched, transfixed, the recent Netflix series *Harry & Meghan*. Although Harry and Meghan (the Duke and Duchess of Sussex) are different from the many interracial, transnational couples that I work with because of the extreme privilege of their positions, the themes in their relationship—such as the meaning of home, family, and belonging—echo the themes in my clients' relationships.

Harry & Meghan is not only a "modern fairy tale" but also a family drama of our times—a tale of transgenerational trauma, the effects of parental separation and divorce on children, sibling rivalries and family estrangements, and the uneasy hold of media and social media on public opinion. The racial, cultural, class, and national differences between Harry and Meghan seem to be subsumed by a consideration of the complex and intergenerational family dynamics of the Royal Family of which they were a part and the wider contexts of Britain and America in the 21st century. Hence, an examination of 21st-century contexts of mass migration, technological advances, and changing social mores and attitudes is essential to an understanding of the intercultural couples with whom we work (Singh, Killian, Bhugun, & Tseng, 2020). Perhaps the tension between traditional and contemporary contexts and values, and the ways in which different actors in the system are positioned and copositioned within these competing discourses are among the most striking features of the Harry and Meghan story.

My fascination with intercultural couples goes back a long way, far before Harry and Meghan's story. My parents were an interfaith couple, my father a Sikh, although estranged from his family for cutting his hair and marrying my mother, who was Hindu and Sindhi. They spoke different languages and had different cultural traditions but were united in the fact that they were both refugees from what is now Pakistan. They created a home together in newly independent India, forged a shared linguistic system comprising mostly Hindi and English, and a hybrid culinary system, with strong Anglo influences.

As a child, surrounded by monocultural couples and families, in a land that was still dominated by arranged marriages and strictures regarding marriage outside caste and community, I was somewhat confused by my "mixed" identity. In my adult life, I found myself drawn to difference and my romantic relationships were invariably across class, religious, national, racial, and cultural boundaries.

When my husband (who is White, English) and I ran into problems, we sought couple therapy from a psychodynamic couple psychotherapist. Although the experience was valuable, little attention was paid to the racial and cultural differences between us. My experiences of racism were dismissed as being "overly sensitive." I realized that our therapist was working from a Eurocentric model of couple relationships, which she assumed was universal. This experience inspired me to set up the London Intercultural Couples Centre in 2016, which was intended to provide a space for intercultural couples to talk about their unique challenges, while acknowledging and recognizing their resiliencies and strengths.

In London, according to the 2021 census, one in four households (22.3%) comprises more than one ethnic group. London, a multicultural city, is not representative of the rest of England, where in 10.1% (2.5 million) of households in England and Wales, two or more ethnic groups were represented. This is an increase from 2011 (8.7%, 2.0 million). The figures are similarly high for other parts of the Western world. In the United States, almost four in 10 (39%) of Americans who have been married since 2010 have been to those from different ethnic/cultural groups, and according to the Australian Bureau of Statistics (2017), about 28% of couples were Anglo-Australian born with overseas-born partners. In other parts of the world, too, the number of transnational and interethnic couples is increasing; for example, in Singapore, one in three marriages is between a Singaporean and nonresident. It is important to understand that intercultural couples mean different things in different cultures—for example, in Italy, it could mean a North–South divide. Furthermore, not every intercultural couple is troubled, and not every concern presented by an intercultural couple has to do with intercultural differences. As with any other group, we have to adopt a "both–and" perspective, understanding that cultural difference is *one* lens through which to view couple relationships and eschewing a tendency to reify and pathologize difference.

The idea of cross-cultural marriages was introduced to systemic family therapy by Celia Falicov (1995), and other authors since then have highlighted the themes and processes present in intercultural and interracial couple relationships. In addition to drawing on ideas from such eminent scholars in the field, as my work at the London Intercultural Couple Centre developed, my collaboration with Janet Reibstein evolved into the *intercultural Exeter model* (Reibstein & Singh, 2021).

Around the same time, I was strongly influenced by Valeria Ugazio's (2013) theory of semantic polarities and positions within families. The theory posits that families and couples construct their conversations through semantic polarities—that is, through opposite meanings, and with all members taking up positions within these meanings. The four semantics that predominate are semantics of freedom, belonging, good, and power. Ugazio and I, with a number of research associates and students in Italy and the United Kingdom, became interested in exploring how intercultural couples negotiate the differences in meaning that may emerge in their conversations, ways of interpreting the world, and interactions. The findings from our small-scale research study seemed to indicate that semantics of freedom, belonging, and power predominate in intercultural couples, and that problems appear to arise when the partners in the couple come from different semantic worlds (Lugli, Kalaydjian, Atkas, Lerussi, & Singh, 2022). Although it is beyond the scope of this chapter to offer an in-depth analysis of the findings from this research, the study has provided a framework for my understanding of the dynamics, processes, and interactions within intercultural couples.

INITIAL ASSESSMENT AND CASE FORMULATION

Ali and Rachel were referred to me by a psychiatrist colleague who specializes in working with perinatal women and refers a number of pregnant women and their husbands/partners to me for couple therapy. At the time of referral, Ali was 35, from a South Asian

(Pakistani) Muslim background, and Rachel was a 32-year-old English woman. Rachel was suffering from symptoms of anxiety and depression, and she attributed her symptoms to the difficulties she and Ali had with his extended family. Although the pregnancy was planned, Rachel did not anticipate such a quick conception and felt immediately plunged into anxiety when her pregnancy was confirmed at 6 weeks.

Ali has a medical background and works as a physician in the area of tropical medicine. He is ambitious and driven. His parents, both doctors, were migrants from India who had come to the United Kingdom in the 1980s to pursue further education and career opportunities. He has a younger sister who is a math teacher in an inner-city London school. Rachel's parents live in the country and, in contrast with Ali's parents, are artists and somewhat eccentric. Rachel studied history of art at university and is currently working at a museum in London. She has two sisters, one of whom is a musician and the other, a social worker.

After my initial conversation with my psychiatrist colleague, I hypothesized that religion played a role in Rachel and Ali's difficulties. I wondered if Rachel had converted to Islam in order to marry Ali and whether one of the current strains in their relationship had to do with the expectations for their child to be brought up in the Islamic faith. My hypotheses were based on my work with many interfaith couples, particularly when one partner is Muslim. Pregnancy is a challenging time for any couple but perhaps even more so when religious and cultural differences come to the fore during this life cycle transition.

I wondered how I should position myself—apparently the couple was happy to be referred to a couple therapist from a South Asian background. They'd had previous experiences of couple therapy with an English therapist and had not found it helpful. At the same time, I was aware that one of the main differences between me and Ali was religion, as I am not Muslim. Furthermore, would Rachel see me as more allied with Ali than with her, because of our shared South Asian heritage?

After an exchange of emails and a brief phone call with Ali (who seemed to be assigned the role of setting up appointments with professionals), I met with the couple for the initial assessment. As they came into my consulting room, I was struck by how beautiful they looked together—Ali presented as dark, sauve, and sophisticated and Rachel as an "English rose"—blond, petite, and visibly pregnant.

Creating a Safe Context to Bring Up Race and Racism

In a chapter I coauthored with Kyle Killian, he offered these wise thoughts: "Love and prejudice can coexist within the same relationship, and it is sometimes the task of the clinician working with intercultural couples to provide a safe context in which the partners can explore the unsaid, without fear of being judged as racist by their partner or their therapist" (Singh et al., 2020, p. 167). I drew on Kyle Killian's words in my early work with Ali and Rachel in order to create a safe space to discuss differences and similarities, keeping in mind the wider contexts of Islamophobia and racism in Britain.

Hence, after a brief conversation about the referral process, pregnancy, and the couple's due date (5 months away from our first session), I started my initial assessment session with Ali and Rachel by exploring racial and cultural difference. I used my own similarity and difference from the couple, saying, "Although I am of Indian origin, I am not Muslim, and there may be many things I don't know and don't understand about Islam, Ali. Please, could I check with you from time to time to see if I am getting it right?" And then, turning to Rachel, I asked, "What does it mean to you to be working with a South Asian therapist? There might be times during the course of our work when you feel that I am more allied with Ali than with you because we share a cultural heritage. Please do stop me at any point if you feel I am not being neutral or not understanding things from your perspective. I am a woman and a mother, and perhaps these shared experiences will help you to feel comfortable working with me."

Rachel and Ali seemed to respond well to my positioning within the complex, intercultural therapeutic system we were creating. Ali talked openly about his experiences of "otherness" and institutional racism, about being stopped and searched at airports, and the racist bullying and harassment his mother had experienced at work. Rachel talked about how she struggled to understand Ali's rage about these issues and felt that it was being directed toward her, as a White person. Although she acknowledged her White privilege, she was deeply hurt by her perception of the way in which Ali's parents and elder relatives positioned her, as a *Memsahib*—a reminder of India's colonial past.

Listening to Ali and Rachel put me in mind of my own experiences of being in an interracial couple relationship. I could relate to Ali's experiences of open discrimination and racism at airports and on the streets and the microaggressions in the workplace. It reminded me of the loneliness of being the only brown face in all-White country pubs, subject to the hostility of staff that may never have encountered an interracial couple. Their arguments echoed discussions I have had with my husband about colonialism and the British empire, discussions that sometimes end in misunderstandings, hurt feelings, and even helpless rage.

When Rachel and Ali had first met online, just before the COVID-19 pandemic, religious differences did not come up between them. Rachel had grown up outside London in a small village in East Sussex and was not used to racial and religious diversity until she moved to London about 5 years ago. Although she now had a few friends who were not White and English, she did not pay much heed to race and racism, and was saddened by the fact that some of her friends and family had been prejudiced toward Ali, because he is Muslim.

Rachel was quick to offer her own experiences of being discriminated as a woman, as an equivalent to Ali's experiences of racial/religious discrimination, and I suggested that she be able to listen to his experiences without feeling guilty or responsible.

Toward the end of the initial assessment, I coached them both in an active listening exercise—for Ali to take on an "I" position about his experiences of racism without blaming or holding Rachel responsible, for her to paraphrase and then have her turn. Ali was able to describe how much harder he had to work than his colleagues in order to prove his worth at work. Rachel was able to express her own anger on Ali's behalf, saying, "I know how clever you are and I feel so angry when this is not recognized. . . . I feel guilty that life is so easy for me and that I am completely accepted at work." This exercise, introduced in the initial assessment, helped them both to slow down, suspend judgment, and genuinely hear each other's experiences. As a homework task, I asked them to practice this exercise at home for 5 minutes every day, starting with something as innocuous as how their day had been.

In line with my initial hypothesis, the presenting problem of Rachel's anxiety and depression was linked to the religious differences between them and their families. Ali's family was liberal, and he described them as more culturally than religiously Muslim. Ali drank alcohol and did not fast during the Ramadan season. Although there was some pressure on Rachel to convert to Islam in order to marry Ali, they both resisted the pressure and did not have to go through a *Nikah* (Islamic marriage ceremony). However, Ali and his family were clear that Ali's children would be brought up within the Islamic faith, which meant circumcision if they had a male child. Both Ali and Rachel recognized, as soon as the pregnancy was confirmed, that they could not hold out any longer; they would have to concede to the wishes of Ali's family. Rachel was prone to anxiety and now began to be immensely fearful of herself and her unborn baby being subsumed within Ali's extended family and religion. She felt that there would be no place for her ties to her own family and culture, and that her identity would be taken over. Ali, on the other hand, felt torn between his parents' expectations and Rachel's. As the only son, he was close to his parents and felt strongly allied to their struggles as migrants to the United Kingdom. He was also close to many of his relatives in Pakistan and India, and wanted Rachel to be accepted by his extended family. He was worried about her mental health and well-being during pregnancy, and wanted to protect her from what she experienced as pressure from his parents.

Visual Assessment Tools

With intercultural couples, especially when English is not the first language of one of the partners, I often employ visual methods such as the cultural genogram and culturegram (Reibstein & Singh, 2021). As part of the assessment, I co-constructed a cultural genogram with Ali and Rachel (see Figure 11.1). Although I use such tools as part of the assessment process, I often revisit them in later stages of the work to understand and unpack emerging themes.

BEGINNING PHASE OF THERAPY

There was an overlap between the assessment and beginning phase (Sessions 2–4) in which I used the two visual techniques of the cultural genogram and culturegram to help Rachel and Ali understand each other's cultural heritage, beliefs, and values.

Cultural Genogram

I was mindful that embarking on the cultural genogram exercise could evoke complicated feelings associated with transgenerational themes, and that it was important to ensure that the couple was prepared to do this. Rachel was at the beginning of her second trimester at the time. She was in good health and stabilized on antianxiety medication. During the course of my work with the couple, I would touch base with my psychiatrist colleague from time to time to make sure that Rachel was not too distressed. The early sessions were held weekly, as the couple was keen to engage and work through their issues before their baby was born.

During the second session, I began by co-constructing Ali's cultural genogram. In doing so, I was mindful that I was anticipating that his cultural genogram would be more complicated than Rachel's. However, my rationale for starting with his genogram was to help the couple grapple with and understand his transgenerational context, as they attributed the problems in their relationship to difficulties in their relationships with Ali's family.

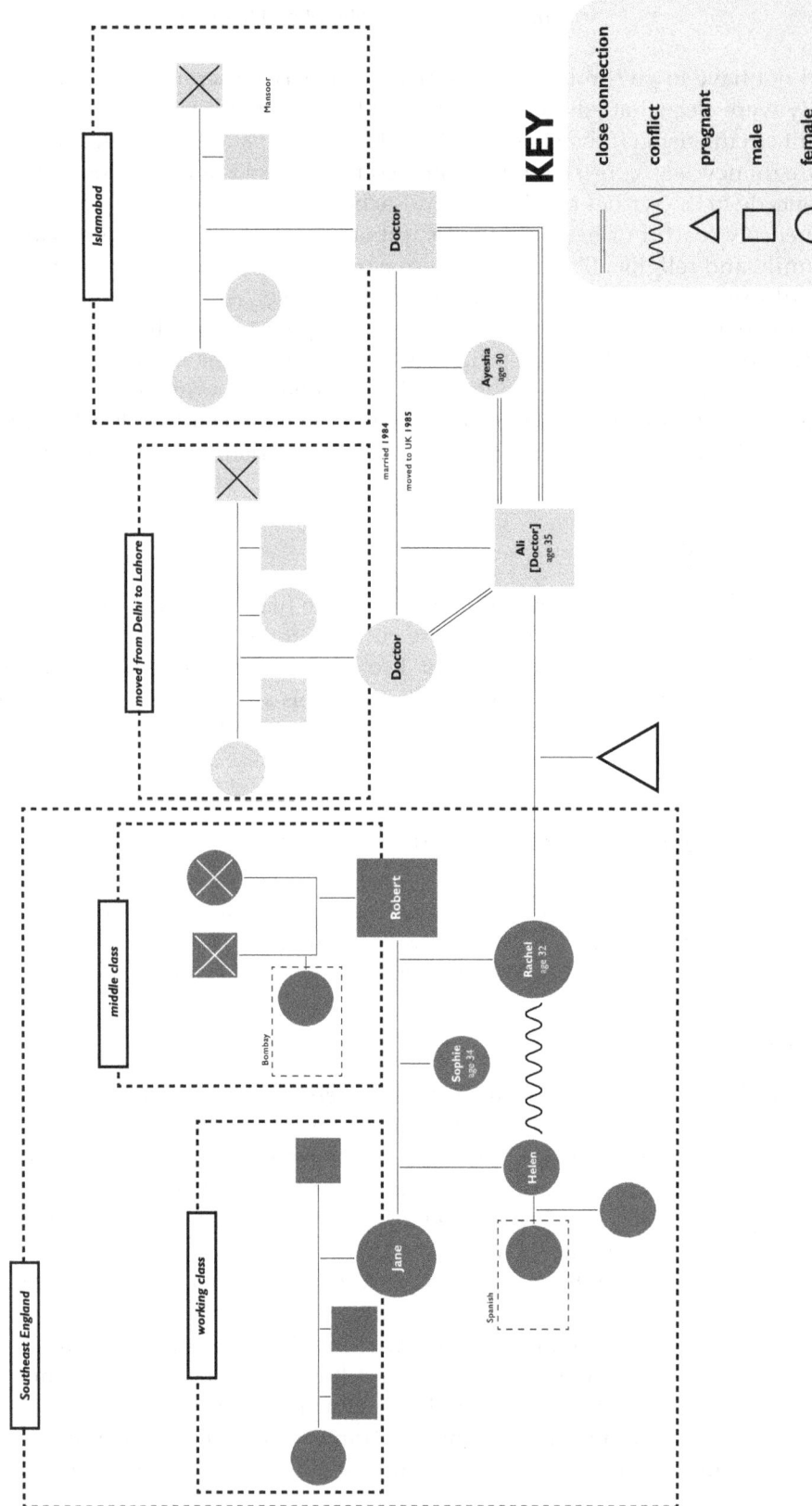

FIGURE 11.1. Rachel and Ali's cultural genogram.

Ali felt closer to his mother and her family than he did to his father's family. His maternal grandfather was a doctor in the British army, and both maternal grandparents had fled from Delhi to Lahore, during the partition of India in 1947. They had started life afresh in Pakistan and had missed their ancestral home, possessions, and friends. Ali's paternal grandparents had not had similar experiences of displacement, as they had always lived in Islamabad. Nevertheless, they had experienced the horrors of partition and witnessed the atrocities committed against friends and neighbors. Hence, both of Ali's parents had been brought up in the shadow of the Partition of Pakistan and India.

Ali's parents met in medical college in Islamabad and, after a period of courtship and with the consent of both families, they got married in 1984. In search of better economic opportunities, they migrated to the United Kingdom together in 1985. Apart from a distant cousin in Birmingham, they had no relatives in the United Kingdom and had created a family and built up a community of colleagues and friends in their new country. They kept in touch with their families back home, and Ali's early memories are of going back to Islamabad, Lahore, and Chandigarh to visit his parents' families. As I was co-constructing Ali's cultural genogram, I used different colors to depict his two sets of grandparents, to denote that although both sets were Pakistani, one set of grandparents was refugees from India and the other had always lived in Pakistan. Ali and his sister had been born and grew up in the United Kingdom. They considered the United Kingdom their home but also had close ties with Pakistan, where most of their relatives lived.

Through co-constructing Rachel's cultural genogram, we realized that home had a different meaning for her than it did for Ali. Generations of Rachel's family had lived in southeast England, apart from a great-aunt, who had grown up during Colonial times in Bombay. Rachel's sisters had always been more adventurous than she. Sophie, a concert pianist, was based in London but toured the world. The other, Helen, had a Spanish partner, and they had a home in Spain. Rachel had a conflictual relationship with her, which appeared to be about her perception of Helen as "bossy." Rachel was deeply connected to both her parents and, as the youngest, had struggled to leave home. Although both parents described themselves as "English," there was a class divide between them. Rachel's mother's family was working class, from the East End of London, where her grandfather ran a grocery store. Rachel's paternal grandfather, on the other hand, was a Vicar, and her paternal grandmother was a schoolteacher. All her aunts and uncles on her father's side were professionals and somewhat conservative. Rachel's father had been talented at art and had escaped to art school in London in the 1970s, where he had met Rachel's mother. Rachel's mother had told her about the struggles of being accepted by her father's family. Her accent and working-class habits were frowned upon, and it had taken her a long time to become "posh."

What effect did it have on me to hear Ali's and Rachel's stories? Although I could relate to aspects of Rachel's stories, having grown up with two sisters, I felt more closely allied with Ali's story. My heart ached for Ali's grandmother, who had gone through the trauma of leaving her home and traveling on one of the many trains that brought refugees from Delhi to Lahore. The image of this train is vivid in my mind as my mother, whose family members were refugees in the other direction (from Pakistan to Delhi) would recount the harrowing story of their escape from Pakistan. I acknowledged that this must have been traumatic for his grandparents' family, sharing that my parents had been refugees, too, without going into much detail.

I explored the theme of transgenerational trauma in Ali's family and asked, "What effect do you think it had on your mother, that her family had to move from India to Pakistan, during the Partition?"

Ali replied, "My mother doesn't really talk about it, but I know that my *Nanaji* and *Naniji* [maternal grandparents] suffered significant losses. They lost a lot of their ancestral wealth, as they had to leave their land and home behind and start from scratch. . . . They began to speak in Urdu, whereas in India they would speak more Hindustani or Punjabi. They always longed for life back in Delhi, saying that the fruit was much tastier, as were the samosas! My mother would talk, though, about how her and my father's early days in the United Kingdom were similar to being a refugee, although she knew there were important differences. Like her own parents, she felt that she had sacrificed a lot to come to this country and settling down here was hard. . . . This affected me, too, in that I felt protective of my parents and would intervene on their behalf. Although my father's family remained in Islamabad, my *Dada* and *Dadiji* (paternal grandparents) spoke, too, about Partition and how traumatic it was to see their friends and neighbors being killed by rival groups on the streets." His story resonated with me. "Yes, I have heard and read accounts of this terrible time in history, too."

I then turned to Rachel and asked, "What is it like for you to listen to these stories?"

"Somehow I start feeling responsible," she said. "I am aware that the British had a part to play in the violence of Partition and I feel implicated. . . . I know it was a long time ago and that it wasn't directly related to anything I or my family did, but I do have a great-aunt on my father's side" (pointing to the genogram) "who lived during these troubled times." (She turned to Ali and continued.) "I sometimes feel your family blames me, as if it's my fault."

Ali reached out to hold Rachel's hand. "Honey, of course my family doesn't think that the Partition has anything to do with you. In our generation and living here in the Western world, we have to go beyond these divisions. You are not responsible for the Partition in the same way that I am not responsible for acts of terrorism that take place nowadays."

I was touched by Rachel's vulnerability and Ali's response. "I feel moved to hear and see how you both are coming together. . . . I wonder what you think it will be like for your unborn child to inhabit two such rich heritages? Rachel, looking at both your cultural genograms together, what do you think some common themes are that your children will inherit?"

She paused and then said, "I am thinking of how difference is not necessarily about racial and religious difference. In my family (pointing to her cultural genogram) my parents are from the same cultural background but completely different with regard to class. So it's been helpful to use different colors, as it makes me realize that differences can exist and can be overcome."

I offered, "So perhaps a theme of belonging and a desire to create a home across differences?" Both Rachel and Ali nod, and we take up this theme in a later session.

Culturegram

The culturegram is a wonderful visual tool. The exercise begins by with partner describing their identity, depicted as a circle in the middle of a piece of paper (see Figure 11.2). Spokes are drawn from the middle circle, each one representing a belief or value. Attached to the spokes are circles in which the partners write about how they have adopted or adapted the belief or value, learned from their families of origin, in their family of creation. I used the culturegram as a visual assessment tool to explore Ali's and Rachel's beliefs and values with regard to religion and gender, as I thought these were the two themes that were most salient to their dilemmas around their co-parenting, in the future. In the culturegram in Figure 11.2, I have depicted two of the spokes used to explore these themes.

With regard to their identities, Ali described himself as British, Asian, Muslim, and a doctor. Rachel defined herself as British, White, English, spiritual, and an artist. From his family of origin, Ali had learned a belief and faith in God and religion (Islam). In his own adult life and family of creation, he adapted this to "Religion and faith can be comforting, but I have no tolerance of dogma." Rachel's family was religious, too; her father's family was Methodist (her mother's family did not identify as religious). She had rejected religion in her adult life but defined herself as "spiritual and tolerant of difference."

Rachel and Ali had received different beliefs about gender. Although Ali's family was seen as an Asian patriarchal family, he understood that women were the mainstay of the family and his mother assumed a powerful role in the functioning of the family. In his own family of creation, he wished for men and women to have equal roles and responsibilities. Rachel, on the other hand, felt keenly the differences in power and social class between her parents. She had learned that men have more power and access to resources than women and wished to balance it out in her own family of creation, so that men and

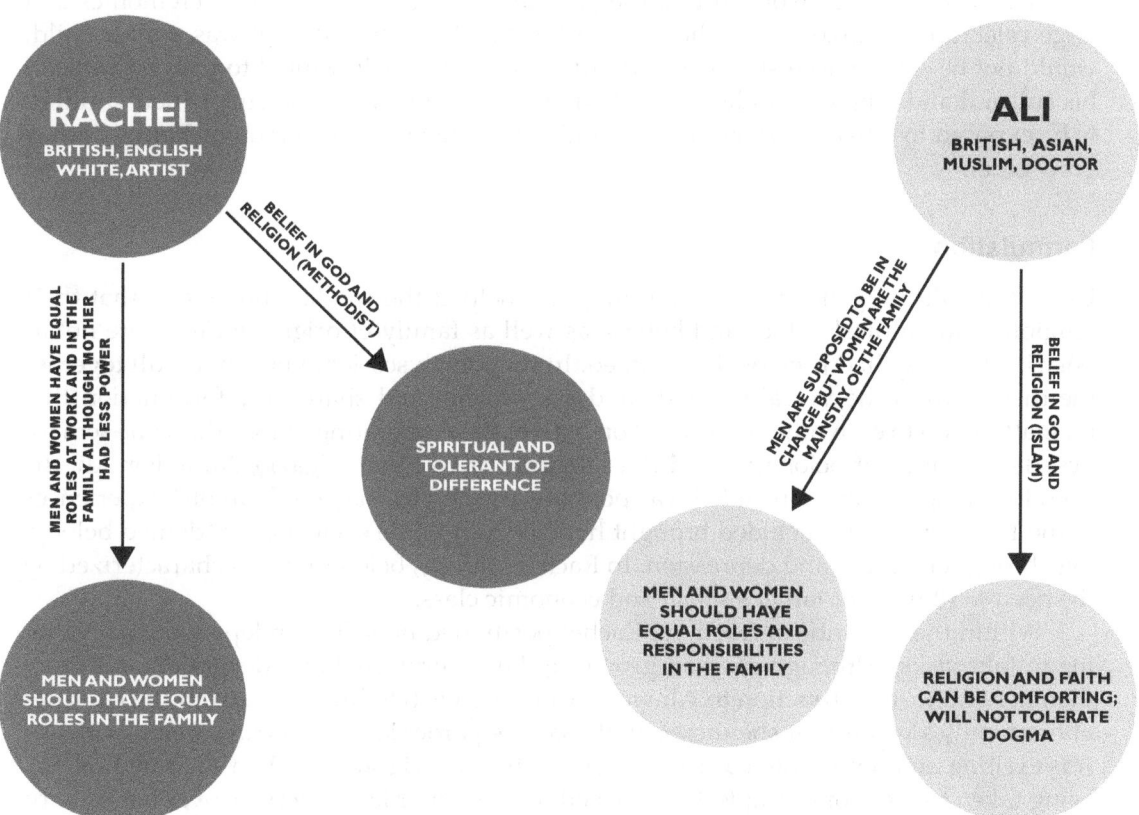

FIGURE 11.2. Two spokes from Rachel and Ali's culturegram.

women have equal roles and responsibilities. Hence, as I pointed out during the session, they had both come to exactly the same belief about men's and women's roles within families from different positions. I helped them to understand that they both had "corrective scripts" or a desire to do things differently from their parents or families of origin. This may have been one of the themes that brought them together.

I used the culturegram to discuss how they would like to co-parent and how they would like to incorporate both their beliefs and values about religion and gender into their joint parenting. Discussing religion was challenging, as it reminded them of how their religious differences had impacted the process of getting married. Rachel and Ali had gotten married during the COVID19 pandemic and the time leading up to the wedding had been extremely stressful for both of them. Rachel had experienced considerable pressure from Ali and his family to convert to Islam and to go through a *Nikah*. Her parents would have liked the couple to marry in the family church, and Ali had been willing to go through both a *Nikah* and a church wedding, but Rachel considered it hypocritical to have either ceremony. She had envisaged and designed a small, secular ceremony and because of COVID restraints, only close family and friends had been able to attend. Ali had talked endlessly to his parents about Rachel's wishes, and they had finally conceded, partly with the hope that they might have a larger celebration with their entire extended families after COVID restrictions had lifted. Rachel became pregnant soon after that. However, she was worried that the pressure to engage in religious ceremonies and large celebrations surrounding the birth of their child (especially if it was a male child) would not be so easy to resist. She could understand that Ali wanted to pass on some of his cultural and religious traditions to their children, but she was keen for their children to be exposed to other traditions as well, and to be able to make their own choices as they grew older.

Formulation

Using the cultural genogram and culturegram helped the couple understand that their religious and cultural values and beliefs, as well as family-of-origin stories, were not as polarized as they had previously assumed. In the fourth session, I began to pull together the themes from the visual methods and assessment, and shared my formulation that their attraction to each other was based on both of them operating within the same semantics: the semantic of belonging and the semantic of freedom (Ugazio, 2013). For Ali, the need to belong and to be included was possibly affected by his grandparents' experiences of the Partition. Being included brought honor (*Izzat*) while exclusion or "denied belonging" brought disgrace and depression. In Rachel's family, belonging was characterized by the need to fit into her father's social and economic class.

Within the semantic of freedom, Rachel positioned herself as independent and willing to take risks. Although she had grown up being protected and dependent, far more than her sisters, her attraction to Ali was part of her wish to break free from the confines of her family's world that she increasingly saw as parochial and narrow. Being with Ali was exciting and represented a risk. However, she was frightened when she saw this risk being taken too far, for example, being asked to convert or losing control over her unborn child's religion. Her anxiety symptoms occurred as a response to this perceived risk and were consistent with the psychopathology associated with the semantics of freedom.

Both Ali and Rachel were able to relate to my formulation. We agreed that our work together would be to help them to understand and respect each other's positions within these two semantics of freedom and belonging. I formed an interview schedule of the following questions, which we agreed to explore together in subsequent sessions:

> Belonging: What will creating your own family unit look like? What language will you use to speak to your child/children and what religious/cultural traditions will you practice?
> Freedom: Will you be able to choose the amount of distance and closeness from each of your families that feels appropriate and comfortable to both of you?
> Which aspects of your religions would you be happy for your child/children to adopt, and which ones would make you less comfortable? How would this be different with a male versus female child/children?

At this stage, I checked out the trustworthiness of the therapeutic alliance and asked, "Do you both feel that I have heard and understood your stories? How would I know if one or both of you do not feel heard or respected? Will you be able to tell me?" They both seemed to have engaged well and indicated that they were finding the therapy meaningful, and Rachel reported already feeling more supported by Ali.

The formulation, hypotheses, and corresponding questions that I outlined earlier highlight the significance of taking on a "both–and" position when working with intercultural and interfaith couples. At one level, a formulation with any couple at a life cycle stage similar to that of Ali and Rachel would be about the renogiation of boundaries, distance, and closeness with both their families of origin. Exploring issues of gender and power within the couple relationship and how such conversations were affected by my position as a female therapist is another salient theme that cuts across all systemic couple therapy. Furthermore, thinking about the effect of external factors such as the COVID-19 pandemic on relationships could be seen as pertinent to any couple or family treated during this time. However, at another level, the impact of racism and the profound differences in values and beliefs between the partners apply particularly to intercultural couple work, regardless of whether the presenting problem is focused on cultural and religious differences (as presented by Rachel and Ali) or whether it is more implicit. The cultural genogram, culturegram, and other visual and representational methods are useful in teasing out cultural and religious differences and beliefs but could be used to good effect with any couple or family.

INTERMEDIATE PHASE OF THERAPY

I seemed to have formed a good therapeutic alliance with the couple, and the work was progressing well until the fifth session, when Rachel and Ali presented as distressed, angry, and upset. The night before the session, Ali's mother had invited them for dinner to meet a relative from Pakistan; Rachel was not feeling well and did not want to go, which had greatly upset Ali's mother, Amina. She had first spoken to Rachel directly, trying to persuade her to attend the dinner, even for a short while. She had then spoken to her son, who had stood by Rachel's side. Ali felt fearful about upsetting either of them and expressed this by his refusal to engage with the issue and by a somewhat uneasy alliance with Rachel. Amina had lost her temper and said that she was disappointed. She had hoped that when Ali and Rachel got married, she would gain a daughter, and now she felt that not only had she not gained a daughter, but she was also losing her son. This interaction resulted in Ali, in turn, being upset and shouting at his parents and sister (who was pulled into this argument) on the phone.

Rachel and Ali both felt themselves to be at an impasse when they came into the session. Rachel was terrified about whether these pleas to meet relatives would become even more pronounced when the baby arrived. She was upset by how Ali's father and sister were drawn into these battles and at how reactive and angry with his parents Ali would become. The shouting upset her—she was pregnant and wanted some peace. Ali felt pathologized by Rachel's comments about his family's way of expressing emotions, which he insisted was culturally appropriate. The couple launched into a heated debate about forms of emotional expression in different cultures, with Ali insisting that Rachel's family was "repressed," and that she was judging his family using cultural yardsticks that did not fit. He was good at debating and could beat Rachel down. I intervened, bringing the couple back from the general and abstract to the particular (Singh et al., 2020). I reminded them of the active listening exercise we had tried in the first session and coached each of them again to let the other know how the episode had made them feel from an "I" position. Rachel was able to own feeling overwhelmed and engulfed, and Ali expressed how torn he felt. He wanted peace, too, and for the competing demands from his family and wife to stop. I wondered what it would be like if he did not join in with his family's communication style and was able to negotiate a solution peacefully with them. Furthermore, what would it be like for him to go and meet his visiting relative without Rachel? He was surprised when Rachel said that she wouldn't mind!

I shared with the couple my hope that working through this complicated situation would provide a template for future interactions after the birth of the baby. Could there be times when Ali could take their child over to meet his parents, without Rachel? What would that mean to her? Similarly, would she and the baby sometimes engage in activities with her family and friends without Ali?

Following this session, which seemed to bring some resolution and much-needed peace, the couple went away on holiday. They came to the sixth session having attended the 20-week fetal ultrasound. They were excited to report that they were expecting a daughter! Rachel was relieved, as it meant that they did not have to think about the issue of circumcision. Coming from a family predominated by girls, she felt that she would be far more comfortable with a daughter, who would fit in better with her family. Ali was happy, too, although he was slightly upset by his parents, who had remarked about how they had been hoping for a male heir to continue the family lineage.

As Ali and Rachel were grappling with the complicated issue of the meaning of their unborn child's gender, I asked them if they would be willing to try the exercise of "internalized other" interviewing. I began by interviewing Ali as if he were Rachel. In order to do this, I asked them to switch seats and to embody or become the other. The following extracts demonstrate the process:

> ME (RS): Okay, tell me a little bit about yourself. How old are you, Rachel, and what do you do?
>
> ALI: (*as Rachel*) I am 32 and I work in a museum in London.
>
> ME (RS): Do you like your work?

ALI: (*as Rachel*) Yes, I really enjoy it, except when I wake up feeling not too well during my pregnancy.

ME (RS): What does Ali (here) do to help you at such times? Tell me about your relationship—what do you value most about being with him?

ALI: (*as Rachel*) He's great fun to be with—he's my best friend. We talk about everything and he (usually!) takes good care of me.

ME (RS): You mentioned that you are expecting a daughter. What's that like for you?

ALI: (*as Rachel, cries*) My tears are of relief, happiness, and gratitude. Of course, I would be happy whatever gender child we were expecting, but it makes our lives so much simpler to be having a daughter. I feel grateful . . .

After checking with Rachel whether Ali's responses to my questions fit for her, I moved on to interview her as if she were Ali. I started by asking her exactly the same questions I had asked Ali—to tell me a bit about himself and what he valued about the relationship with her.

ME (RS): So what's it like for you, Ali, that Rachel will be giving birth to your baby daughter?

RACHEL: (*as Ali*) It's awesome! I am so happy.

ME (RS): What's it like for your family?

RACHEL: (*as Ali*) They are excited, too. However, I wonder if they are also slightly disappointed, as they would have liked our first born to have been a son . . .

ME (RS): Ali, what do you think it's like for Rachel that your family might be feeling slightly disappointed? Or wait, lets ask Rachel (*turning to Ali as Rachel*). Rachel, what is it like for you that Ali's family is feeling slightly disappointed?

ALI: (*as Rachel, starts crying*) It makes me feel so undervalued. It's difficult carrying a baby, and then to feel that she won't be good enough is so difficult . . .

After I had finished interviewing the partners as each other, I made connections with the wider family on both sides. Rachel realized that her outrage was not only from a feminist perspective but also on behalf of her mother, who had not borne a son. Ali could appreciate and explain his mother's position as a professional Muslim woman who had had to work doubly hard to excel in what she saw as still being a "man's world." Although she had provided both Ali and his sister, Ayesha, with equal opportunities, Ali had always been aware of—and felt somewhat guilty about—his special privileges as a male child.

As I interviewed the couple about the gender of their soon-to-be-born daughter, I was aware of my own associations to their conversation. Like Rachel, I am one of three daughters and was deeply aware of the meaning, for my mother, of not having a son in the cultural and historical context of India in the 20th century. I am the mother of two boys and have often longed for a daughter. I did not divulge any of my inner conversation to the couple, as I did not think it would be helpful.

The couple seemed to have found the "internalized other" interviewing extremely helpful and made reference to it in subsequent sessions. Both were touched by how well their partner seemed to know and understand them. Rachel was particularly moved by how open and vulnerable Ali had been when he was being interviewed as her and was struck by the fact that he had cried during the interview, which apparently was rare for him!

We went on to talk about practical matters, the name of their baby and cultural/religious birth rituals. They had decided to name their daughter Aliya, and her second name would be Margaret, after the aunt who had lived in Bombay. They agreed that they would have both a Christening and observe the Islamic practices of shaving the baby's head and whispering the Muslim call to prayer in her ear.

CONCLUDING PHASE OF THERAPY

Something significant seemed to have shifted after the internalized other interviewing in the sixth session. I saw the couple for only three further sessions, spaced out every 2–3 weeks. This was partly because, entering the third trimester, Rachel was becoming too uncomfortable to attend in person; in fact, one of the concluding three sessions was online. The work in these later sessions comprised revisiting, consolidating, and planning for the future. Mostly, I was in a holding pattern, aware that I did not want Rachel to become overly distressed close to her due date. In consultation with my psychiatrist colleague, the couple had decided that Rachel would continue on her antianxiety medication in order to avert postnatal depression. The couple was attending and enjoying prenatal classes to prepare for the birth and postnatal care.

Which Is the Primary Dyad?: The Therapist's Dilemma

During the eighth and penultimate session, Rachel reported yet another row between herself and Ali, this time to do with whether his parents (who lived in a London neighborhood quite far from the couple) should move closer to them after Aliya's birth. Rachel, whose parents lived outside London, did not want her in-laws as neighbors, whereas Ali thought it would be wonderful to have his parents' support. He explained to Rachel that his primary loyalty had always been to his parents who, in turn, had been close to his grandparents (especially his maternal grandparents) to help them with child rearing. In Rachel's family, on the other hand, her parents had sought to forge a nuclear family together, and their primary attachments had been to each other, to the exclusion of their own parents and even children. Rachel and her sisters had left home to go to university, allowing her parents a chance to become even closer. Although she had remained connected to her parents, she thought that marrying Ali had allowed her to finally leave home and to maintain a healthy distance from her family. She was quick to judge Ali's reliance on his parents.

Given that Ali and Rachel seemed to be coming from two different belief systems about the construction of the couple relationship and attachment to their respective parents, I revisited the culturegram and asked them to draw an additional spoke to explore their notions of who the primary dyad in the family ought to be. Rachel drew a spoke from the circle and wrote, "The couple is the primary dyad" to indicate that this was a belief that she had received from her family of origin. By contrast, for his additional spoke, Ali wrote, "Parent–child relationships are the most significant." During further discussion, he adapted this belief: "My loyalties lie with my parents, as well as my wife and daughter." Depicting their opposing beliefs in visual form together starkly demonstrated the differences that might well be irreconcilable and could create ongoing conflict in the future.

For me, the conversation about the primacy of the couple dyad represented a real dilemma and brought up for me the splits in my own cultural identities. At different stages of my personal and family life, I have experienced the joys and benefits of connections with extended family and community, as well as the rewards of my primary loyalty being to my partner. I am keenly aware of the pitfalls and cultural connotations of deeming one a better or more superior way of relating; they are different, but not more or less.

However, in this case, I coached Ali to try and persuade Rachel of his loyalty to her and to Aliya, perhaps even to the exclusion of his parents, sister, and extended family. When working with intercultural couples, I see one of my tasks as "translating meaning" (Reibstein & Singh, 2021) between one partner and the other, or helping them to understand and empathize with each other's cultural values and beliefs. Hence, positioning myself as a cultural broker, I helped Rachel, in turn, to understand why, as the elder son of migrants to the United Kingdom, Ali's relationship with his parents was so important to him. I suggested that, over time, she might learn to trust and rely on Ali's parents, value their input as grandparents, and even want them to live closer by.

In the ninth and final session, Rachel said that she had observed a further shift in Ali's behavior. He seemed able to support her and stand up to his parents more. The couple felt they were pulling together well and getting ready for the birth of their daughter. We reviewed our work together and decided to stop, with the proviso that they could get in touch after the birth, if needed. They had been practicing the active listening exercise at home and reported that their communication had improved greatly.

A couple of months later, they contacted me to let me know that Aliya had been born, at a healthy 7½ pounds. The entire family was doing well. I did not see Rachel and Ali again. In the following year, Ali contacted me to let me know that he and Rachel were still getting on well and to ask if he could give my contact details to his parents, who were seeking couple therapy! I referred them to a colleague, in case he and Rachel ever wanted to come back to see me. I did not think that they would come back but wanted them to have the space in case they did ever need it.

FURTHER REFLECTIONS AND IMPLICATIONS

Forming and fostering a secure therapeutic alliance with both Rachel and Ali seemed essential to the success of my work with them. In order to build a good working relationship with intercultural couples, I tend to spend longer in the beginning phase, creating a safe context in which to talk about race and racism. Using and unpacking visual assessment methods (which can be revisited later in the work) helps partners to feel understood and to understand each other better.

Rachel seemed to engage well with me, and I could identify with her experiences, some of which reminded me of what I had been like as a young woman. With Ali, I felt an immediate affinity, perhaps based on our shared cultural heritage. My dilemma was whether my affinity with Ali positioned me to redress the balance by working even harder on my therapeutic alliance with Rachel, thus running the risk of alienating Ali. Speaking to my supervisor and coauthor, Janet Reibstein, who is American and Jewish, about my alliance helped me to continually interrogate the neutrality of my position. I realized that when working with clients from a similar cultural background, I could more readily make assumptions and lose curiosity, and Janet's outsider position also helped me to retain cultural humility.

When I look back on my work with Rachel and Ali, I am mindful of the way in which I positioned myself, in particular during the concluding part of the work, when I seemed to be pushing Ali in the direction of adopting more "Western" notions of how the couple is constructed. Although the intervention seemed to have created a powerful shift for the family system, I wondered what influenced me to position myself in that way.

One obvious reason for my positioning was that Rachel was pregnant and suffering from anxiety and depression. She had always had a somewhat nervous temperament and during her first year of university had struggled with a similar episode of anxiety and depression. I hypothesized that leaving home—whether in the guise of going to university or getting married and having her first child—created considerable anxiety for Rachel. My consideration of the effects of my interventions on Rachel meant that I did not want to challenge her or perturb the couple–family system too much. Her pregnant state and attendant mental health difficulties evoked a protectiveness in me.

A second possible reason for my positioning is because I felt strongly allied not just to Ali but to Amina and wanted to position myself as different from her. Amina and I were of a similar age and life cycle stage. My older son is almost exactly Ali's age, and I have the expectation of becoming a mother-in-law and grandmother in the next few years. Like Amina, I am a migrant and a professional woman. In addition, my parents, like Amina's, were refugees during the Partition of India. Without ever having seen Amina, I realized, early in the work, that in order to have a therapeutic alliance with Rachel, I would have to be sufficiently different from Amina, which would probably mean being more westernized. This would be helpful for Ali as well, who might have sought Rachel out in order to achieve some distance between himself and his parents.

When I look back on the work, I wonder what effects my therapy had on Ali's extended family. Did Amina want to see me to complain about my work? Did she feel as if she had lost her son? Should I have agreed to see Ali's parents or Amina separately for at least a session? On balance, I still uphold my clinical judgment in not agreeing to see Ali's parents, as I expect I may see Ali and Rachel again in the future, perhaps when she is pregnant with their next child.

What might I have done differently? In retrospect, I might have shared my dilemma, saying something like the following:

> "Rachel, I hear that you think that partners' primary loyalties lie with each other and that you, Ali, think that the couple relationship ought to be embedded within the extended family. Neither position is right nor wrong. From Western models of mental health and family therapy, as well as some of my own personal experiences, I agree with you, Rachel. On the other hand, from an intimate personal knowledge of South Asian extended families, I agree with you, Ali. I would like you both to talk about and negotiate the amount of distance and closeness from each of your families that feels suitable to each of you. This is in light of understanding and seeing (pointing to the culturegram) your different values and beliefs. Can you respect each other's values and find a middle ground? What would that look like?"

This intervention would have made my dilemma transparent and facilitated the partners to own and work through their own impasse, thus preparing them for working through similar situations in the future without me.

Focusing on this dilemma highlights the delicate balance between self-awareness, self-reflexivity, transparency, and self-disclosure in the therapeutic process. It makes me think of the moment-by-moment decisions we make as therapists to disclose or not disclose aspects of ourselves, depending on when we deem it helpful and when we do not. These decisions are often intuitive; for example, I have no certainty about whether I made the right decisions to reveal my own parents' experiences of the trauma of the Partition, and whether I made the right decision to withhold the information that, like Rachel, I grew up with two sisters and therefore understand the nature of gendered sibling rivalries and competition.

From a self-reflexive position, exploring transgenerational themes in Ali's family reawakened my curiosity about the transgenerational trauma and loss in my own family. It has led me to find out more about my parents' experiences of the Partition and to wonder whether their interfaith relationship provided each of them with a protective distance from—as well as a shared understanding of—transgenerational trauma and loss. These are ideas that I wish to take up in future research about the resiliencies and protective factors in intercultural and interfaith couple relationships.

Rachel's and Ali's stories highlight the complex and intersectional nature of racial, cultural, religious, and class differences. It reminds me not to make assumptions about cultural and religious differences. It confirms to me that "Whiteness" is not a monolith, in that Rachel's family comprised parents from different class backgrounds that could be as much of a barrier as racial differences. Ali's family, on the other hand, was different from many of my Muslim clients, in that his family did not cut him off, or threaten to cut him off, despite the fact that Rachel did not convert to Islam. Therefore, Ali and Rachel did not have to confront the pain of not being accepted by his family, and their negotiations with Ali's family could be made from the safe position of knowing that they would always be a part of the family. In this important way, their story was different from my father's, who was disowned and disinherited from his family on religious grounds.

This brings to mind my theoretical understanding of the semantics that drew Rachel and Ali together—the semantics of freedom and belonging (Ugazio, 2013). They sought each other out because they were both interested in difference, exploration, and adventure. However, from a semantic of belonging, they both valued the creation of shared worlds in which they and their children could belong and be accepted. In previous generations, their parents had striven to belong and create homes, either in a country or in a social class that initially must have seemed alien and alienating. My work with Rachel and Ali was about helping them to create hybrid worlds for themselves and their children, bringing together valued aspects from both their cultures.

What about the semantics of power? The dynamics of power and powerlessness were constantly alive in Rachel's and Ali's experiences. For Ali, experiences of racism, discrimination, and Islamaphobia underpinned his professional and personal life. Rachel, although being from the White majority in the United Kingdom, which had always been her and her family's home, could easily feel powerless in the context of Ali's professional extended family, where she had the experience of being outnumbered and judged as not good enough. It was no wonder then that she needed Ali's unswerving loyalty, just as he needed her to be able to hear his experiences and feelings of powerlessness and vulnerability in British society.

And as for the therapeutic system the three of us created together, the theme of power cut across our interactions and relationships. Although I could invoke the power of my status as a therapist and of my age, being from Ali's and Rachel's parents' generation, Ali had the power of being the only male in the room and the status of his profession as a medical doctor. The history of the relationship between Hindus and Muslims meant that Ali and I were each positioned and copositioned as "the Other," yet determined to go beyond these narrow categories and embrace our shared cultural heritage. Rachel had the power of being the only White, English person in our therapeutic triangle, rendered even more complex in a shared history of relationships between the colonizer and colonial subjects. We were all three keenly aware of our positions and were able to refer to them in ways that promoted trust and safety in the therapeutic encounter.

I used a range of interventions, both empathic and behavioral. The internalized-other interviewing appeared to have created the most change. I promoted the idea of separate cultural spaces (Falicov, 1995) and coached Rachel and Ali in clearer communication. They had both grown up in the United Kingdom, and English was their first language so, unlike some of the other intercultural couples with whom I work, they had similar communication styles. This, however, sometimes belied the subtle and profound differences in their value and belief systems that came to the fore through the use of visual methods such as the culturegram.

I would like to think that the process and specific interventions of my work with Ali and Rachel would fit for couples in which the partners are from a range of different religious backgrounds, faith traditions, or have different relationships to their shared religious background. It may also have implications for couples from different cultural and class backgrounds or nationalities, and could resonate for clients who, in previous generations, have been subjected to political upheaval and trauma.

The process and interventions I've described here could also be relevant to any couple negotiating the significant life transition of having their first child together. Returning to the narrative of Harry and Meghan, pregnancy in interracial couples especially can evoke a number of fears and fantasies. These could center around the appearance of a mixed-race child and how they will be welcomed by the extended family. Pregnancy can be an emotional and fearful time, but also a time of dreams and hopes that bind partners together. I hope this account of my work with Rachel and Ali points to the richness of working with intercultural couples—especially those confronting critical life transitions. Therapists can experience deep, meaningful rewards in helping intercultural and interfaith couples to forge unified bonds that help create secure, resilient, mixed-race interfaith children, protected and far removed from the effects of intergenerational conflict and trauma.

REFERENCES

Falicov, C. J. (1995). Cross-cultural marriages. In N. S. Jacobson & A. S. Gurman (Eds.), *Clinical handbook of couple therapy* (pp. 231–246). New York: Guilford Press.

Lugli, V., Kalaydjian, J., Atkas, M., Lerussi, S., & Singh, R. (2022). Do intercultural couples come from different semantic worlds?: Report on a research study funded by the (AFT) David Campbell creative fund. *Context, 180*, 38–43.

Reibstein, J., & Singh, R. (2021). *The intercultural Exeter couples model: Making connections for a divided world through systemic behavioral therapy.* Hoboken, NJ: Wiley.

Singh, R., Killian, K., Bhugun, D., & Tseng, C. (2020). Clinical work with intercultural couples. In K. Wampler & A. Blow (Eds.), *Handbook of systemic family therapy* (Vol. 3, pp. 155–183). Hoboken, NJ: Wiley-Blackwell.

Ugazio, V. (2013). *Semantic polarities and psychopathologies in the family: Permitted and forbidden stories.* London: Routledge.

CHAPTER 12

Affirmative Therapy for Queer Relationships[1]

REBECCA HARVEY

> *Editors' Comments*
>
> Rebecca Harvey offers a compelling narrative of therapy with persons in LGBTQIA+ relationships—informed by the unique challenges they face, as well as broader issues of social justice embedded in a traditional White heteropatriarchal society. While the chapter focuses on relational therapy for LGBTQIA+ clients, the couple described by Harvey—a White, 32-year-old, nonbinary queer person and a 38-year-old, cisgender, African American lesbian—wonderfully illustrates how multiple facets of social location (e.g., race, sex, gender, class) intersect in complex and mutually amplifying ways.
>
> Evident in this narrative are the common elements essential to effective therapy and illustrated throughout many of the chapters in this *Casebook*—building the therapeutic alliance, disrupting negative interaction patterns and promoting alternatives, attending to both individual and relationship histories—but observe the unique aspects of each of these in the context of affirmative therapy for queer relationships. For example, creating safe refuge in the therapeutic setting requires explicit, empathic acknowledgment of sociopolitical oppression and minority stress that queer persons endure on a daily basis. Long-standing survival strategies are challenged through "difficult dialogues" that attend not only to developmental influences from family or other early salient relationships but also the broader ecosystem that fostered "losing relational strategies" that now undermine authenticity and vulnerability. Listen as Harvey shares with the reader her

---

[1] The words we use to describe ourselves and our relationships are inherently personal, political, culturally located, and constantly evolving. For LGBTQIA+ people (lesbian, gay, bisexual, transgender, queer or questioning, intersex, asexual, and other diverse gender and sexual identities) this is particularly important, because specific language raises critical issues about power, privilege, agency, and inclusion. When working with clients or students, my intention is to use the labels they prefer to name themselves, their relationships, and their identities. I sometimes use LGBTQIA+, while other times I use the term "queer" as an umbrella term for anyone or any relationship identifying as not traditionally heterosexual. Similarly, I try to limit use of the word "couple" in my writing and focus more on relationality and relationships to highlight alternative ways people can imagine and structure their partnerships.—R.H.

> own thoughts and feelings influencing her decisions about when and how to enact specific interventions. Note also how she shares with this couple selective elements of her own experiences as a way of "nurturing queerness" and inspiring the partners to recognize "what's real, possible, and even imaginable."
>
> Harvey reminds us of the power and privilege we hold as therapists—regardless of our own unique position across various facets of social location—and summons each of us to practice liberation as a relational process. Her case narrative wonderfully illuminates some of the core values and specific therapeutic elements in pursuit of this ideal.

My introduction to the idea of therapy occurred when, as a teenager, I was dragged kicking and screaming by my parents to a psychologist. My parents, who had divorced after a tumultuous marriage, never agreed on anything. But when they realized that my sullen mood and surly attitude had graduated to include cutting behaviors, they agreed I "needed help." In retrospect they were, of course, right. I was navigating my gender-nonconforming teenage years and emerging queer sexuality in the wake of their calamitous divorce and a sometimes-perilous childhood. Unfortunately, this was prior to LGBTQIA+ affirmative therapy so the help I needed was not the help I got. As a result, I focused early in my career on developing affirmative theory and interventions that nurture queer youth and their parents (Stone Fish & Harvey, 2005). How therapy could affirm couples was largely a mystery to me then. I was busy living out my own romantic misadventures—managing shame and dodging vulnerability during the hatefulness of the 1990s version of the culture wars. There was near silence in psychological literature at this time about LGBTQIA+ relationships. It felt a lot like trying to build a plane while flying it.

Effective relational therapy for LGBTQIA+ people must acknowledge the complicated isomorphic effect of sociopolitical oppression or *minority stress* on relational processes. Queer people experience relationships against the backdrop of a nauseating roller-coaster ride of cultural advances in social acceptance and legal achievements, and then setbacks, reversals, and violent backlash against our community. We've become used to all aspects of our most intimate lives used as cannon fodder in political battles in which our well-being is beside the point. For many, this has created a disembodied experience in which our sanity, morality, fitness as parents, and the validity of our romantic relationships are regularly judged, debated, and censured, often by people we know and institutions we respect. Simultaneously, we must navigate legal, physical, and psychological threats, all while trying to build our lives, fall in love, create families, and parent our children.

The relative health of any relationship is developed and maintained within the context and pattern of relational process. Thus, I focus on tracking and intervening in the process between partners rather than seeing any one person or issue as the problem. But interpersonal process is learned and practiced within the larger sociocultural systems in which it is embedded. Just as problematic family dynamics are unwittingly passed from generation to generation, so too are problematic patterns of domination replicated from the larger White heteropatriarchal culture and filtered into relational processes. And while queer people live on the margins of White heteropatriarchy, we do so to differing degrees. Intersections of social location multiply so that racism, sexism, religiosity, classism, and heterosexism intersect in unique ways and with various effects, so that even people very much in love do not have the same experience of being LGBTQIA+. In addition, queer people are more likely than those who identify as heterosexual to develop cross-cultural intimate relationships (Gates, 2012). This makes it imperative for clinicians to understand how complex intersections of racial, gender, and sexual identities interact within interracial or intercultural relationships (Coolhart, 2023) and are part of presenting problems that on the surface seem wholly disconnected.

Intimacy requires justice. Partners can be intimately connected only to the degree that they believe that authenticity, and thus vulnerability, has value, is reciprocal, and won't be used against them in an already unjust system. Meanwhile, all levels of society are imbued with racism, sexism, heteronormativity, religiosity, and classism that promulgate injustice and invulnerability. This has psychological consequences. As we experience ubiquitous oppression and injustice, we learn to expect this and re-create it in order to survive—even when those conditions hurt us, when at our core we value something different, and even when it disconnects us from what or who we cherish. Clinical work that ignores this will simply encourage LGBTQIA+ people (in fact, all people) to accommodate themselves to power imbalances and relational expectations created in the image of White heteropatriarchy that, by definition, seeks control and domination—not collaboration and intimacy.

I assume that every human being has had to maneuver through embodied experiences of domination, false empowerment, coercion, or neglect. In response, we learn three types of survival strategies to protect ourselves: (1) *attack strategies*—these include responding forcefully to any perceived threats with coercion, control, aggression, belittling, or gaslighting, and often include prioritizing individual needs to the detriment of others or the relationship; (2) *compliance strategies* in the face of threats that include minimizing one's own individual needs or consistently accommodating to and focusing on the needs of a partner; and (3) *exiting strategies* such as withdrawal, freezing, or hiding when threatened. This may include evasive maneuvers such as avoiding hard conversations, distancing from strong emotions, or avoiding commitments altogether. Importantly, these strategies are learned when we are young, are practiced repeatedly, and are encouraged by our families and communities, both overtly or covertly. Strategies are established and entrenched long before we have adult resources and cognitive abilities to see and understand the detriments of responding in such a manner. Real (2018) refers to these as *first consciousness* or *adaptive child* responses. As such, they are instantaneous, urgent, and feel justified given the protection they offer from chronic threats of powerlessness and isolation. But what feels momentarily protective can become enduring, habituated responses that, over time, harm relationships.

My clinical work with LGBTQIA+ relationships (couples or polyamorous relationships) has been an evolving theoretical fusion of feminist and Black feminist critique, queer theory, and systems theory, specifically relational life therapy (Real, 2018). My overarching aim is to lessen domination (das Nair & Thomas, 2012) and support each person to develop a quality of presence in their relationship with themself and their partner marked by compassion, justice, curiosity, and an increasing capacity for intimacy. I work to create refuge from sociocultural oppression (Harvey, Murphy, Bigner, & Wetchler, 2022; Harvey & Stone Fish, 2015; Stone Fish & Harvey, 2005). I utilize *difficult dialogues* to teach and practice authentic, effective communication skills. I nurture new, queer ways of understanding how survival adaptations create destructive relational processes, and

I encourage change and transformation. My work with Nadine and Alex illustrates this approach.

INITIAL ASSESSMENT AND CASE FORMULATION: CREATING REFUGE

My initial contact with Alex and Nadine came by way of a colleague. Nadine had been the driving force into therapy, and she was the one who made the initial call to me.

> "Alex and I have been together for 10 years, married for 3. I'm 38 and Alex is 32, and I think the age difference might be insurmountable. I want to settle down, buy a house, have children; Alex seems less sure. I thought after we were married things would be better, but they've actually gotten worse. Alex is spending more and more time at work and socializing, going out at night. We simply can't talk productively about having a child or really about anything. All of our conversations about our relationship explode. I find myself angry, sad, and lonely. I'm worried we're drifting apart."

I could hear Nadine's confusion that getting married hadn't seemed to help in the way she thought it might, and I sensed her growing hopelessness. On the other hand, they'd been together for 10 years and had committed to one another. That counted for something. I was curious how Alex would describe what was happening. I was also interested in understanding the dance between them. What drew them together? What seemed to get in their way now? From the limited information I had, it appeared they identified as an interracial, same-sex lesbian couple. Nadine had already identified age as a potential factor in their interpersonal dynamics. What other intersections of identity would be salient? But without asking directly, it was impossible to know.

When beginning a new case, I send out paperwork requesting basic client information. I specifically ask about preferred pronouns, gender identity, sexual orientation, relationship status, and demographic information, including race, religious background, and whatever social or community affiliations about which clients want me to know. I'm beginning right away to assess for potential sources of power imbalances that can interfere with connection and intimacy. I also ask for a list of all the people in their life they consider family either by blood, marriage, or families of choice—close friends, former lovers, partners, and others in the LGBTQIA+ community that traditionally have been important for queer people who may be disconnected from rejecting families, churches, or communities once important in their lives. Finally, I also ask about health or family issues, past and present, including any issues with substances, anxiety or depression, aggression or acting-out behaviors, illness or hospitalizations, as these issues may need to be addressed prior to or conjointly with relational therapy. When I receive Alex's and Nadine's paperwork, I learn that Alex identifies as a White 32-year-old nonbinary queer person who uses she/they/them pronouns, whereas Nadine identifies as a 38-year-old cisgender African American lesbian who uses she/her pronouns.

During the initial 90-minute consultation, I answer any questions they have, and I work to understand how each person describes the problem for which they're seeking help. I begin tracking the process between them and what it feels like for each of them to be in the relationship. I rely a lot on my own feelings in the room and what I feel when I'm around them. But I don't get married to my stories. My initial ideas and feelings are simply data that inform ongoing assessment. I use these early ideas to ask more focused questions. Those answers then allow me to craft increasingly nuanced interventions unique to these people and their specific relationship with one another. When I meet with Alex and Nadine, what I notice right away is that Alex seems withdrawn and slow to answer. Alex's large frame, 6-foot body sinks low and tight into the couch like they're trying (unsuccessfully) to disappear underneath the cushions. I can't tell if it's exhaustion, self-protection, or resignation. In contrast to Alex's low energy Nadine comes in hot—highly energized and taking charge. She's as quick to answer as Alex is to hang back and take the temperature of the room. While Alex holds back with awkward silences, Nadine jumps quickly to conclusions, often negative ones, like she's preparing herself for heartache. I begin to wonder in what context they learned these relational styles and how it helps them navigate around the intersections of their lives.

I ask them to tell me how they met and what drew them together. This is both an assessment and an intervention, as I'm hoping to hear their history and observe how they interact. Alex smiles and says, "Well I think in our case, opposites attract."

They're laughing and I say, "Well I could guess, but I want to make sure I understand. How are you opposites?" I'm wanting to hear and adopt their language.

Nadine says, "Well, I'm small and femme and Black. And Alex is White and masculine and large."

I continue, "I'm curious about how you've discussed these differences, being femme or masculine and White or Black, and how you think these identities affect your relationship—would you be willing to pursue this as we get to know each other?" Nadine readily agrees. Alex says little, which I'm coming to suspect is on brand for them. My intention here is to invite the direct discussion of intersectional identities early on.

I then ask what else is important for me to understand as I get to know them? I wait a moment and Alex follows with "I've always stuck out in a crowd and have always hated it. I don't quite fit. I'm masculine but not a man. Most people assumed I was a boy. I used to think of myself as a masculine woman and a lesbian. But . . . well let's just say I make a very ugly girl." Alex says this with a laugh, but I sense hurt. Alex is referencing how their experience is threatening to others invested in heteronormativity. Alex hurries on, "But these days—well, I don't think of myself as a proper man or a proper woman, I guess I'm a masculine queer person." We talk about the limitations of common language for gender and how this affected Alex's sense self. I share that it sounds like Alex grew up not feeling valued or protected. Alex laughs, saying, "That's an understatement." I thank Alex for being so forthright with me and for sharing their preferred language. I also clarify whether it feels right for me to use they/them pronouns when referring to them, and Alex agrees that it does. Nadine then talks about her experience as a BIPOC person (Black, Indigenous, and People of Color), how often she feels underestimated, and how that has affected her sense of self. I express my hope that therapy will not replicate these negative experiences in the larger world, and I encourage both of them to let me know if it ever does. Here, I want to invite direct discussion of intersectional identities, as I believe these have played an important role in their development as people and in their relationship. I am hoping to create a refuge in therapy from how these identities may have been discussed, misunderstood, or ignored in the past.

Next, I learn that Nadine and Alex met at work in a large multinational company.

Nadine, a lawyer, was already advancing in the company when Alex started there as an intern. Since then, Alex has worked their way up in the IT/software department of the company, obtaining an MBA along the way. Alex and Nadine readily acknowledge that their personal relationship has helped them both be more successful in their careers. They often strategize about work together and over the last 5 years have worked on many successful shared projects, although sometimes those projects become sources of conflict. I ask them to help me understand from each of their viewpoints what brings them to therapy. Alex mentions feeling worried, stuck, and dissatisfied with the constant tension between them; Nadine yearns for emotional closeness and for Alex to be more communicative, but admits that no matter how many times she asks, it doesn't seem to happen. I notice that they both stay rather vague and sense that I could be more helpful with specifics. So, I ask for a description of a recent example of a conflict between them. Nadine defers pointedly to Alex, who tentatively begins.

"Nadine just always seems unhappy, dissatisfied, and angry. At first, I thought that getting married would satisfy her. But now she's totally focused on having a child. She just keeps forcing this conversation, creating tension, like she's trying to wear me down. She knows I'm not sure about this."

Nadine interrupts, "Right, you're not sure. But you knew I wanted this when we got together. You *know* this has always been important to me."

Alex counters, "And you knew I wasn't sure. Besides, that was 10 years ago. A lot's changed in that decade. I honestly don't know if I want to bring a child into this world and into a queer family. It's getting harder, not easier, these days."

Nadine inserts an eyeroll, and her frustration is palpable. "It's arguably the *best* time in history for us to have a family. You're just saying that because *you* don't want a child. We have marriage equality and more legal protections than ever."

Alex counters, "Yeah, and we have the Pulse nightclub, trans hatred, and extremists of all kinds targeting us and doing their best to undo those very protections you're talking about."

Nadine bursts out with her frustration, "Shit . . . this is important to me and you never really show up for this conversation. Maybe we just aren't meant for each other." Nadine moves into hopelessness, and Alex seems lost and overwhelmed. I can feel the escalating tension between them in my body. My heart rate increases. My stomach drops. I sense Alex feeling cornered and wanting to flee, while Nadine's desperation is palpable. I remind myself that these are their feelings, not mine, so I can get some distance.

Then I interrupt, as this isn't going anywhere good. "So, if this conversation were happening at home, what would happen next?" I learn from them that this conversation is frequent and typically escalates to yelling on both of their parts, then devolves into a chilly standoff that can last for days. I ask them to notice what's happening in their bodies right now as we talk about this. Nadine flatly describes feeling disconnected and mostly numb, while Alex says that heart and mind are racing. I ask them what they know about caring for themselves when they're in this state. Both indicate that when they're in emotional distress because of an argument, they mainly separate and focus on something else, usually work or TV. I explain that it makes sense that their urge is to disconnect from these unpleasant feelings, but I wonder if they could also learn to pay attention to what's happening inside their bodies in moments like these and actively calm themselves rather than simply disconnecting from their experience as they wait for the feelings to pass.

I introduce some basic breathing techniques, and we practice in the room together. We spend some time talking about how activities they already enjoy such as walking, swimming, painting, and sewing could be used in difficult moments as forms of self-care. I also introduce some other options such as taking a shower, stretching, yoga, and meditation. I'm aiming to help each of them develop coping skills, so that when they feel threatened or disappointed, they know how to identify and care for their own feelings. As they learn to tolerate distress and practice doing so, they can slow down automatic responses that harm their relationship.

As we near the end, I summarize what I've heard and check in with them for accuracy. I'm struck by what a good team they make, and I tell them so. They're both loving, intelligent, and successful. Nadine's vibrancy and generosity complement Alex's kind, thoughtful, laid-back style. Clearly, they care deeply about each other and about the work they do together. I share with them my admiration for their having built such a solid foundation for their relationship. And I offer my understanding that as an interracial, queer couple, they built this foundation despite the personally and politically threatening environment they've been navigating. This speaks highly of their commitment and resilience. I share my view that they're at a crossroads, and that this isn't evidence of some fatal flaw but rather a sign that they already know how to do hard things together. If they want to continue working together, I believe that I can help. My intent is to offer hope and a clear way forward in therapy that is both realistic and positive. Both Alex and Nadine feel affirmed by the idea that what's happening between them is evidence of their resilience and maturation as a couple, a thought that hadn't occurred to them. Nadine offers, "Well I never thought that our arguments could be seen as a good thing."

Alex agrees, saying, "That's about the last thing I'd thought you say."

Given this response I go a little further. "You both describe frequent debates like the one I witnessed today. The battle lines get drawn, evidence and data points get tossed around in order to convince one another who's right and who's wrong. Whatever the issue is, I'm guessing that the process you engage in when you argue is similar. Your minds are battling, but I don't think you can feel what is in each other's hearts. I'd like to help you each learn to slow down and do something different. But you'd both have to be willing to take a look at how you're participating and focus less on what the other is doing." They agree and we make a second appointment.

In the initial stage of treatment, I work to create a refuge using all the traditional hallmarks of joining with clients: empathy, validation, attentiveness, and an affirming, strengths-based view of their relationship. This is critical for LGBTQIA+ clients, who must wade through negative messaging about themselves daily. But even more than this, I'm carving out space where their difficulties become located not only in themselves but in their families of origin and in the sociocultural world. At best, that larger world minimizes LGBTQIA+ relationships—leaving queer people to imagine and build relationships that are hard to envision because they never were really supposed to exist. When this can be named and known, it can create freedom and hope. So I flag the interracial identity of Alex's and Nadine's relationship, and ask directly about their differences (racial, sexual, gender) as a way to introduce intersectionality and begin to make these topics accessible for us to discuss in therapy. I also highlight what they've accomplished and reframe their struggles as signs of their solidarity as a couple—recognizing that in the wider culture the validity of their relationship is constantly under siege.

BEGINNING PHASE OF THERAPY: DIFFICULT DIALOGUES

During the next session, the tension is thick right from the beginning. Alex and Nadine had a disagreement earlier in the week about a work project that is still hanging icily in the air. Nadine explains that on these shared projects, they combine Alex's technology expertise with Nadine's legal expertise, and while it has been professionally very successful, it has often led to conflict in their personal relationship. Nadine mentions that practical and important considerations of scheduling and team communication tend to overwhelm Alex, who avoids handling them, which means they tend to fall on Nadine, who is naturally outgoing and good at logistics. "I guess I'm just supposed to take up the slack as usual," Nadine gripes. I wait to see what Alex will do, and they are quiet for a long time.

Eventually, I ask, "So Alex, Nadine thinks you're avoiding these tasks. Is that how you see it?"

Alex's words come slowly and carefully, "She is just so good communicating with everyone. I know it will get done right when Nadine handles it." Nadine seems to perk up at the affirmation Alex offers. She clearly enjoys the validation, but her resentment is palpable. Alex seems well-meaning but at best clueless about how their avoidance effectively hands responsibility for these tasks over to Nadine, who is evidently willing to keep trying to balance doing everything, even when it isn't good for her. I will come back to this, but first I'm hoping to understand better the pattern in which they get stuck. In this still early phase of therapy, my goal is to slow down, track relational process, provide empathic direct feedback, and introduce feminist ideas of relating that challenge traditional White, heteropatriarchal assumptions about marriages as a way to help partners reimagine how they might interact differently with each other.

I ask for another example of when they feel disconnected. Nadine says, "Well, like the most recent example was when we tried to discuss children this week. It went *really* badly. You know, I just don't think Alex was ready for a real marriage. They didn't date much prior to our relationship and I worry that Alex just doesn't want to be tied down." I notice Nadine overstepping, telling Alex about Alex and, as if on cue, Alex sinks lower into the chair and seems to want to disappear.

I slow Nadine down so she can notice her own feelings and behavior. I reflect, "So you sound worried that Alex doesn't want the same things as you do. Is that it?" Nadine agrees that she's worried about this. I continue, "In that conversation about having children when you get worried, how do you respond?"

Nadine says, "I try harder to get Alex to see my point. And when that doesn't work, I just give up and go take care of myself on my own."

Alex jumps in here saying, "Yes, that is so frustrating! She follows me around the house telling me how I feel. How I *feel* is rushed, criticized, and misunderstood! And after she doesn't get her way, she's cold and distant. She tends to go off and make quick decisions that affect me without including me."

I ask Nadine if she knows what Alex means, and she acknowledges that she does but feels justified: "Alex clearly doesn't want to be dealing with me, so fine, I can be on my own."

I reflect back to Nadine, "So if you're going to have to be alone, at least you'll be fine on your own?"

Nadine agrees. "What else is there to do?" I summarize here, noting that I can see how worried Nadine is, and I highlight that when worried, she sometimes responds by overstepping, as though telling Alex how they feel, or criticizing their response might bring Alex closer. Nadine is a swimmer, so I use a swim metaphor and suggest she "veers into Alex's (swim) lane" and gets less of Alex, not more, when she does so.

I return to Alex. "So, what kinds of decisions does Nadine make without you?"

"Well, at work she might schedule meetings on our projects without letting me know. I can get caught off guard, because someone I supervise knows about a meeting before I do. Or when we moved recently, she made arrangements with a moving company that involved me, without even checking with me."

Nadine responds, "That's not true! I do check. It just takes you forever to decide, and you often *don't* decide and just never get back to me."

I ask Alex about this. They reply, "I guess that's true sometimes. I just feel anxious about decisions, so I put off deciding."

I say, "And then you just forget to communicate to Nadine about that?" Alex admits this is true. I turn to Nadine, "So that must get pretty frustrating not to know when or even if Alex is going to give you an opinion."

"Yes!" Nadine responds, "it's so completely frustrating. I feel unimportant and all alone. I just want to move on with a decision and get away from the loneliness of it."

Alex counters, "Sometimes you don't tell me what's going on or even ask me for a response. Or you know I'm not going to want to do something, so you purposefully don't ask and just decide without me."

Nadine says, "Well when I do ask, you don't respond, so what am I supposed to do?"

I notice Alex and Nadine getting stuck again in a back-and-forth exchange that goes nowhere. I want to interrupt the unproductive grind between them and instead have them communicate through me, so I can assist the process. I say, "So is this how it goes at home?" They agree that this is what many of their recent discussions are like. I ask Alex and Nadine how they feel right now, after having had this disconnecting experience in the session. Nadine identifies feeling lonely, angry, and hopeless, while Alex feels sad and numb. I ask, "So, at home, what would happen next?" Alex says that at home they would emotionally disconnect from Nadine, and wait until it all blows over. Nadine agrees and says she would do something similar, though she would lead more with anger. After a few days of tension, when mainly they would not communicate, Nadine would usually be the one to insert some discussion about family or weekend plans to help chill the frost in the air. But, as I say to them now, "Waiting for a disagreement to 'blow over' isn't the same thing as resolution, which requires attention and skills to repair."

Here, I focus on slowing, tracking, and understanding the interactional cycle between Alex and Nadine. I ask for multiple examples and look for patterns that persist even when the content of an argument changes. I want to understand how they argue, what they're each experiencing during those arguments, and how each person understands their own responses and behavior. I check in frequently to make sure they're confident that I'm getting what it feels like to be in this relationship both on a good day and on a bad one. I do this because, as a systemic therapist, I see their interaction pattern as my main client. Before a pattern can be changed, we must have a shared understanding of what it is and how they both contribute to it. From their description, I hypothesize that Alex has developed a first consciousness response to criticism that involves avoidance and disconnection, as they often simply wait for tension to pass. When Nadine expresses wanting something different, Alex might then respond with passive aggression and more withdrawal. Nadine is threatened by feeling ignored or unimportant and has developed an attack strategy that entails pushing hard for what she wants, but when that fails to engage Alex, she can become emotionally remote, critical, and rigid.

I've realized the importance of informing clients about how I see what's happening and how I imagine I can be helpful. I say, "I can feel the tension! What I notice is that you're each responding to what's happening between you in ways that aren't helpful. Are you interested in some feedback about what I think is happening?" Alex and Nadine's agreement here is crucial, and I do not want to continue without it. If therapy is to be a refuge, then, as a therapist, I want to collaborate with rather than dominate clients. Gilligan's feminist ethics of care (1982) guide me, as I want to challenge traditional ideas about relationships, starting with how I relate to clients. Therapists can have brilliant ideas and clinical interventions, but when these are disembodied from the relationships we build with clients, missing what's most salient and pressing for them, then our help becomes focused more on solving problems than on care or concern for them as whole people on a journey. Asking directly helps me assess whether the refuge we've built so far in therapy can move toward more honest and relational dialogues. If I've joined, understood, and tracked well what is happening, then Alex and Nadine are likely to feel respected and engage in what I offer. If one or both balk or seem disinterested, then I have more joining and tracking to do before we continue.

Once they agree to feedback, I offer a direct, compassionate, down-to-earth assessment of what I notice about how their defenses are interfering in their relationships. When they indicate interest, I continue. "It sounds to me like you both come heavily armored to your interactions these days. Alex, you come expecting tension, on the lookout for Nadine's criticism and anger, and ready to withdraw at the first sign of it. While, Nadine, you come to these same interactions expecting to be disappointed and thus already urgent, critical, and ready to push through Alex's defenses. Alex, the more you avoidantly withdraw, the more you, Nadine, urgently criticize. As the tension rises, you both get locked into doing more of the same. On the one hand, Alex, you don't want to be misunderstood or told how you feel, yet you shut down and emotionally disappear, leaving Nadine little choice but to decide on her own what's happening. Nadine, you don't like the lonely feeling you often get in the relationship with Alex, yet you often choose to 'go it alone,' blaming and criticizing Alex for your decision to do so. You're both successful at empowering yourselves in these difficult moments but not so good at empowering the relationship. So, we have to slow it down and change the pattern." They are both quiet. I definitely have their attention.

In this session I'm gently and consistently encouraging Alex and Nadine to shift their attention inward, paying attention to what they're experiencing and how they're responding to one another. Instead of continuing to "work on" one another or even the relationship, I'm hoping to help them focus on the only thing they have legitimate power over—themselves and how they behave in their relationship. This means inviting them to care for their own vulnerable feelings rather than making their partner responsible for "making" them feel uncomfortable. It also means inviting them to let go of the illegitimate claims of power that are often expected and encouraged in White heteropatriarchal social structures, including coercive control, manipulation, punishment, retaliation, withdrawal, and stonewalling, or what Real (2018) calls "losing relational strategies." These strategies are encouraged and modeled at every level socioculturally. And that is why in difficult moments, it feels natural for Nadine and Alex to focus on the reactive or off-putting behavior of their partner and feel compelled, even entitled, to their defensive posturing in return. To do otherwise would mean tuning into their own vulnerable feelings in a world where they often feel maligned and their vulnerabilities are used against them.

To counter this, I offer a view of their relationship as an ecosystem in which they're both inhabitants. As such, they each have a responsibility to care for it, themselves, and one another. They decide whether they nurture it or whether they pollute it. I say, "Committed relationships can become entrenched from time to time in difficult patterns. You're each responding with losing relational strategies that might have helped you before but aren't helping your marriage."

Nadine says, "But I get so frustrated. I just want Alex to change, now!"

I respond, "Can you slow down your response and instead be more curious and empathic with yourself?"

Alex offers, "How do we do that in the middle of yelling at each other?"

"Great point," I say. "Let me teach you how to take a time-out."

I provide them the basic rules of time-outs, along with a resource, so they can read more about it.

> "Time-outs are simple but also hard to do. During a time-out, you're agreeing to interrupt a conversation as soon as it escalates to a point you can no longer be open or productive. Responsible time-outs require an agreement about precisely when you'll check back in with each other. Usually, this is 20 minutes but it can be longer depending on how long one or both of you need to calm down and get out of the 'flight–fight–freeze' space. When you reconnect, don't revisit the difficult topic. Instead, decide together when a good time would be to try again to discuss it. And then simply resume your day. When either one of you requests a time-out, it should be honored right away. Remember, this is a way you're committing to take care of your relationship, yourselves, and one another."

We practice recognizing signs that a conversation is going badly (heart rate, breathing, volume, as well as the urge to criticize, withdraw, etc.). They practice requesting a stop in the action before they're so upset that they can't make this request in a moderate way rather than a punishing or challenging one. This gets them laughing as they imagine trying to say kind, calm words through gritted teeth and deep breaths. I laugh along—sharing a funny story about a recent time I struggled to ask my partner for a time-out. I do this to normalize how hard this actually is to do and to give them permission not to be perfect or even good at it right away.

INTERMEDIATE PHASE OF THERAPY: NURTURING QUEERNESS

The next time we meet, Alex and Nadine seem notably warmer and more at ease with each other. I notice this out loud to them and ask them what's changed. Nadine says they've been practicing time-outs, which led to a joint decision to not discuss having a child right now, since that conversation kept escalating. "How's that going?" I ask.

Nadine laughs, "It's going great for Alex; they never want to talk about that anyway. I think we both needed a break from the tension."

"Fair enough," I remark, "but just to clarify, you're both making a choice that suits you, Alex, and perhaps the relationship, at least in the short run, but is not good for you, Nadine, in the long run, right?" Nadine agreed that was true. "So, it will be important for you to know and communicate to Alex when you need something different—or Alex, for you to check in to inquire how this is going for her." I say this because both Alex and Nadine have learned well the cultural expectations that encourage some people (especially those in devalued positions, BIPOC, femme/female, etc.) to accommodate to the needs of others (especially those in empowered positions, White, masculine/male) rather than vice versa. I sense this dynamic is playing out between them, contributing to their problematic pattern and interfering in the equitable, intimate relationship they both want.

As I noted earlier, I think of therapy in four overlapping phases. I'm consistently assessing whether there is enough refuge to sustain whatever difficult, honest conversation is salient. If I think that there is, I lean into that discussion as I did here to *nurture queerness* (the third stage) or, in other words, a shift in the (White heteropatriarchal) status quo. So I overtly mark Nadine's accommodation and offer alternative pathways in which Nadine is invited to pay attention to her needs and advocate directly for them. Meanwhile, Alex is invited to take a turn accommodating Nadine. I consider this a first-order change. In this stage, I also try to understand current survival strategies in the context of families of origin.

In subsequent sessions, we talk more specifically about where Alex's chronic feelings of being overwhelmed and their withdrawal strategy came from: growing up queer, nonbinary, and poor in a single-parent, Catholic home. Alex stuck out from a young age—Dad had been physically abusive, dominating the household before leaving and essentially being uninvolved after that. Mom was anxious, demanding, and alternately loving but then verbally abusive. As the oldest child, Alex had responsibilities to care for two younger siblings and often felt overwhelmed and ashamed of their powerlessness, queerness, and poverty. Alex learned to cope by staying under the radar, passive and frozen, in order to do damage control. Alex finally left home for good at 17, when their mom became verbally and physically aggressive when Alex came out. This sheds new light for Alex (and for me) about their exiting strategies.

When I check in about how things have been between them, Alex uncharacteristically offers, "Well I want to share how shocked I was to realize how often I get overwhelmed and have the urge to emotionally disconnect. I think I process way slower than Nadine. I regularly feel rushed and overwhelmed, and I just never paid attention to that." Alex who is usually quiet, is speaking up. This is a change in their earlier pattern and something for which Nadine has hoped.

I want to encourage Alex, so I say, "Brilliant—now you're noticing what you'd prefer in your intimate communications. So, next time, when things are feeling fast, how could you advocate for this?" Alex tentatively decides they could simply ask Nadine to be less critical. Instead, I direct Alex to use "I" statements and start with owning their feelings of being overwhelmed.

But Nadine looks increasingly troubled, and she responds fiercely, "So in short, I have to be less intense and critical, and Alex has to stop withdrawing and hiding. But sometimes things have to be decided quickly. Where do you think I'd be if I politely waited around hoping people would notice me?" There's an edge to what she says, almost a challenge, and I catch a reactive part of me that wants to argue with her.

I take my own advice: Slow way down and get curious. "So, Nadine, what just happened for you?"

Nadine takes a deep breath and says, "I'm furious and so impatient! I don't know if I can slow down or if I want to." I offer, "I could imagine a thousand reasons that as a cis female, BIPOC lesbian, you might feel impatient and furious right now. What if you trusted your impatience and your fury?" Nadine seems disconnected and says tersely, "I wouldn't know where to begin." I ask Nadine to begin wherever makes sense, perhaps when she first noticed being furious or first worried about being labeled as angry. So far, we've been focused mainly on recognizing and disrupting survival strategies. At this point, we continue to shift the status quo by addressing the underlying experiences and vulnerabilities that fuel those old strategies.

Nadine describes a childhood household full of both love and tension. Her parents have been together for 45 years. Their marriage wasn't particularly happy, but happiness seemed beside the point. They had met after both sets of her grandparents had moved from the South to the same northern city during the 1960s. They shared southern roots, the experience of racism, migration, and a strong desire to improve their economic prospects. Her father, a mechanic, doted on her as the youngest daughter, who was intellectually gifted and mechanically inclined. But he was also remote and emotionally disconnected. He stayed scarce when tensions at home got high, as they regularly did. And although he could be warm, he rarely expressed emotions—preferring quiet calm or stony silence when angered. Nadine's mother, a homemaker who was perpetually frustrated, worked as a legal secretary until Nadine's brother was born. She loved her children, and though she wasn't warm or affectionate, she was reliable, well-organized and attentive to their day-to-day needs. Her mother, like Nadine, was gifted—brilliant even. She had aspired to be a lawyer but couldn't afford the schooling. She seemed frustrated with her life, resentful of her husband's freedom and career, and was often quietly seething. There was a lot of pressure on them as African American, working-class people to "do good and look good doing it." Perfection, or close to it, was expected of all of them, especially in public. It was unsafe to do otherwise. Her mother was controlled and contained in public, but in private her moods could veer wildly, and she sometimes lashed out verbally and physically toward her children, especially Nadine. Nadine's theories on why her mother seemed to target her varied. Maybe her connection with her father was threatening to her mother? Maybe her mother sensed the truth about her sexuality? Whatever the reasons, she couldn't live up to her mother's standards for "lady-like behavior" despite wanting to please her. From the time she was small, Nadine had always felt distant and disconnected from other children, including her siblings. She felt like she had to hide that she excelled at school, or keep separate her diverse and eclectic friends, or later, hide that she was a lesbian, as she understood how threatening that would be to her family.

Nadine's academic interests continued to lead her away from her working class BIPOC roots into a highly visible, professional job surrounded mainly by upper-class, White, cisgender, heterosexual folks with their good intentions and microaggressions. We discussed how she learned to be careful and controlled as a survival strategy, first around her parents, then later around White friends, lovers, or coworkers, protecting herself by protecting them from having to talk directly about race or sexuality. It was a difficult needle to thread, especially regarding race. She had to be driven and intense to plow through the low expectations others seemed to have of her or the way White people seemed to not see her if she remained patient or compliant. On the other hand, if she was too driven, then she was seen as angry and difficult. Instead, she was always meticulously curating herself, judging how "real" she could be in any given moment, learning to tone down anything too queer in some spaces or too Black in others; too mouthy or too mousy, and always with a sense of growing urgency that she had limited time and limited options, and she had to make the most of them. And now she felt that same urgency about having a child.

With this information, Nadine's loneliness and intense need for emotional connection take on new meaning. I ask her if she protects Alex the way she protects other White people, and she admits she does.

Alex protests, "We do talk about race all the time. I do get it. The same things happen to me at work. People misgender or microaggress because of my queerness."

Nadine responds by reporting that Alex can talk comfortably in the abstract about racism, but whenever it gets local or personal, Alex's first response is to minimize Nadine's experience, particularly when they talk about her experiences at work. Alex is very quiet.

"What would you like Alex to do instead?" I ask.

"I want to talk about race, and I want Alex to listen to me and believe me," Nadine says simply.

I asked Alex directly, "Are you willing to discuss race differently than you have in the past?" Alex agrees. "Can you start by not equalizing her experience with race and yours?" Alex indicates willingness but looks like a deer in the headlights.

I forge ahead, directing them back to our previous conversation about their work conflicts. I ask Nadine how she thinks race plays a part. Nadine describes a team of people they're currently working with on a project. Nadine experiences two members of this team as openly hostile to her because she's a Black woman. Nadine recounts how these two individuals routinely question her decisions and challenge her authority. Despite successfully co-leading this and other projects for years with Alex, she overheard these two coworkers dismissing her contributions to other employees: "At least she [Nadine] diversifies us."

Nadine said, "And when I tried to talk about it with you, Alex, you said, 'They do that to everyone. They're not racist, they're just assholes.'"

I turn to Alex, who looks stricken. I want to help Alex remember to breathe and slow down, so I check in, ask if they need a minute, and we breathe together for a moment. Then I say, "Do you remember what Nadine asked you for?"

Alex replies, "To listen and to believe her."

I respond, "Good, so can you do that right now?"

Alex says a little stiffly, "I am listening. Please tell me more."

Nadine continues. "Do you know how many times people have pulled that shit with me? I know when I'm being targeted. I know when it's about race. How can you even say that to me?"

Alex breathes, hesitates, and responds, "You're right, you're right. I discouraged you from talking about it. I was worried it would escalate out of control. I felt overwhelmed and didn't know how to help."

Nadine responds, "You can help by acknowledging what is actually happening at work and say so *to them. That's* what would help!"

I'm thinking about Alex's pattern of avoidance and withdrawal in light of what Nadine is saying. "Alex," I say, "how are you feeling right now?"

Alex replies, "Feeling pretty shitty."

"Yes, that sounds about right. I think you feel bad because you really love her and you know she's right. You haven't showed up for her." I continue, "I don't want to pile on, but I have some hard feedback for you that I think is important. Are you ready to hear it?" Alex agrees to hear me out. I ask them to reflect for a moment on the early disagreement they had about the team project. "If I have this right, you get anxious about team scheduling and logistics, and then disappear, leaving Nadine to manage communication with racist, hostile team members. Do I have it?"

Alex nods, letting in what I'm saying. I continue, "That's pretty tone deaf, no? Do you want to keep disappearing on her like that, having Nadine fill in the gaps for you while you skate by using your charm and privilege? I think you can do better. You're this beautiful strong masculine queer person! How can you show up for her? Support her? Protect her?" This important conversation is difficult and tender, and it invites both of them to shift from first-order to second-order change. If first-order change can be thought of as only a change in behavior, second-order change is a shift in process— specifically, a shift in relational rules and expectations. So instead of avoiding vulnerability by shouldering it all on her own, Nadine is talking openly about the very real reasons for her fury and impatience. Instead of commands or critiques, she's leading with specific asks and effectively requesting what she wants. This requires a fundamental shift in her relationship with herself. Similarly, Alex is managing the intensity of a fight–flight–freeze response differently and choosing to do something different by staying present. Nadine's directness invites Alex to understand how their withdrawal strategy unintentionally intersects with their White privilege causing them to fail to show up and effectively support Nadine's experience with racism.

CONCLUDING PHASE OF THERAPY: ENCOURAGING TRANSFORMATION

Clients often return to previous stages of therapy as they face crisis or life transitions, and this is what happened with Alex and Nadine. I worked with them solidly for a couple of years. As they built a new way of relating to one another, therapy moved into more of a maintenance of the second-order relational changes they had made. We spent time encouraging the transformations they had made by recognizing old survival strategies as they came up, exploring the fears and vulnerabilities that fueled those survival reactions, and translating those into specific, reasonable, current requests for each other. Much of what we talked about was the kinds of topics that bring all people, from all walks of life, to psychotherapy from time to time. And we also addressed issues specific to queer, BIPOC, and gender-nonconforming people: internalized homophobia and shame, differences in levels of "outness," and protecting themselves and their relationship from minority stress and microaggressions. They got better at having hard, respectful conversations. They wrestled on and off with the idea of having children without pursuing it further than that. Their positions on the issue did not change, and, inevitably, when Nadine turned 41, she became desperate to become a parent. Alex had remained noncommittal on the topic—unable to make a clear decision one way or another, preferring to avoid a decision altogether. So, they returned to therapy to address the stalemate directly.

At one point during yet another fraught conversation in session, things escalated. Alex asks Nadine to slow down. Nadine, frustrated and impatient, gets tangled up with the part of her that forges fiercely ahead and begins yelling emasculating insults at Alex, perhaps as an attempt to shame them out of paralysis. Alex physically recoils and Nadine responds, "I know, I know I'm the angry, scary Black lady."

I interrupt her quietly and steadily until she stops speaking. "Nadine . . . (long awkward pause), Nadine . . . (another long awkward pause). Can I stop you?" Finally, Nadine looks at me. "Let's breathe for a minute, okay?" After a minute or two, I ask Nadine if she's ready to hear me. She nods. "You have important things to say, but you stopped actually saying them about 5 minutes ago. Meanwhile Alex has already stopped listening to you. Can you feel that?" After another long pause, we talk about what she feels in her body. "Right now, do you hear Alex asking you to slow down?" Nadine agrees that she does. "Your fierceness has helped you be successful in a world that doesn't want you to be. Sometimes it serves you. But right now, it's not helping you communicate effectively with this person you love. So, what do you want to do?" Nadine looks confused. "Do you want a suggestion?" She nods. "Just stop. Or if you can't, then take a break. Get some water. Go for a walk. I'll walk with you, if you'd like. Just be with this part of yourself that feels so threatened and desperate rather than letting it run you." Nadine expresses a willingness to try and decides to take a walk on her own and come back to this conversation the following week.

In sessions I have the power of a therapist and the privileges of a White person and a middle-class, educated professional. So I have a responsibility to manage my own survival strategies, particularly with minoritized people, queer, trans, and especially BIPOC folks. In this session, I was working very hard to manage my own reactivity. I was uncomfortable and unsure as a White-bodied person how to both honor Nadine's anger and challenge her behavior. I could feel Nadine's urgency, and I resonated with her. I had always wanted to have children, and because of my own shame and insecurity, it took me a lot longer than I wanted before starting the process. This lit some fire in me, and I became reactive to both Alex's passivity and Nadine's escalating fury. When I was breathing with Nadine, I was trying to calm all of us, especially myself. If I had continued without recognizing and managing my discomfort, shame, and grief about the losses in my life, then I would have intervened from a place of domination rather than collaboration—exactly the opposite of what I strive for and value.

As we revisited this conversation over the next few weeks, I supported Nadine as she apologized for the insults she had lobbed in Alex's direction. And I coached Alex to reassure Nadine that they knew the conversation was important and was willing to make headway. Alex shared that they had felt pushed into getting married by Nadine, sensing that she was doing it to appease her family more than anything else. Alex was afraid the decision to have children was a repeat of this. Nadine responded openly, admitting that she had pushed for marriage as way to legitimize herself in the eyes of her parents. She believed that, once married, her parents would finally see her and her heterosexual siblings as equally valid. Alex asked Nadine directly whether she wanted a child for the same reason. Nadine asked for a week to think about this. When she came back, she reported that in the past, this may have been a major part of her desire to be a parent, but that was no longer true. She felt sure that they would be good parents, and instead of trying to convince or argue with Alex, she simply asked, "What would becoming a parent be like for you?" Alex had a lot of worries and fears about being a gender nonbinary parent and felt overwhelming dread at the thought.

When I asked Alex what they were most afraid of, they responded, "That my being nonbinary or us being queer would harm the child or that they would be ashamed of me."

I laughed gently. "Are we talking about your shame or your future, potential, as-yet unborn child's shame? The poor kid isn't even conceived yet."

We were, of course, talking about Alex's shame, which once again had gotten its hooks into Alex's life—overwhelming their resources and convincing them as queer and nonbinary that they should not be a parent, that they did not belong. Hemphill (2021) proposes that shame is the internalization of oppression and becomes an "emotional ritual" (p. 43) for the marginalized, a practice that helps ensure safety and belonging. As queer folks, we are fed a steady diet of shame, living as we do in families and communities that mostly don't share our queer experience and thus simply don't want to or don't know how to protect us. Instead, we must learn to protect ourselves. And the more intersections of marginalization that we must navigate, the more danger we are in. So we study what the world finds so unworthy about us. We study so that we can learn to be enough of ourselves to survive but not so much that we no longer belong. Shame becomes a protective barrier keeping queer people from stepping too far out of bounds, forgetting ourselves or the limits of what this world will allow us to be. Shame persists for queer people, because it's the price we pay for any shred of safety and belonging in the White heteropatriarchy in which we live.

It is this internalized shame that had frozen Alex in place—and after 2 years we've arrived back at the original disagreement that brought them to therapy. But this time, they were better prepared. Alex no longer needs to withdraw in shame and isolation to manage feeling threatened. Instead, they summon the strength and skills to stay connected to self and to reach out to Nadine. And Nadine, no longer feeling alienated from Alex, now uses her fierceness to be steady and calm.

We devoted additional time in sessions to addressing their fears and vulnerabilities about parenting: Is queer parenting bad for children? Is having a nonbinary parent confusing? The research is ongoing, but evidence suggests that the opposite is true and that children thrive in LGBTQIA+ households (Goldberg & Allen, 2013). Alex asked what becoming a parent would mean for their identity, and would the child be ashamed of having a nonbinary parent?

"Good questions," I said. "Parenting is going to affect both of your identities in unpredictable ways and, as to the second question, your child will likely be ashamed of you for any number of reasons! Welcome to parenting!" There were moments like these in our time together that I shared stories about my own journey as a queer parent and how I'd realized that the same things I had been taught to be ashamed of were actually sources of strength for me. I ask them, "What unique gifts will you bring to parenting because of your queer and nonbinary identities?"

Alex smiled and said, "I hadn't exactly thought of it like that before—but, yes, I think I know something about how to protect a child but allow them to be free."

FURTHER REFLECTIONS AND IMPLICATIONS

I still see Alex and Nadine from time to time as they now navigate being queer parents. They're loving partners to one another and good parents to their children. Their relationship has inspired them to mature and their love to deepen in ways they had not imagined before they accomplished it. As Haines (2019, p. 833) writes, "Social conditions have everything to do with defining what is real, what's possible . . . and even what's imaginable." I've used the phrase "White heteropatriarchy" throughout this chapter to describe these current social conditions. As a professor and clinical supervisor, I worry that when I use this term, my supervisees believe I'm describing something merely philosophical, wholly disconnected from their day-to-day lives. Actually, I'm trying to impress upon them something very concrete: There are psychological and relational consequences of White heteropatriarchal assumptions that are not adequately considered by clinical theories or supervisory models, because racism, sexism, classism, heteronormativity, in fact, domination itself, are so commonplace and familiar. It's our job as therapists to understand how oppression plays out in intimate relationships and to intervene in the harm and disconnection that result. But there is by far more cultural tradition and expectation to actively avoid discussions of racial, gender, and class power imbalances than there are sustained and effective examples of how to do this well.

Just as human behavior cannot be adequately understood outside the family context, neither can it be understood outside of a broader social context. The problematic coping strategies Nadine and Alex employ in their most difficult moments are not only representations of their experience in their families of origin but also their sociocultural context. Power differentials are routinely weaponized between loved ones—such as when Alex, blinded by White privilege and scrambling to avoid conflict, discounts Nadine's experience of racism and gaslights her; or when Nadine, threatened and believing she must make something happen, uses emasculating insults to try and coerce Alex into action. It is one thing to have these very human reactions, but quite another thing to live in sociocultural realities that expect, justify, and encourage them. This atmosphere permeates family life, routinely encouraging unhealthy relating and making it difficult to develop healthier attitudes and behaviors.

Therapy and therapists are not immune to this process. In my work with Alex and Nadine, I sought supervision, because I could feel myself shutting down in stressful moments, relying on old coping mechanisms learned in my family as a White, working-class, queer woman: Avoid conflict, stay quiet, don't make waves. These strategies are born out of my unique intersection of oppression and privilege. Silent shutdowns might masquerade as "professionalism" but would not have helped Nadine and Alex, or addressed the racism or heteronormativity in the room. To accomplish that, a therapist must be willing to push their own growing edges and be honest with themselves about how their unique intersectional vulnerabilities affect their work. Yet precious little clinical training teaches clinicians how to do this. Few theories offer effective ways to challenge entitled, racist, sexist, classist behavior or even name them for what they are. Most advise against doing so, claiming objectivity and neutrality as professional moral high ground. But neutrality and objectivity only conserve the racist, sexist, classist status quo, and thus the relational harms these inflict.

Other systemic theories are "strengths based"—where strengths are defined by White heteropatriarchal standards that value individuality and status over collaboration or relational ethics. From this viewpoint, Nadine's "go it alone" defense in the face of Alex's withdrawal, or Alex's ability to stay unemotional and logical as Nadine experiences microaggressions at work, might be viewed as strengths and go unaddressed or even be encouraged. Focusing only on the positives can easily cause missed opportunities to identify problematic relational processes such as those I outlined with Nadine and Alex. Finally, there are also systemic theories that encourage vulnerability in clients without a clear road map for how a therapist should address intersectionality or establish transparency about the use of power in sessions. To effectively invite marginalized people to be more vulnerable requires explicit acknowledgment of the invisible protections of privilege, the invisible burdens of oppression, and a nuanced understanding of the way shame operates specifically for queer and BIPOC folks in White, heteropatriarchal contexts. It also requires the patient development of shared understanding and language about what queer clients uniquely stand to lose and gain with increased relational vulnerability and authenticity.

Like many queer people, Nadine and Alex have been made to feel ashamed for the ways they transgress the framework of White heteropatriarchy and the binaries of gender, race, and class. These binaries have serious limitations, especially for healthy relating. What is often disallowed in mainstream context is space to freely inhabit a fuller range of the human experience. We can be masculine or feminine. We can have individuality or togetherness. We can have agency or be accommodating. We can have one or the other, but without equity, we cannot have both.

Queer folks have learned to be lesser versions of themselves in order to procure a sense of safety and belonging. Despite this, queer relationships have been on the vanguard of alternative ways to structure romantic and sexual relationships for a long time. There are gifts that come from living on the margins. It can inspire one to be more flexible, scrappier, and less entitled. It allows for the creation and celebration of chosen families, employs the creativity of a whole spectrum of gender roles, and inspires a definition of family that isn't limited by blood or marriage or monogamy. This allows for affection and commitment to be maintained and community to be preserved even long after traditional marriages or romantic relationships end.

Therapy is inherently a relational endeavor—one would hope, a useful navigation of ways of being and thinking about the world between therapist and clients. It can and ought to be a refuge nurturing queer and BIPOC people to be fuller versions of themselves, seeing their differences as important and necessary in a world organized around disempowerment and domination. To do this, affirmative therapists have to summon the courage to envision relationships, families, and communities outside White, heteropatriarchal imagination and to practice liberation as a relational process in their own lives. The more power, privilege, education, money, or status we have in this society, the more responsibility we have to do so. Other ways of relating can be imagined. This reimagination is at the heart of the work I do these days with my clients, with my students, and in my own life.

REFERENCES

Coolhart, D. (2023). Therapy with queer couples. In J. L. Lebow & D. K. Snyder (Eds.), *Clinical handbook of couple therapy* (6th ed., pp. 512–530). New York: Guilford Press.

das Nair, R., & Thomas, S. (2012). Race and ethnicity. In R. das Nair & C. Butler (Eds.), *Intersectionality, sexuality and psychological therapies: Working with lesbian, gay, and bisexual diversity* (pp. 59–88). West Sussex, UK: Blackwell.

Gates, G. J. (2012). *Same-sex couples in Census 2010: Race and ethnicity.* University of California at Los Angeles Williams Institute of Law. Retrieved July 19, 2023, from *https://williamsinstitute.law.ucla.edu/wp-content/uploads/ss-couples-race-apr-2012.pdf.*

Gilligan, C. (1982). *In a different voice: Psychological theory and women's development.* Boston: Harvard University Press.

Goldberg, A. E., & Allen, K. R. (Eds.). (2013). *LGBT-parent families: Innovations in research and implications for practice.* New York: Springer.

Haines, S. (2019). *The politics of trauma: Somatics, healing, and social justice.* Berkeley, CA: North Atlantic Books.

Harvey, R. G., Murphy, M. J., Bigner, J. J., & Wetchler, J. L. (2022). *Handbook of LGBTQ-affirmative couple and family therapy*. New York: Routledge.

Harvey, R. G., & Stone Fish, L. (2015). Queer youth in family therapy. *Family Process, 54*, 396–417.

Hemphill, P. (2021). The wisdom of process. In T. Burke & B. Brown (Eds.), *You are your best thing: Vulnerability, shame resilience, and the Black experience* (pp. 43–53). New York: Random House.

Real, T. (2018). *Fierce intimacy: Standing up to one another with love*. Louisville, CO: Sounds True.

Stone Fish, L., & Harvey, R. G. (2005). *Nurturing queer youth: Family therapy transformed*. New York: Norton.

CHAPTER 13

Couple Therapy with Older Adults
*Navigating Challenges
and Building on Opportunities*

DOUGLAS K. SNYDER

Editor's (JLL) Comments

In this chapter, Doug Snyder focuses our attention on working with older adult couples. Couples bring universal processes to an intimate relationship, but distinctly different issues accompany various stages of the life cycle. Snyder highlights that being older can be both "the best and worst of times" for couples—not only an opportunity to find meaning in life and enjoy what has been learned over a lifetime but also the unique stresses of growing older and the challenges of decline and mortality.

    This case focuses on two major passages in older couples. The first is retirement of one or both partners from the work activities that have organized much of their lives. While this may conjure up free time on the beach, for many couples, retirement represents a life crisis of reshaping their lives. The second passage involves mental decline—a problem now so frequent in the very old. Snyder wisely and empathically helps this couple cope with both of these passages.

    Snyder's therapy exemplifies the best of pluralistic integrative practice, which draws systematically from concepts and strategies from specific approaches. Note the orderly progression from assessment to case formulation, to making informed choices about intervention. He models how experienced therapists ask assessment questions in a way that is open ended, efficient, and caring. Note as well how the therapy moves smoothly between work with the couple and one or the other partner, and from directing skills such as communication and problem solving to exploring how family-of-origin experiences (here so long ago) continue to shape present experience. Snyder's interventions change at various choice points based on what emerges as most useful for the couple, while he strives to remain an empathic witness through their life voyage.

    Snyder also provides a master class in how skillful therapists recognize and speak to their own internal process, in relation to both the couple and personal countertransference. Snyder's inner dialogue highlights the importance of the interface between the couple and the therapist.

Upon reflection, my interests in older adults likely evolved from early childhood. I was the youngest of three children. My father was also the youngest of three, and my mother the second-youngest of nine. I was nurtured by a large extended family—with cousins close to my parents' age, and uncles and aunts approaching the age of my grandparents. I was both cuddled and coddled shamelessly!

The broad age span of an extended family afforded me numerous opportunities to witness remarkable diversity in how my elders engaged both the challenges and opportunities of later life. Such individual differences in how older adults navigate aging were further illuminated early in my clinical work. Some of my older adult couples rediscovered and built upon the very best in themselves and their relationship; others stumbled and teetered on the edge of despair from immense strains and the anticipated decline in their quality of life.

Now, upon entering my 70s, the fulfillment I gain from working with older couples no longer flows solely from a genuine but perhaps dispassionate caring I felt in earlier years but, rather, from an emerging and keen awareness on a deep personal level of life's finiteness and my own determination to make the best of what time remains. Movies with aging characters—as with Katherine Hepburn and Henry Fonda in *On Golden Pond* (Rydell, 1981) and their narrative of reconstructing relationships with adult children— have more profound meaning for me than when I first watched them in my 30s. (Even citing this film—a favorite among my generation but now 40 years later—brings home the passage of time.) And more recent portrayals of couples confronting end stages of life—as with Helen Mirren and Donald Sutherland in *The Leisure Seeker* (Virzi, 2017)—now provoke uncomfortable but vital conversations with my partner about how we would choose to live and die.

How privileged I am to continue to learn and to share with aspiring therapists some perspectives on working with older adult couples! The need for couple therapists to have both clinical and cultural competence in working with older adults is apparent from even a casual glance at the demographics for this group (U.S. Census Bureau, 2018, 2020). Worldwide, the total number of people 65 and older is projected to more than double from 730 million in 2020 to nearly 1.6 billion by 2050. In the United States, the percentage of population 65 and older comprises the fastest growing age group. By 2030, older Americans will make up 21% of the population; beginning in 2035, adults 65 or older will outnumber children 18 or younger for the first time in U.S. history. By 2060, nearly one in four Americans will be 65 years or older, and the number of those 85 or older will triple.

So how does life change for older couples? To borrow phrasing from Charles Dickens in *A Tale of Two Cities*, it poses the best of times, the worst of times, or—more often—a mix of both. For some couples, partners' deepened knowledge of themselves and each other promotes a tempering of negative reactivity—fostering reflective rather than reflexive responses to potential triggers and facilitating more compassionate perspective taking. For couples in long-term relationships, having weathered numerous trials and tribulations together can promote a secure attachment and comfort from anticipating that "whatever life throws at us, we'll face it together." Some couples experience increased resources of time and money that enhance their quality of life and opportunities for leisurely pursuits. For many, recognizing one's own mortality promotes efforts toward completion of "meaning"—whether through volunteering or other ways of giving back to the world, or strategizing specific ways of disbursing gifts to persons, organizations, or social causes important to them. For some older couples, life now provides opportunity to reconstruct relationships within the extended family—for example, by making repair with adult children or with siblings and moving past earlier enduring conflicts or estrangement.

At the same time, older years pose significant challenges—sometimes inevitably, other times unevenly. Most obvious are the challenges to physical health (e.g., decline of the immune system and decreased muscle mass), as well as cognitive functioning (most noticeably the learning and recall of new information and cognitive processing speed). Older adults may contend with multiple losses including work-related or social identity, decreased mobility and related social isolation, or the death of friends or family members. Financial strains may increase and adversely impact numerous facets of life. Just coping with everyday tasks may become overwhelming. Sometimes the challenges arise from within the relationship itself—just as they might for younger couples, but with greater risks of entrenchment. The cumulative toll from years of neglecting one another or taking each other for granted, creating separate and increasingly distant lives, may render it difficult for partners to find their way back to an intimate and joyful union. Enduring conflicts around adult children, differences in core values, or virtually any other aspect of a couple's relationship may contribute to chronic bickering or episodic flareups that perpetuate partners' avoidance and resentments.

My clinical work with any client reflects a pluralistic approach—that is, one that recognizes the usefulness of multiple theoretical perspectives and draws on constructs and therapeutic strategies from across theoretical models by tailoring interventions to a given case at any given moment based on their clinical relevance and potential utility. In my previous writings (e.g., Snyder, 1999), I've advocated a pluralistic approach to couple therapy involving six levels progressing from building a collaborative alliance and managing initial crises through strengthening the couple dyad and promoting relevant relationship skills, to addressing cognitive components and developmental sources of relationship distress. These last two levels encourage partners to look inward to reflect on the meaning they give to events in their relationship, to deepen their understanding of enduring maladaptive relationship patterns often rooted in family-of-origin experiences, and then to harness such understanding to offer more compassionate responses to their own and each other's distress.

When working with older couples, I'm also informed by a contextual developmental model that integrates individual, relational, and broader sociocultural perspectives on older couples' strengths and challenges (Knight, 2023). I work toward interweaving a narrative approach throughout the therapy—helping partners to coconstruct a shared understanding of "who" and "how" they've been as a path toward restoring and building on the best in themselves and their relationship. Later life affords us opportunities to pause, step back and see the bigger picture, reconcile ourselves to previous mistakes or make amends, and be more mindful and intentional as we write the final chapters of our lives. Jed and Annie, the couple described in the following pages, exemplified this work in ways that continue to inspire me.

INITIAL ASSESSMENT AND CASE FORMULATION

The initial contact came by email, as it typically does nowadays, in my small clinical practice:

"We were referred to you by Dr. Barrington. We've been married for 47 years, through thick and thin. But lately we've been arguing more. My husband just turned 72, and he seems more irritable than usual. I'm 69 and get tired more easily. We've been snapping at each other more, and neither of us is happy with how it's going between us. Dr. Barrington suggested maybe you could help us communicate better."

"Gosh—47 years," I thought to myself. I'm always struck by the levels of commitment and tenacity reflected in such long-term relationships. That duration is no mean feat. Rarely are such couples' histories free of challenges or even times of teetering on the brink, yet somehow the partners find ways of managing or working through those periods—some better than others, some more damaged than others—and their perseverance provides me an opportunity to speak to that determination as a testament to their character.

My initial consultation with couples always begins with some version of the following script:

"I'd first like to take some time today just to get to know some about each of you as individuals—who you are, a bit of your history, how you're doing, and anything else you'd like me to know about you. Then I'm going to ask the two of you why you're here—what you're struggling with as a couple, what's working and what's not, and how you've already tried to deal with things. Finally, before we stop today, we need to decide together whether we'll meet again and, if so, responsibilities we'll each have in trying to make things better. How does that sound to you?"

I never learn as much as I'd like in that initial session—each revelation begs for more. But I quickly acquired enough information to discern remarkable strengths in both partners, and I hoped that we would find ways of working together.

They had attended the same small, rural high school—Jed was a senior when Annie was a freshman. But they had only known each other in passing and had never dated. After high school, Jed began working in the parts division of a local car dealership and eventually progressed to manager of that division. He had excellent organizational skills and had run a "tight ship" as a manager but was generally liked and respected by his parts staff. Annie had gone on to college and obtained a teaching certificate. The couple were reintroduced during her sophomore year in college and started dating casually but, after a year, were in an exclusive relationship. They married shortly after Annie graduated from college. Annie had taught at a nearby elementary school for 40 years before retiring at age 62. Jed had continued working for several years past that, retiring at age 68, four years earlier. He would have worked longer if he could—it had been his life—but he found it increasingly difficult to adapt to the evolving technologies for tracking and maintaining inventory, especially when his dealership merged with another and he faced an entirely unfamiliar line of vehicles, as well as completely different software system.

These were hardworking and conscientious folks, I thought to myself. Each had been successful and respected at work. How had they partnered together at home? What had they done best together, what had they struggled with, and what was making it more difficult for them now? Older couples have so much history—both individually and in their relationship—that I can't always discern what will become relevant in our work together. I listen not only for histories of trauma, but also for stories of resilience that speak to their character. I wasn't surprised that Annie and Jed might be struggling with the transition into retirement and the challenges of shifting roles and identities. I've always found it ironic that the literature is replete with studies and couple-based interventions addressing the transition to parenthood, yet generally devoid of analogous research and interventions for couples transitioning to retirement.

"Tell me about your earlier years at home," I asked. "Did you have children together? How did you manage as a team back then?" I wasn't just seeking information. I phrased my prompt, hoping it might promote positive memories and an opportunity for Jed and Annie to connect.

"We have two children and four grandchildren," Annie shared, smiling. Their son Toby and his wife had a daughter and son of their own, now 14 and 11. And their daughter Ellie and her husband had twin daughters age 8.

"And how's everyone doing?" I asked—a general prompt to see where it might take us.

"Everyone's fine," Annie said. But her smile faded slightly and I could sense the tension between them as Jed stiffened but remained silent. Clearly, there was more to this story, but I was unclear about whether to pursue it now—wondering whether it related to the couple's struggles and also uncertain of Jed's level of comfort in the session or his comfort with me.

"Do you have much contact?" I asked—another ambiguous prompt to gauge their readiness to engage the topic further. The query provoked several moments of silence before Annie continued.

"They each live about 10–15 minutes from us. I try to see them as much as possible—at least every week. I retired at 62, in part so I could have more time with our grandchildren—I had to work while our own youngsters were little—and Ellie's twins were just a year old and she needed all the help she could get!" A smile, then a pause, and the smile faded. "Jed doesn't get to see them as often."

"We don't need to get into that," he injected. "We're here about us, not them."

It was another choice point for me—whether or how to follow-up. My impulse was to accommodate Jed's discomfort. We could always return to the topic and, for now, facilitating a collaborative alliance with both partners was my higher priority.

"That's fine," I said. "If we continue to meet after today . . . [another nod to Jed's discomfort by conveying that I had no presumptions at this point regarding his commitment to further sessions] we can always return to this if it seems relevant. For now, talk with me more about what's going on with the two of you. What are you struggling with at home?"

With some couples, I might have looped back to my previous question about their early years—how they had been drawn to each other and what they had done well together. Devoting time to that question sometimes informs me as to whether a couple has ever created a healthy relationship. And, occasionally, the recounting of earlier good times fosters a collaborative alliance and reassures partners that I won't restrict our focus to their struggles and neglect their strengths. If we continued to work together, I'd want to return to that question, in part to discern previous paths for connecting that might inform opportunities moving forward. But for now, I wanted to understand better why they were here and how they each hoped I might be helpful.

The couple shared a variety of concerns—some common to distressed couples, such as recurrent difficulties in discussing differences. Other challenges were common among couples transitioning to retirement, such as reshaping identities that had been grounded primarily in work or navigating new relational dynamics precipitated by extended time together on a daily basis. Jed had thrived as a manager at the car dealership and was accustomed to being in charge. Annie was also accustomed to managing her own classroom and, in addition, had assumed the role as primary manager on the home front—particularly as it had involved their children. She bristled when Jed now tried to assume control of decisions in their home—ranging from how to organize forks and spoons in the drawers to whether to repair or replace a major appliance. Jed, in turn, felt increasingly like an outsider with no place of his own.

Jed and Annie also had different visions of how they wanted to embrace the newfound freedoms of retirement: She wanted as many opportunities as possible to be with their grandchildren, while he had hoped they would take advantage of an RV they had purchased a few years earlier and travel about the country for weeks or even months at a time. Differences in this regard were entangled with tensions they experienced around their adult children, which, for now, remained opaque to me.

As we approached the end of our session, I shared my initial impressions and invited their thoughts in return. I commented on their strengths, both as individuals and as a couple—their conscientious and hardworking nature, their respective leadership qualities, and their inherent commitment reflected in 47 years of marriage. I contextualized some of their struggles as common challenges of transitioning to retirement, validating the distress each of them was experiencing but placing this squarely within a normative framework. I expressed optimism that they could work through these challenges with some guidance promoting constructive conversations. I also shared that it was clear to me that they were struggling with concerns around their adult children, and that I was open to helping them in this regard as well, but we could decide together down the road whether they wanted to pursue those issues with me. Privately, I had no doubt that we would need to address these concerns. But typically, my top priority in any first session is to have a second one—to gain a foothold and create a safe place to work on relevant issues agreeable to both partners for now, and then tackle more difficult or contentious issues as partners' trust in me and in each other evolves.

They both seemed relieved by a formulation that normalized their struggles. I sensed that Jed recognized my deference to his discomfort with exploring dynamics regarding their adult children during this first session, and that Annie recognized I had clearly discerned this issue and would likely reintroduce the topic down the road. I was glad when they both agreed to an initial trial of four to five sessions I had suggested. I felt connected to both partners from the beginning—admiring their character and likely identifying with some of their struggles—and I hoped for the opportunity to facilitate a difference in their lives.

BEGINNING PHASE OF THERAPY

"We argue about the dumbest things," Annie bemoaned early in the next session. "I just don't get it. We didn't argue like this in the past. I'm tired, and it's wearing me down."

"They may be dumb things to you, but they're not to me," Jed countered. "Why can't I have some say so about how we do things? Why does it always have to be your way?"

"It never mattered to you before. Why now?" Annie continued. "I'm not one of your underlings at the dealership! I don't need to be told the *best* way of doing things" (*placing air quotes around "best"*).

And so there we were, off and running.

Couples can argue about all sorts of things, for all kinds of reasons. But when recurring arguments revolve around what appear—at least on the surface—to be nonsubstantive or even trivial matters, both our theories and clinical experience guide us to look for underlying influences. For some couples, those influences involve enduring struggles around autonomy and control. For others, such arguments may be the surface residua of unresolved hurts or resentments. For some couples, such differences reflect the failure of one or both partners to differentiate preferences from values—assigning disproportionate emotional weight to issues or situations that, when evaluated from a more dispassionate perspective, don't merit the subjective importance attached to them.

Annie and Jed told me they hadn't engaged in such bickering earlier in their marriage. So what had changed? I decided simply to ask them. "Can we pause for a moment? I hear that this way of arguing is fairly new, that you didn't have it earlier in your marriage. What do you think could be going on? You probably have better insights than I do. Can you help me understand better?" Inviting partners to step back and join me in a stance of "detached curiosity" sometimes helps to unlock their entrenched perspectives and soften the conversation.

"Well, for one thing, we're together a lot more now," Annie offered. "Jed never had the time or energy to deal with mundane things at home before, and that was fine with me. (*Looking at Jed*) Your work was exhausting, and I didn't mind managing things at home. (*Then returning to look at me*) But now, it seems like he wants to manage things at home like he did at work—everything being done 'just so.' And it's driving me crazy."

Annie paused and I turned toward Jed—creating opportunity for him to respond. He looked at the floor and seemed to be weighing his words. When he spoke, it was in a softer tone than before. "Sometimes, I just don't know what to do with myself." He took a deep breath and paused again. (*Looking at Annie*) "I just feel shut out. It's your space, not mine. There's no space I get to claim as my own, except maybe the garage. There's no place that's even really 'ours' in terms of what's there, how it's organized, how we use it . . . " Jed's voice trailed off and he looked away, I suspect because he didn't want either Annie or me to see the sadness in his eyes.

I wanted to reflect and empathize with that feeling, in part because Jed had taken the risk to be more vulnerable in the moment, and I suspected that was difficult for him. I wondered how far I could go in joining with Jed in the moment without losing Annie, but then decided the risk of that was low. From the beginning, she had seemed more comfortable and trusting of me and our conversations in session.

I eased ahead. "No space of your own or perhaps even to share. A guest—a welcome guest to be sure—but perhaps feeling more of an outsider than an insider." I paused to see how that landed. Jed gave a slight nod and continued to look away; Annie offered no objection. "I suppose that could feel a bit lonely at times," I continued. "Or maybe even a bit confusing." I wondered if he might walk with me a bit further.

"And she's got the kids and grandkids—all of them."

"And you don't?" I asked. I waited a few moments in silence. Annie alternated looking at me and at Jed, before I continued. "Do you feel ready to share a bit more about what's going on?"

He replied that he wasn't—at least not yet—and Annie seemed disinclined to push Jed further, so I redirected the conversation to the topic of separate and shared space, which seemed a more comfortable level of engagement for both partners in the moment. The subsequent conversation reflected my shifting to a more psychoeducational and solution-focused approach. Both Annie and Jed described how their respective experiences of the home space had evolved, and Annie acknowledged how Jed could feel like a bit of an outsider to decisions regarding that space. I wondered aloud (as a means of offering a "soft pitch") whether there might be some value in thinking about areas of their home where Annie might have primary "decisional prerogative" (adopting a consultative model of inviting input from Jed), areas where Jed might have such decisional authority (consulting with Annie for her input), and other areas where they would pursue decisions together using a more collaborative shared approach.

Many couples achieve such a mix of decisional models easily and implicitly, in part because they permit a level of efficiency in managing daily life. Indeed, Annie and Jed had done so earlier in their marriage across many facets of their lives, including how they managed finances, parenting, leisure time, and so on. Those models, whether implicit or explicit, now needed to evolve as the couple transitioned through the challenges and opportunities of retirement. Annie and Jed welcomed the pragmatic approach I offered, and readily agreed to my suggestion that they coconstruct a chart prior to the next session identifying the various areas of their home for which they had implement unilateral, consultative, or collaborative decision making. The idea of creating a chart appealed to them both, especially Jed.

I sensed an opportunity to resurrect an unanswered question from our initial meeting: How had they connected early in their relationship? What had drawn them to each other, and how had they created joy together? They then shared that it had just seemed "natural, good, and so right" from the beginning. Besides their physical attraction, they had enjoyed each other's company, shared important values, and generally just played well together. "What happened?" I asked, hoping to convey both by facial expression and tone of voice my sense that some of their playfulness had slipped away.

"Life got busy," Annie replied softly, and Jed offered a brief nod of agreement.

The next session began on a more positive note. Their discussions about areas of their home and their respective wishes to have influence had been constructive, and had brought clarity and some resolution to the more poignant differences they had experienced in this regard. They had discovered the usefulness of scaling all on their own by asking, "How important is this to you on a scale of 1 to 10?" Low ratings had encouraged mutual concessions; higher ratings by both had prompted negotiation and taking turns.

"Gosh, it sounds like a genuine shift in tone in your home—nice for you," I offered. "How will you maintain that, and what could get in the way?"

"I want to talk about how we never spend any time together," Jed ventured. "Annie seems content with how things are, but I'm not."

"I've learned how to create my own happiness, Jed. It's not that I don't want to spend time with you, but I need to be able to have time separate from you and, yes, that includes times with the grandchildren. Sometimes you join me, and that's great. There are times you won't, and that's fine, too, so long as it doesn't stop me." There was a long pause before Annie continued, "I worry about you. You don't have friends you hang out with. You and Toby still barely acknowledge each other, after all these years. That has to stop. It hurts you both."

This was my opening. I wanted to find a way of inviting Jed into the conversation without provoking further retreat. "Jed," I spoke softly. "That sounds like a voice of concern, not an accusation." I was hoping to impact the meaning he would give to her words.

"I know this is a difficult topic for you, and I've wanted to respect that. But *I'm* concerned for you as well. Can you let me in, just a little?" Knocking gently works better than pounding insistently. And Jed opened the door.

I recalled just a bit of history about his own family that he'd shared during our first session, but I wanted to know more. What roles and values did he witness growing up? Which did he take in, which did he reject, and how did these play out in his and Annie's marriage? Various approaches to couple therapy point to the importance of illuminating developmental experiences that influence how persons engage in their subsequent intimate relationships. Oftentimes (albeit not always) the experiences of greatest influence are those from the family of origin that inform values, expectancies, apprehensions, and coping strategies that inadvertently undermine relationships as a partner or parent. What had happened between Jed and his son to rupture their bond? What continued to block repair? And what in Jed's history contributed to this?

I adopted a conversational style using soft inquiries, brief reflections, and short pauses to create space for Jed to share the narrative at his own pace and in his own way. He recounted how his father had struggled to manage a small family ranch, and his mother had been a homemaker. In a family with three children, money was always tight. Their home was stable but constrained in emotional expressiveness—with chronic economic stress and intermittent tensions between his parents. Jed worked hard, loved Annie and their children, but ruled with a stern approach. He had wanted more for their son and was furious when Toby had not gone on to college to get the business degree Jed had hoped for him. Toby had always been held to the high expectations of his father, whether in school or athletics, and had never felt he measured up. When Toby turned 21, his and Jed's relationship blew up—each shutting the other out of their life. In the past 22 years, it had never really healed, even after Toby had established his own ranch and developed a close-knit family with his wife and two children. Jed longed to have a stronger relationship with his one grandson, Mason, but that hadn't been possible given the lingering alienation from Toby.

"I'm sorry," I said. Jed continued to look toward me but seemed at a loss for words. "It must be difficult," I tried again and waited.

"It is what it is," he offered with resignation. And, again, we sat for a while in silence.

"What would you like him to know from you? If you had the opportunity to open up with Toby, what would you say?"

"I'm not going to apologize for wanting a good life for him, better than I had." And then he stiffened. "Besides, why I should be the one to try to change things? He could come to me just as well."

He was a proud man but also a wounded one, and I debated how much he would let me push. I opted to leverage our closeness in age. "So here's the thing, Jed. You and I are old enough to know that our days are limited. We can feel it in our bones when we get up in the morning, and at night when we crawl into bed. Knowing our time is limited is both the curse and the benefit of growing older. Younger folks can never know this in the same way. So you have to take the lead. Don't let you and Toby squander what time remains."

It often strikes me how some of my older clients—whether in individual or couple therapy—yearn for some kind of reconciliation with their adult children but seem at a loss for how to pursue this. I always affirm their wish and then collaborate around possible steps forward. So now I paused, trying to gauge how this had landed. He continued to return my gaze in silence but his face had softened, so I tried again. "What would you want him to know from you?" From the corner of my eye, I could see Annie watching intently but remaining silent, allowing the space for Jed's and my conversation.

"I'd want him to know he's done a good job," Jed finally spoke. "And that Cammie and Mason are amazing, and I wish I could have more time with them."

"Anything else?" I wondered aloud—another ambiguous prompt to see where it might take us. But Jed shook his head, and I recognized that we had probably gone as far as we would that day. "Okay, that all sounds pretty good. But I'm wondering what you're hoping he might say in return?"

He paused and then replied, "Maybe just 'thanks' or a nod."

"That would be perfect," I said, intentionally lowering the stakes. "Nothing dramatic, just nudging the needle. Maybe a slight thaw that would loosen things up a little and perhaps make things just a bit more comfortable for everyone." He nodded, so I continued. "So, perhaps this week sometime, create an opportunity when the two of you are off by yourselves. Go slow, keep it low key. The wording you just suggested is perfect. Don't expect a reply—he may need time to process it before he can respond."

And that's exactly what happened, they let me know, when we met 2 weeks later. Jed had accompanied Annie on her next visit to their son's home, and he'd found an occasion to join Toby outdoors as he repaired one of the fences. Jed shared with Toby that he was proud of him—not just for what he'd accomplished with the ranch but, more importantly, for how he and his wife were rearing Cammie and Mason together. Jed and Toby had each made a nod toward a thaw, Toby offered a one-word "thanks," and their time since then in the same space had been just a bit more comfortable, nudging just slightly but meaningfully beyond civility. The longterm trajectory was unclear, but they had effected an inflection. I was not only glad for them but also relieved, because such efforts toward rapprochement don't always succeed. When that's the case, I encourage patience, stepping back but remaining available, managing sadness or hurt when approaches are rebuffed but continuing to look for opportunities to create even the slightest movement or inflection.

In the weeks that followed, Annie and Jed pursued the inflection they'd created in their own relationship. Our conversation from an earlier session, when I'd asked about how they had connected "back in the early days," prompted them to rediscover things they had enjoyed together early on, before their children had arrived—some board games they'd retrieved from a spare bedroom closet, reruns of shows from 40 years earlier that Ellie had shown them how to stream on TV, or an occasional evening stroll when the weather was cool enough. Jed expanded his workspace in the garage, tinkered with repairing small engines for lawnmowers and chainsaws (his own and some neighbors'), and even entertained the idea of starting his own small engine-repair shop. Their exchanges at home became warmer as Jed felt less resentment toward Annie during the day, and she found him more approachable in the evening. They acknowledged at times still getting "snarly" with each other, but we worked at recognizing these "regrettable incidents," pausing and stepping back, and then returning to the table to express regrets and reboot. They now were disposed to say to each other, "Our time together is short. Let's not squander it by bickering over the small stuff." They even reached a compromise around Jed's wish for them to get away together—taking short trips during the week but reserving weekends for time with their grandchildren.

We met only a few more times before the three of us sensed that we had done what we needed to do together. Life wasn't perfect, but it was substantially better. Interactions at home and with family were warmer. We agreed to suspend our sessions "for now," with the understanding we could always resume, but with no presumption that we would do so. It was bittersweet for me and perhaps for them as well. I felt sad to say good-bye but glad for the time we'd worked together.

INTERMEDIATE PHASE OF THERAPY

Sometimes couple therapy has discernible beginning, middle, and end phases. Other times, it waxes and wanes, with periods of working together, times apart as couples consolidate their gains and move on with their lives, and then further times of working together as new challenges emerge. That was the nature of my relationship with Annie and Jed, and 2 years after suspending our prior work together, I received the following email:

> "I hope you remember us. Jed and I benefited a lot from our time with you, but lately things haven't been going so well. We're both confused, and I'm worried. Can we set up a time to meet with you again soon, please?—Annie"

"It's good to see you again," I said as we sat down together the following week. Annie smiled, but Jed's gaze was somewhere else. He didn't seem upset or resistant—more like aloof. "Talk with me about what's going on," I invited them both, with alternating glances toward each.

"I don't know where to begin or exactly how to describe it," Annie began. "We've tried to avoid nitpicking since we last saw you, you know—not sweating the small stuff, but lately it seems like it's crept back in anyway. We'll agree on something, but then it doesn't happen, and when I remind Jed, he says we never had the discussion. Or he complains that I've moved something and he can't find it, and then we'll find it where we always keep it. (*She turns to Jed.*) You're not sleeping well and you seem restless during the day . . . and not very happy with me." (*She begins to tear up.*)

I waited to see how Jed might respond. He turned toward me but remained silent. I thought it best simply to leave space until he was ready. He turned toward Annie.

"I just never seem able to get it right, and you don't seem happy with me, either. I'm not losing my mind. But you say we've discussed something when I don't recall that at all. Or I'll say or do something that's not quite right somehow, but you won't just let it go. What difference does it make? I don't need your correcting me all the time." And then he paused, looked into the distance, and seemed to pull into himself. A heavy silence settled on the room.

I have a list at home with two columns: On the left are normal, age-related memory changes, and on the right are symptoms that may indicate dementia. I use this when teaching undergraduates about disorders of aging but probably keep it accessible to reassure myself when I forget earlier conversations with my partner, confuse the names or ages of my grandchildren, walk into a room and can't recall what I'm looking for, or struggle to find the right word that seems on the tip of my tongue. Multitasking invites mistakes, and learning new tasks (e.g., saddling a horse after a lifetime of suburbia) requires an unreasonable number of trials. For many, such is the life of aging. Still, it beats the alternative, we remind ourselves.

I told them about my list—partly as a way of normalizing their struggles, partly to promote empathic joining, but also as a way of providing information about cognitive changes, so we could explore what seemed to fit within normal limits versus cognitive slippage of potential concern. "So, what do you think?" I asked—another one of those ambiguous prompts to see where it might take us. They agreed that most of the memory changes they'd noticed were in the left column—Annie had them as well, but Jed more so. Neither of them got disoriented in familiar situations, were unable to follow directions, or had difficulty performing routine tasks. Jed had begun to repeat phrases and stories in the same conversation but, so far, that was the sole symptom in the other column suggesting concern. And his effectiveness in repairing small engines in the shop he'd expanded in his garage continued.

"Well, there are two strategies that might help," I offered. "The first is to become better behavioral engineers." They gave puzzled looks. "It's about finding effective prompts. Some folks use their smartphones—I'm still a sticky-note kind of guy." They laughed and nodded. "We just need more frequent and visible reminders of when and how to do certain things. Like a note on the mirror reminding you what time you're leaving Saturday morning to visit the grandchildren. Or a tab on the steering wheel to remind you to disconnect the chains from the RV before driving off." They laughed again, but none of us ventured to share details of some of the *really* dumb things we'd done.

"And the second strategy is one you're already familiar with. Use scaling and don't sweat the small stuff. Assign a number from 1 to 10 to indicate how important something is once you've stepped back and can view it from a larger perspective. If either of you forgets something at a level of 3 or lower, or uses the wrong word or misstates details of one sort or another, let it go. Lower the stakes and make it safe to ask each other for help. You're in this together; you each have a caring partner. Protect that. It's so much better than aging alone." They nodded in silence, but their softening was apparent. Annie took Jed's hand, and he placed his other over hers.

I considered whether to encourage neurocognitive assessment for Jed and gently inquired further about any symptoms that would have elevated my concerns—difficulty executing simple tasks, getting lost, showing poor judgment, or becoming hypervigilant. Had Jed appeared receptive to pursuing diagnostics of any sort, I would have provided him and Annie information on how to do so. But, at least for now, none of those more worrisome indicators seemed present, and Jed appeared closed off to further discussion, so that's where we left it. It was another instance of my debating internally when and how much to push Jed. He was already defending against Annie's fears about cognitive decline and perhaps his own fears as well. Providing information about age-related decline, as well as dementia, seemed the right balance for now, and I trusted they would engage me in a similar discussion if it became relevant down the road. We met a few more times, mostly to fine-tune their approach to coconstructing prompts for themselves and each other. But the most important impact of our earlier conversation was their explicit intention to "make it safe" to have lapses, make mistakes, and ask for help. They drew on their best as caring and gracious partners.

And for another year that was better than just good enough—it was genuinely good on a deep level. But then Annie—always the one to initiate our work together—sent another note:

> "We need your help discussing something that's come up. Jed's really been struggling and went to our family doctor to see if there were some sort of memory pill to help.

His doctor wants him to see a neurologist, but Jed doesn't want to go. I know he's frightened, but so am I. When can we see you?—Annie"

The terror of dementia. None of us wants to grow old while gradually losing awareness of everything and everyone around us. By the time we reach middle age, virtually all of us have experienced it in one way or another—a parent or grandparent, a distant relative or the relative of a close friend, in film or on TV, or news accounts of persons in the public eye. My grandfather suffered with dementia, as did both my father and mother. My mother's dementia progressed for 6 years before she died. My father's was cut short by a life-ending stroke. Hence, my list.

Something about Jed had changed, that much was clear. I trusted Annie's attunement to his progressive struggles, and she was alarmed. By her account, Jed was also—reflected in his wish for medication to help his memory and his fear about what further consultations with a neurologist might reveal. My decision a year earlier not to push Jed into further diagnostics was no longer a viable option. Could I harness his trust in me to engage his fears and help him confront whatever it was that he was now experiencing?

We greeted each other with a familiar warmth but spent the first few moments in silence when we met the following week. "Can you share with me where things are at?" I prompted. "This is hard stuff, I'm sorry."

"She deserves better," Jed began after some further silence. "I never wanted to be a burden."

"For better or worse, Jed," Annie whispered. "In sickness and in health."

"You deserve better," he repeated. We returned to silence for a few more moments.

"Jed, what do you know so far?" I asked. "Annie shared with me that you saw your doctor, and she recommended you meet with a neurologist. Where are you with that?"

"What's the point? There's not a cure; it is what it is." I debated how hard to push, unsure how determined Jed was not to get further consultation, not wanting him to experience me as siding with Annie against him, but hoping as well to have influence. I'd held back a year earlier when we met—perhaps a mistake on my part—but now, I felt I had no choice. I trusted that he would at least hear me out, although I had no expectation that he would give weight to my opinion.

"So, here's the thing, Jed. I don't know if there's a cure for your memory struggles or not, or whether there are interventions that could help slow the progression or manage the symptoms. My sense is that we don't know yet whether you're experiencing early signs of dementia or, if you are, what type of dementia you have or how rapidly it's likely to progress. But that's the sort of information that could be useful—not just for you, but for Annie as well. I get it—you don't want to squander the rest of your good time being consumed by fears about something you can't control. But if it *is* early dementia, you also don't want to squander your opportunity to complete various things that are important to you."

"You mean like a bucket list? I don't care about that."

"No, more than a bucket list. If it heads in the direction you fear, then you need to make some preparations for Annie's sake while you still can. Figure out what needs to get done, so she doesn't have to deal with it later on her own. Care for her while you still can." I paused to gauge how he was taking this in. He appeared pensive, not shut off, and so I continued. "In some ways, Jed, knowing if your time is limited gives you an opportunity to reach decisions about how you want to confront the ending of this life. How do you want to leave? What would you wish to leave behind, and to whom? Who would you want to say good-bye to, and how do you hope to be remembered? Not everyone gets the chance to do that, Jed, but you may." Tears appeared in their eyes, and the lump in my own throat made me pause.

We sat together quietly for a full minute, which seemed like an eternity. Then Jed broke the silence. "So, what do I do now?" He had opened the door and was inviting me in.

"For now, arrange an appointment with a neurologist. See if your doctor's office can expedite something within the next couple of weeks. Make sure Annie goes with you, so that she can ask questions of her own and keep track of the information you both get. And let's get back together as soon as possible afterward."

When we next met 3 weeks later, they confirmed the diagnosis—all the evidence pointed to progressive dementia, most likely of the Alzheimer's type. Alzheimer's occurs in about 5% of persons over age 65, and doubles in prevalence with every 5 years of age. People age 65 and older survive an average of 4–8 years after a diagnosis of Alzheimer's disease. At age 70, persons with Alzheimer's are twice as likely to die before age 80 as those without the disease. Jed was now 75, and his symptoms appeared to have been progressing rapidly over the past 6 months.

Annie returned to the conversation we'd had a few weeks earlier. "We've been talking about the things you mentioned," she said. "We can only have those conversations for 15 or 20 minutes at a time; otherwise, they just feel too overwhelming. The legal and financial preparations seem the easiest. We're updating our wills. We've started to explore how to get some home health care, if it comes to that. I've shared this with Toby and Ellie, with Jed's permission." There was a long pause, and I wondered what might be coming next. Jed and Toby's relationship had thawed, but there was lots of unfinished business there. "Could you see them?" Annie asked. "Jed and Toby, without me?" I looked toward Jed, who gave just the slightest nod.

As couple therapists, our passion is all about helping partners heal their injured or broken relationship. But relationships in need of healing or reconstruction come in all forms, and the healing of Jed and Toby's relationship was as important to Annie as it was to either her husband or her son. It was an opportunity to reconstruct that relationship in ways that could have enduring benefits for Annie, Toby, and the entire family long after Jed was gone. And so, of course, I agreed.

Toby appeared different than I had imagined when he and Jed met with me a few weeks later. He seemed older than the young man I had envisioned, although, by this time, he was approaching 50. He was several inches shorter than Jed, and had a gentler face and easy manner. Our session began a bit awkwardly, none of us knowing exactly how to begin. I thanked them for being there and acknowledged the various challenges of their situation that had brought us together. I shared with Toby my conversation with his dad about the opportunities occasioned by knowing more clearly that one's time is limited. I asked Toby if he remembered the day when Jed had approached him almost 3 years earlier to narrow the gulf between them. He did—vividly. "What did he say, exactly?" I already knew what Jed had said, but I wanted to resurrect that moment in the here and now, to see whether I could harness any of the thawing that had emerged in that exchange.

There was a long pause. Jed waited and looked toward Toby. Toby returned his gaze and, without looking away replied, "He said I'd done a good job." We sat there for a few moments.

"Hmm . . . a bold moment." I paused as they turned to look at me. "Bold to offer, and bold to accept." We sat together a while longer. "And what would you want him to know from you?" I asked. It was the same prompt I had used with Jed years earlier. I wondered now what Toby might do with it.

"I'd want him to know he did a good job, too." Then, turning to Jed, he said, "Better than good. I am who I am because of you and Mom—both of you. I learned from you how to be strong, how to keep moving when I didn't think I could put one foot in front of the other." And so they each opened the door to the other. Each spoke of regrets, and what he would do differently toward the other if he had the chance to do it over. They both expressed gratitude for having found better ways to be with each other, and their determination to do more during whatever time was left. They wanted to take Cammie and Mason camping together. Jed wanted to teach Mason how to repair small engines. They wanted to do so many things together, knowing full well they wouldn't have the opportunity to do them all.

There was little for me to do during our session. Mostly, I listened. Sometimes I asked questions to promote recollections of good times. I celebrated with them. I thought of things I wished I'd done differently with my own sons, but I tried to keep those thoughts from intruding into this moment. Eventually, our time came to a close, and I shook hands with each of them as they left my office. Toby and I held our grip longer, and his eyes conveyed that the conversation with his dad had been special for him, and perhaps a recognition that there'd be fewer opportunities for similar exchanges in the months ahead.

I never saw Annie and Jed as a couple again. Annie would send me a brief update by email every few months—letting me know how Jed was doing, how his dementia had progressed, how she was trying to cope, or how Ellie and Toby had been providing support to her or their dad. These were challenging times for all of them. I always replied to her notes, assuring her that she and Jed remained in my thoughts. I encouraged Annie to take care of herself—to embrace the support from family, close friends, or fellowship she experienced in her community. I directed her to resources for caregivers of family members with Alzheimer's disease. And I always invited her to stay in touch with me and to give my regards to Jed, who, she assured me, remembered who I was and some of the things we'd discussed.

CONCLUDING PHASE OF THERAPY

> "Could I schedule a session with you? Just me? You know us, who we were. Jed's still at home but barely aware of anything around him. I need help figuring out how to get through this, but I don't want to burden Ellie or Toby.—Annie"

Sara Honn Qualls (2003) describes the reorganization that occurs in a couple's dynamics following the onset of cognitive impairment. Caregiving partners sometimes describe it as a kind of "limbo" or intermediate state—partnered but not partnered. In addition to the logistical burdens, caregiving partners may feel guilt about taking over the other one's privileges and roles. Physical intimacy frequently declines as the other no longer initiates or responds to small expressions of affection such as hugs, kisses, or smiles. After the initial emotional upheaval from the diagnosis of progressive dementia and the eventual restructuring of roles, the strains of caregiving may dominate. Caregiving partners often find meaning from the commitment and opportunity to give to their loved one, but inherent practical and emotional challenges almost always permeate daily living. Guilt may arise from sharing the caregiving role with others. Frustration and grief over losing one's partner a little more each day may surface intermittently in surprising or confusing ways. Ethical dilemmas abound—as in "What would he want if he could decide for himself?" "When can I step back and take care of myself?" "How do I let go? He said he was ready for death and wanted to die at home."

Annie described nearly all these experiences when we met a week after I received her note. "Sometimes, I just feel so angry—not at Jed, but at life. We spent 45 years as passing ships in the night, just trying to keep things afloat and take care of business. We kept telling ourselves that our time would come. And then, when it finally did, it got torn away." She started to weep, and we sat quietly for a while.

"It's unfair," I reflected. "Tragic, and unfair." I paused for a few moments, then continued, "But you were more than passing ships in the night, weren't you? You created a home together and reared two remarkable children with remarkable families of their own. What else do you treasure about the life you shared? I know there were hard times, including times when neither of you was particularly happy. But somehow you persevered together. How did you do that? As you think back over the past 50 years, what do you value the most?"

I knew that Annie's challenge was to revisit the narrative of the life she and Jed had created together—acknowledging the struggles and disappointments but finding meaning in those to celebrate what they'd done best. Those recollections might help sustain her not only now as Jed gradually slipped from her life, but also after he was gone and she was challenged with the task of moving on without him. I invited her to share some of those memories with me.

"Could we do that together?" she asked. "It feels a little strange to do that without Jed here, but I think it could help." I assured her that we could. I invited her to bring pictures of them as a couple to our sessions—photos from their courtship and wedding, baby pictures of Toby and Ellie, mementos from their travels together, family portraits over the years. And I said that she could do the same with Jed. It didn't matter whether he understood or responded. All that mattered was her wish to include him in the narrative, celebrating together the meaning she was rediscovering. She was free to laugh, cry, hold his hand, lie next to him—whatever brought her comfort.

And so that's how we spent our time together the next few months, every 2 weeks, reconstructing and celebrating the narrative of Annie and Jed's life together. We also worked through the hard times—the years they'd spent consumed with work in and outside their home, too often emotionally detached or succumbing to their frustrations with one another. We grieved the lost opportunities—both then and now—but each time returned to a place of understanding and gratitude for the life they'd shared. And eventually, Annie was ready to move on, and it was time for us to stop.

Two months later, I received her text. I had told her that when the time came, she was welcome to reach out. She shared in the text that Jed had passed quietly in the night at home as he had wanted. Ellie and Toby had come to be with her and to plan arrangements. "Might you be able to come to the memorial service?" she wrote. I called her soon after receiving her text. I needed time first to experience my own grief before I could call. I said it would be my privilege to attend the service, and I thanked her for inviting me.

When the day arrived and I entered the small country church where the service would be held, Toby spotted me and came over and gripped my hand, inviting me to sit with the family up front. I was deeply moved and fought the lump in my throat before responding, "Of course. I'd be honored."

I never saw Annie, Toby, or any others of their family again following that service. But each year at the holiday season, Annie sends me a card with a picture of their entire family, with a single word, "Thanks." And each time I whisper "thanks" in response.

FURTHER REFLECTIONS AND IMPLICATIONS

It's been several years now since Jed's passing. I think of him and Annie from time to time, although less often now than before. I have other couples similar in age—some just beginning to address evolving roles as they transition into retirement, others contending with various health issues, some immersed in reconstructing relationships with estranged adult children, and others—like Jed and Annie—facing cognitive decline and the certainty of diminished remaining time together. In various ways, each confronts an array of challenges and opportunities. Some couples are more resourced than others—whether financially, or in terms of physical and emotional health, or support from their family and community. Differences in resources and constraints often influence the changes that couples can effect in their lives.

I had an advantage in developing a therapeutic alliance with Annie and Jed. There was a higher baseline of trust when we first met, based on our similarities in age, ethnicity, and even our living circumstances. (I shared that I had recently moved to the country in anticipation of retirement.) Those similarities made it easier to join empathically around growing pains (literally), grandchildren, the loss of our parents or older siblings, and even our foibles and missteps. I struggled at times with when and how much to share. I never disclosed my family history of Alzheimer's disease or how my parents died—it was too much to disclose while Jed and Annie were so vulnerable and already anticipating the end. I struggled at times to manage my own emotions—monitoring my experience in the moment to facilitate empathic joining, but making sure that the focus remained squarely on them, without distraction by my own intrusive memories.

What would I have done differently given the chance? With some couples, I might have devoted more time to enhancing decision-making or solution-focused skills, but Annie and Jed didn't seem to need this—often discovering strategies on their own that worked well for them. With younger couples, I might have worked more on emotional expressiveness and responsiveness skills, but there's empirical literature (limited and not particularly recent) that older couples often experience less gain from those interventions. I never pursued early developmental histories with either Annie or Jed, but I might have had there seemed to be a reservoir of attachment injuries continually sabotaging their efforts toward change. I debated whether to suggest a separate session with Jed and their daughter Ellie after his Alzheimer's diagnosis was confirmed, but from all indications, their relationship was mutually warm and working just fine.

I wish I had pursued the opportunity to meet with Annie and Jed together just a few more times after that special occasion with Jed and Toby. I would have wanted to help them reminisce about the best times in their marriage, celebrate the goodness and make peace with the disappointments, and exchange appreciation for one another. I'm glad that Annie later sought the opportunity to do this for herself, but I regret I didn't initiate those conversations with the two of them together, while perhaps it could have made a difference for Jed as well. I was guided by the couple's own goals and readiness for change, as these evolved and morphed over the various occasions of our work together. Perhaps we accomplished what was needed—nothing more, nothing less.

I'm keenly aware that the challenges and opportunities of older age are no longer abstractions in my life but rather firsthand experiences I've either encountered already myself or through close friends and families. I'm also acutely aware that the opportunities and challenges faced by older adults covary with important markers of social location and marginalization—for example, that I enjoy better physical health because I can afford better nutrition and better health care, and that those advantages come in part from having been privileged by growing up in a home with two parents—both college-educated and engaged in professional lives—and hence, afforded countless opportunities for educational and professional development of my own. All of which is to acknowledge that cultural competence in working with older adults necessarily intersects with cultural humility derived from self-reflection.

That's an observation I'm eager to share with my junior colleagues and supervisees. Just as I strive to achieve a modicum of cultural competence with minority or underserved populations different from myself—knowing that I can never relate on an intimate level to their own experiences of marginalization but striving to understand as best I can—I wish for this newest generation of couple therapists to do the same in engaging older adults. There are too many of us seniors to rely only on aging therapists! Be curious, respectful, humble—acknowledge what you don't know, share what you do, and pursue a collaboration that merges your respective experiential knowledge and skills sets. My hope is that you may feel as privileged as I have.

REFERENCES

Knight, B. G. (2023). Therapy with older adult couples. In J. L. Lebow & D. K. Snyder (Eds.), *Clinical handbook of couple therapy* (6th ed., pp. 454–471). New York: Guilford Press.

Qualls, S. H. (2003). Aging and cognitive impairment. In D. K. Snyder & M. A. Whisman (Eds.), *Treating difficult couples: Helping clients with coexisting mental and relationship disorders* (pp. 370–391). New York: Guilford Press.

Rydell, M. (Director). (1981). *On golden pond* [Film]. Van Nuys, CA: IPC Films.

Snyder, D. K. (1999). Affective reconstruction in the context of a pluralistic approach to couple therapy. *Clinical Psychology: Science and Practice, 6,* 348–365.

U.S. Census Bureau. (2018). *The graying of America: More older adults than kids by 2035.* Retrieved October 1, 2023, from *www.census.gov/library/stories/2018/03/graying-america.html.*

U.S. Census Bureau. (2020). *An aging world: 2020.* Retrieved October 1, 2023, from *www.census.gov/library/visualizations/2020/demo/aging_story_map.html.*

Virzi, P. (Director). (2017). *The leisure seeker* [Film]. Milan, Italy: Indiana Production Company.

CHAPTER 14

Couple Therapy with Young Adults
Navigating the Transition to Parenthood

ERICA A. MITCHELL

> ### *Editors' Comments*
>
> Erica Mitchell offers us a glimpse of couple therapy at an important stage of life—the transition to parenthood. Much research and clinical experience converge to suggest how important a time this is in the life cycle of couples. It represents the time of a predictable decline in relationship satisfaction as a couple experiences the multiple stresses of vast physical changes in one partner, the hopes and worries about a new child, sleep deprivation, new wrinkles on relationships with extended family, financial strains, and immense pressures about time. Gendered patterns, often carried over from families of origin, can emerge in ways that lead to misalignments between partners. The terrain for conflicts emerging even in heretofore well-functioning couples is in place. Prior vulnerabilities—either from individual histories or suboptimal interaction patterns (e.g., the demand–withdrawal cycle exemplified in the couple described here by Mitchell)—may contribute to challenges rising above a couple's usual threshold of tolerance or abilities to navigate.
>
> Mitchell brings a highly useful positive frame to this transition and how its challenges can be negotiated and harnessed as opportunities for growth. She helps this couple with a marvelous integrative set of methods attuned to the needs of those going through the transition to parenthood. Notice how she frequently brings psychoeducation about what are normal processes during such a time and the couple processes that can be put into place and help. She also provides a wonderful example of using the enactments that can occur around conflicts as opportunities to engage in the core interventions from emotionally focused therapy to help solidify the base of attachment between the partners. Within that framework as her theoretical base, she also integrates a developmental perspective that fosters partners' deeper understandings of themselves and each other.

I became interested in family transitions from a very young age. As an only child from my biological parents, I became a member of a blended family at age 10, following my mother's remarriage. During this time, there was a lot of transition, bringing both excitement and strain to our family system. I became specifically interested in the transition to parenthood (TTP) during graduate school; I was working clinically with couples who were experiencing it and began to weave this into my research. My true passion for supporting couples during this transition, though, came after I had my first child. In my own experience, it struck me that the conversations and preparation around having a baby focused exclusively on the birthing process and newborn care. While these are important and should be included in education, I felt that information about expectations for the adults and the couple relationship was also essential but was missing. During the postpartum period, I noticed that people were asking about the baby and how I was "feeling" (physically, that is); very few people asked about my partner or our relationship. As a couple therapist, I knew how important our individual well-being and our couple relationship were during this transition for the future of our new baby and our family.

The TTP may be one of the most difficult transitions couples navigate during their relationship. Relationship quality declines during this time, evidenced by increases in negative communication and conflict, and decreases in sexual satisfaction (Doss, Rhoades, Stanley, & Markman, 2009; Rauch-Anderegg, Kuhn, Milek, Halford, & Bodenmann, 2020). The TTP is also associated with increased stress, anxiety, and postpartum depression (PPD) and greater risk for intimate partner violence (Epifanio, Genna, De Luca, Roccella, & La Grutta, 2015; Kan & Feinberg, 2011). PPD occurs for new mothers and fathers; poor couple relationship quality is both a consequence and a risk factor for PPD (Faisal-Cury, Tabb, & Matijasevich, 2021). Despite the myriad challenges during the TTP, this transition is often glamorized by society and the media, depicting happy mothers with healthy babies and supportive partners. This can lead to unrealistic expectations about this transition with regard to personal well-being, expected changes in the couple relationship, and division of household labor. Welcoming a new child shakes up the family system and requires renegotiating roles and responsibilities; this is a common source of conflict for couples. Moreover, the intense sleep deprivation that new parents experience negatively impacts their ability to regulate their emotions, thus leading to more conflict. Most couples also find they have less time to focus on their relationship, which often leads to increased strain on the new family system.

Millions of parents experience the TTP each year, and a majority encounter challenges. As is the case with other types of family-based stressors, some couples navigate this transition well, while others experience much more distress and often go to couple therapy. The timing of entering couple therapy as it relates to the TTP also varies widely; some couples, like the couple in this chapter, seek therapy before their child turns 1 year old, while other couples may not go to therapy until their children are much older, in some cases not until they are empty nesters. In my clinical experience, many couples who present several years after the TTP can trace some origins of the distress and disconnection in their relationship back to this transition.

I have advanced training in emotionally focused therapy (EFT; Johnson, Wiebe, & Allan, 2023), and it is my preferred approach. EFT guides couples in digging deep to acknowledge each partner's unmet attachment needs, repair attachment injuries, and foster greater connection. EFT includes three stages: (1) assessment and deescalation,

(2) changing patterns of interaction, and (3) consolidation and integration. Couples can move through these stages fluidly during treatment.

INITIAL ASSESSMENT AND CASE FORMULATION

Vivien called to request couple therapy for herself and her husband, Henry. She described reasons for seeking treatment as "communication" and "general unhappiness in the relationship," which she followed with "Well, I guess you would say unhappiness for me. My husband doesn't seem to be bothered by the same things that I am, maybe because I'm always doing everything for everyone." My immediate perception was that she was overwhelmed and likely burnt out in her relationship, but at the same time seemed motivated to seek help. Vivien went on to share: "We have an 11-month-old daughter, Charlotte, and ever since she was born, our relationship has been getting worse. I don't know what to do." I validated her distress and conducted a brief risk assessment; Vivien denied all indicators of risk. During the intake session, I want to get to know both partners, hear their relationship story, and understand their presenting concerns. I then schedule two individual sessions to get to know each partner better and assess for any contraindicators to couple therapy (e.g., substance use, relationship violence).

Vivien, a 26-year-old, White cisgender female, had earned an associate's degree and currently was providing full-time care for their daughter, Charlotte. Henry, a 27-year-old, White cisgender male, had earned a high school diploma and, immediately following graduation from high school, enrolled in the military, where he served for 8 years. Henry had left military service 2 months ago and was employed full time as a security guard, working various shifts on a rotating weekly schedule. Vivien and Henry started dating in high school; they had been married for 5 years and had recently relocated back to their hometown following Henry's exit from the military.

Initially, the couple said they were struggling with communication; they described themselves as "fighting all the time." Upon digging a bit deeper, I learned that most of their day-to-day (yes—they described fighting daily about this) was around parenting and navigating their roles and responsibilities now that Henry had returned from deployment and they were taking care of Charlotte. They each described the other as "getting mad easily" or "having a short fuse." Henry explained: "Like this morning, Vivien asked me to finish feeding Charlotte breakfast, and when I asked her one simple question, she got mad and said she always has to do everything herself, and then she went off to take a shower. We haven't talked about it since."

Henry and Vivien also disclosed feeling completely consumed by parenthood. When I probed more, Henry said that before Charlotte, they would go out frequently as a couple, but since becoming parents, they hadn't done this at all. Vivien added, "Even now, we have people who can babysit for us, and we still don't spend any time just the two of us." They also mentioned a lack of intimacy in their relationship, which they described as "rarely having sex anymore." Vivien further shared about the strain on their relationship while Henry was in the military, and particularly during times of deployment. They thought civilian life would be "so much easier," but that wasn't proving to be true. Additionally, Henry and Vivien weren't on the same page with regard to having more children. They both had always wanted to start a family someday, but when Vivien proposed getting pregnant a couple of years into their marriage, Henry wanted to wait until he was out of the military. While Vivien understood this, she longed to be a mother and felt that they had waited so long already to start their family. Charlotte was born while Henry was on deployment; he didn't return home full-time until she was 3 months old. They described this initial transition as very stressful; despite my gentle prompting, they did not elaborate much further on this. I decided to leave this alone for now to revisit during their individual sessions. As I was just getting to know Henry and Vivien, I wanted them to take the lead on what they shared. I'm also very aware that sometimes things are too painful to revisit in the presence of one's partner; thus, some partners feel more comfortable sharing in individual sessions. I got the sense that their TTP had been a painful experience, and they needed more time to fully unpack it in therapy. Surprisingly, given their conversations early in their relationship, now that Henry was no longer in the military and had a full-time job, he was ready to discuss having more children, but Vivien didn't feel their relationship was ready for another child. This prompted them to come to see me; they were at a crossroads with this decision, and Vivien believed couple therapy could be helpful for them in navigating this challenging time.

I wrapped up our intake session.

"We have a few minutes left, and I want to thank you for being here and sharing your story. You've endured many challenges in your relationship, from moves to deployments, to your daughter being born. I believe the transition to parenthood is one of the most difficult transitions couples face, and many couples I work with come to therapy for just that reason. It's difficult for couples to prioritize their own relationship when they have a new baby. Just being here today shows your commitment to your relationship. I'd like to schedule individual sessions with each of you. It's important for you to know though that I don't hold secrets; the information you share with me in our individual meetings will likely be brought back into our couple sessions. If there's information pertinent to your relationship that you haven't shared with your partner, I'll encourage and support you in doing so."

After Vivien and Henry left my office, I found myself taking a deep breath. They had experienced so many transitions in their relatively short relationship and were clearly distressed; I knew we had a lot of work to do. Despite the multiple transitions they faced, Henry and Vivien seemed most distressed around the issue of parenting and the disconnection that had been building in their relationship since Charlotte was born. I followed their lead and made this the focal point for treatment. I felt a lot of empathy and admiration for both partners around this issue. Vivien navigated this extremely difficult transition largely on her own, and despite having "made it through," she desperately wanted support and connection from her husband. On the other hand, Henry missed the early parts of this important transition and felt unsure about his role in his family.

Despite seeming slightly withdrawn during the initial conjoint session, Vivien was very expressive during our individual session. She described how hard it had been to take care of Charlotte on her own until age 3 months. She also expressed anger toward Henry for not helping take care of Charlotte the way she needed. Vivien is the oldest of three children, and has maintained close relationships with her parents and siblings. It was difficult for her to relocate when Henry was in the military; she felt lonely and sometimes resentful that they had moved so far away from family and friends. As much as Vivien wanted to have more children, she was unsure whether it was possible based on how things were in their relationship. She described herself as having an internal conflict in which sometimes she was critical of herself for setting this expectation of wanting a stronger marriage before having another child. During this session, I witnessed more of Vivien's pain due to feeling disconnected from her husband and having to "do it all." I believed unpacking this pain with Henry present would offer an avenue for change and connection. Although Vivien largely functioned as a caretaker in her family of origin, she felt lonely and angry at Henry for not being there for her in the way she needed him to be. I was able to validate these feelings, and continued to build an alliance with her.

Henry was engaged during our individual session and told me, "While I'm not the biggest believer in couple therapy, my wife and my daughter are everything to me, and I'm here for them." He quickly followed that up, expressing fear of losing them if, according to Vivien "things didn't change," but acknowledged that he "doesn't really understand what she needs." He described how difficult it was for him to be absent for the first 3 months of Charlotte's life and, while he was so happy to have her, he felt some resentment toward Vivien for not waiting to start their family. He also shared his frustration with the constant conflict and feeling like he can never get it right when it comes to Charlotte. Henry is an only child. His dad was in the military for over 10 years, and he lived in different places during early childhood; thus, being in the military and moving around a lot at this stage of his own life seemed normal to him. During our individual session, I continued to experience Henry's commitment to his marriage and his family. I gained a clearer picture for how lost he felt navigating conflicts around parenting, but how desperately he wanted things to be better. I also sensed an openness from him to engage with me that wasn't quite as apparent in the first conjoint session; I suspected that this might not continue with Vivien present.

Due to issues with child care, Vivien and Henry brought Charlotte with them to the second conjoint session. Vivien seemed distracted and was less engaged during the session, which I believed was due to caretaking responsibilities for Charlotte. While I was surprised that they brought her and found it more difficult to engage with them throughout session, especially with Vivien, I wanted to respect their decision and child care limitations; I worked hard to keep us focused on their relationship. From prior experience, I also knew that it's common for couples to bring a young child with them from time to time and still have a productive session. Additionally, as a parent myself, I know how difficult child care can be, and I felt empathic toward their circumstance.

This session focused on exploring the couple's patterns of interaction. In addition to Vivien appearing distracted with taking care of Charlotte, both Vivien and Henry were very quiet during this session. It seemed that some of the reservation about opening up that I'd experienced from both partners during our first conjoint session had returned in this session when they were in the room together again. Vivien presented as a burnt-out "pursuer"; she had spent many years in this role—further amplified during their TTP—and was now tired of pursuing Henry for connection. Henry presented as a "withdrawer"; he would exit their exchanges when things became too overwhelming, leaving Vivien frustrated and unsure when he would return. This pattern was often initiated when Henry did not follow through on something Vivien had asked him to do, frequently related to parenting or household responsibilities. This triggered Vivien's fears of "I don't matter" or "I'm not important to him," and she would become angry and critical. This criticism triggered Henry's fears of "I can never get it right" and "I'm useless"—and he would withdraw, because he felt there was nothing he could do to please Vivien or make the situation better. I presented this conceptualization of their cycle. Both partners were slightly more engaged during this conversation and reflected that it was helpful to name this pattern that they had been in for so long.

Before wrapping up, I checked in with the couple on their child care situation. Based on Vivien's decreased engagement in this session and my prior experience working with couples with children present, I felt it would be difficult to do more emotion-focused work with Charlotte there. I shared this with them and also explained that my clinical recommendation would be to meet weekly, at least in the beginning. Although the couple agreed with the value of weekly sessions, paying for child care every week on top of therapy would be a financial burden for them. We agreed to meet every other week, without their daughter. While this wasn't my preference, I feel it is important to meet clients where they are and to work within their circumstances.

Initial Formulation

Vivien's and Henry's cycle is a common pursue–withdraw pattern. Their presenting concerns align with common challenges for TTP couples. The TTP presents a renegotiation of time and division of household labor—what worked for a couple before having a baby won't necessarily work after baby arrives. Henry's deployment coinciding with Charlotte's birth forced Vivien to, as she put it, "do it all on my own" for those first couple of months, and what she discovered was that she fell into a routine and a certain way of doing things. When Henry returned home, she expected that having him present would relieve her stress—and to a degree it did—but Henry also found it difficult to integrate into the routine that Vivien had established. He often felt like he didn't have a clear place in his family, thus resorting to a more hands-off approach. While the circumstance of his deployment was unique, I often hear fathers express a similar sentiment of not knowing where they fit in after baby arrives.

What also struck me as unique were the many other transitions they experienced alongside the TTP, or the "transition within transitions," as I described this to the couple. They experienced the transition of Henry returning home when Charlotte was 3 months old; whereas Vivien already had a couple of months of parenthood experience, this was brand new for Henry. Within months, they moved; moving and an employment change for Henry occurred simultaneously with the TTP. The couple resonated with the "transition within transitions" description. Vivien commented, "I'd never thought about it that way. Sure, Henry's deployment was really stressful, but I thought becoming a parent and moving back to be closer to our families were positive things."

I clarified, saying, "Those are both positive things, but even positive changes are still transitions and are often stressful." It was clear to me why this couple was stressed, overwhelmed, and having frequent arguments. I believed it was important to normalize this from the outset of therapy to help them contextualize the distress they were experiencing.

I also felt hopeful for this couple. Vivien's initiation of therapy and desire to improve their marriage signaled a commitment to their relationship, and Henry had so vulnerably shared his fears of losing his wife. I reflected this commitment to them. Vivien responded with a look of disbelief. When I invited her to share what she was feeling, she replied, "It just doesn't seem like he cares that much; if he did, we wouldn't be here."

I validated her uncertainty and turned to Henry, "I hear Vivien's uncertainty. Could you turn to her and share your commitment to your marriage with her now?" Although he was hesitant, he turned to Vivien and said, "You and Charlotte are everything to me. I don't want to lose you. I'll do whatever it takes to make this better." Vivien started to cry. While we still had a lot of work to do, this exchange was one to take hold of. I believed an important connection happened for this couple in that moment, and I suspected that this occurred in a way that it had not in a long time.

Through these initial sessions, I witnessed the pain both partners experienced around the challenges of the TTP. I believed that Henry saw Vivien's pain and distress, too, but I didn't think Vivien was able yet to see Henry's pain—and this would be an important goal for treatment. Henry's fear of not being good enough and Vivien leaving him was evident, and he was clearly committed to his marriage. However, Vivien's experience of "doing it all" that had been exacerbated during the TTP left her feeling fearful that she didn't matter, resulting in resentment and criticism. Henry and Vivien resonated with the conceptualization of their cycle, which gave us something on which to build. I believed that if therapy could help them see the other's pain and connect with their fears, Henry and Vivien could regain the connection they had lost through the TTP. Also, as a relatively new parent myself, I resonated with the struggles this couple was experiencing around navigating new roles and household responsibilities. In some ways, working with this couple took me back to my own feelings of distress, and I found that tapping into that helped me connect with them.

BEGINNING PHASE OF THERAPY

I began our next session by reflecting on the moment of connection I witnessed at the end of the prior session, and invited Henry and Vivien to share how this felt for them. Vivien reported mixed emotions, "It was really nice to hear that I still matter," which she followed up with, "I don't understand why he couldn't just tell me that without having to come to therapy." I validated this, "Sometimes partners experience each other differently in here than they do outside of therapy. In fact, this is one of my hopes for couples—that they can take new experiences in here and replicate them outside of therapy, too." This seemed to resonate. Henry then looked at Vivien and said, "I didn't know I had to tell you that you matter to me, I thought you already knew." We explored this further. Vivien said she used to be confident in that, but since Charlotte was born, their relationship changed and she often feels unsure whether she really matters to him.

During these sessions, I was attuned to my alliance with both partners. In general, I built a strong alliance with them through validating their experiences, and normalizing how each can have different experiences of their relationship, but these differences don't negate either partner's lived experience. Each partner also approached therapy in different ways, which presented individual challenges to working with each of them. For example, Vivien felt she had tried so hard during the past year in her roles as mother and wife, and she was sometimes unwilling to try anymore. Thus, I expected more resistance from her in engaging with Henry in session, and responded to this resistance accordingly—slowing down and working through each moment of resistance as it came. Henry was more withdrawn toward the beginning of treatment and had more difficulty accessing his emotions; thus, my prompts to do so would sometimes lead him to feel frustrated. When Henry appeared frustrated, I would name this, and we would process his feelings—including his frustration with me—in the moment.

I often began our sessions by checking in with Henry and Vivien about the past 2 weeks. Inevitably, an issue had arisen during the time between sessions—usually around parenting—that we framed in the context of their pursue–withdraw cycle. I also worked to slow them down, so they could more deeply process their emotions. Processing these in session allowed the other partner to witness this, and to slowly create more connection between them. The issues that arose between therapy sessions provided further evidence of the couple's cycle, and over time, the couple used this language to talk about these events. As I worked to slow them down, I was also intentional about asking them to speak directly to one another. Although this was uncomfortable at first—and I sensed resistance from them—over time, Henry and Vivien seemed more comfortable with this process. To help with this, I provided some psychoeducation: "Talking to me can be helpful, and in the beginning of therapy, I'll facilitate more of the dialogue, but over time, I'd like for the two of you to spend more time talking directly to each other. I'm only with you for 1 hour, but the two of you spend much more time together. Therapy is a place where you can practice having these new kinds of interactions with each other."

This rationale seemed to resonate, and although it didn't immediately remove their discomfort, I think it helped them understand the reasoning behind this. Much of my work with them focused on the here and now, but because we were often identifying attachment-based needs in their relationship, I frequently brought up the origins of these needs. For example, Henry shared that while he was appreciative of all Vivien had done to care for Charlotte, when he returned home from deployment, he didn't feel like he had a place in their home or their family. He reflected, "It reminds me of how I felt as a kid, like I didn't have a place. I hadn't felt like that in years, but since Charlotte was born, I'm not sure where I fit in anymore."

Vivien was quiet for a few moments, then looked at me and said, "I didn't know that. I mean, I knew he felt like he didn't fit in as a child, but I didn't know he felt like that now." I encouraged her to turn to Henry and tell him this; she did, and this created a beautiful moment of connection.

Henry and Vivien brought Charlotte to the next session. Again, I was surprised by this; I expected they would let me know ahead of time if they had a child care issue, and perhaps we would reschedule. I felt unsure what we could accomplish in session with Charlotte there, and worried that Vivien would be distracted and disengaged. Vivien's parents typically watched Charlotte during their sessions, but her mother was in the hospital, and they didn't have another child care option. Because we were already meeting biweekly, they didn't want to skip this session, because that would mean a whole month in between. I validated the difficult situation that they were in, and acknowledged the financial limitations that made it difficult for them to arrange alternative child care. In that moment, I felt that reiterating the challenges of having sessions with Charlotte present wouldn't be helpful; instead, I decided to reframe this and commended them for continuing to prioritize their relationship despite contextual challenges.

During that session, we spent a lot of time processing Vivien's feelings around her mother being hospitalized, which I learned was a result of a chronic illness. One of the reasons Vivien wanted to move closer to her family was to help care for her mother. She had been unable to provide much of this while living so far away, and she felt an immense amount of guilt. However, Vivien was finding it difficult to help her mom and also care for Charlotte. This further contributed to her resentment toward Henry for not stepping up and taking more responsibility for caring for Charlotte, so that she could have more time to help her mom. During this session, it seemed the responsibilities Vivien had in caring for Charlotte in that very moment made it difficult for her to stay engaged in processing this with me. Eventually, she seemed frustrated as she exclaimed, "I'm really trying to talk about this, but it's hard when I'm also taking care of Charlotte." I remained silent and turned my gaze toward Henry. Despite Vivien's comment being directed toward me, this exchange seemed to reflect a common interaction outside of therapy, and I wanted to see how it unfolded without my intervention. A few moments later, Henry stood up and went to sit on the floor with Charlotte.

I asked Henry what happened for him in that moment, and he replied, "She clearly needs to talk about this without being interrupted, and since we're not paying you to take care of Charlotte, I figured I was the only other one to do it." He said this in a lighthearted way that made me smile, and Vivien chuckled. I commented that he heard that Vivien needed to process her feelings around her mother's illness without being interrupted, and he felt he could support her. He confirmed this. I then asked Vivien how she felt when Henry stood up and moved to the floor with Charlotte. As opposed to just saying "when he did this," I intentionally described the specific actions that Henry took.

Vivien responded with mixed emotions: "It was nice to see it . . . (*looking at Henry*) and I appreciate you going to sit with her. (*Vivien looks back at me.*) But I'm also frustrated I had to ask him to do this. I was clearly flustered, because I wanted to talk with you about my mom, but I kept getting distracted. I just wish that I didn't have to ask all the time—that he would just pick up on my cues that I need help."

Vivien's response offered an opportunity to process what it's like for her to ask someone else for help, and she described this as "uncomfortable" and a "sign of weakness." She went on to explain that as the oldest of three children, she was designated as a caretaker in her family from a young age. Both her parents worked outside of the home, and she was responsible for caring for her younger siblings. She didn't feel she could ask for help when she needed it; she just had to "figure it out." I reflected aloud how hard it must have been for her to care for her siblings when she was just a child herself, and how lonely it must have been for her to feel like she couldn't ask for help.

Following this reflection, Henry looked at Vivien and said, "But you're not a child anymore, and I'm not your parents. I want to help. I just feel like I don't know how or when I do try, I end up doing it wrong." This created an opportunity for further processing around asking for help and what each partner needed in this.

While this session began with my own feelings of uncertainty about how much work we could do with Charlotte present, what I found was that her being there offered a real-time opportunity for the couple to navigate one of the biggest challenges in their relationship—parenting. In hindsight, it allowed Vivien to experience Henry in a different way, and for me to guide them in processing this in the here and now. While this didn't change my opinion regarding our ability to continue our work with Charlotte consistently present, it did offer me a chance to see how effective work could still take place and reinforced the importance of being flexible and working within my couple's circumstances.

The couple attended the next session by themselves. Vivien shared that her mother had been released from the hospital and was doing much better. Vivien felt relieved but then continued, "That's the good news. On the other hand, Henry and I got in a huge fight last night. We haven't really talked about it, so I guess we should talk about it in here today."

I replied, "Sure, why don't you tell me what happened. I'll likely be slowing you down and linking it back to your pursue–withdraw cycle."

Vivien looked at Henry, who returned her gaze but stayed quiet. She continued: "It was the same thing we always fight about. I went over to my parents' house last night to check on my mom. Before I left, I told Henry that Charlotte needed a bath—we'd been outside a lot that day—he said 'Okay,' so I assumed he was going to take care of it and I left. When I got home, I asked about their night and her bath, and he told me, 'I didn't give her a bath.' I couldn't believe it—the one thing I asked him to do—I was so furious."

I interjected, "Vivien, I'm going to pause you here for a moment. Tell me more about that anger you felt."

Vivien replied, "Well it was just the same old thing—I ask him to do something, he agrees, but then he never follows through."

I said, "And that makes you angry."

She replied, "Yes, it makes me so angry, I feel like I could explode."

I responded, "Ah, I see—so angry you could explode. And often when we feel angry there's something driving that anger. I wonder what was underneath your anger in that moment?"

She exclaimed, "It just feels like I don't matter to him. If I really mattered, then he would have done what he said he was going to do and give her a bath."

I replied, "Okay, so I hear that you felt like you didn't matter. Can you turn to Henry and share that with him?"

Vivien addressed Henry, "When I came home last night and you said you hadn't given her a bath, I felt like I didn't matter."

Without any prompting, Henry replied, "You do matter to me. I already tried to explain to you . . . "

I interjected, "Henry, I'm going to pause you for a moment. You said something important just now, 'you do matter to me' and I want to make sure Vivien heard that. Can you tell her that again and stop there?"

Henry turned to Vivien, "You do matter to me. You matter to me so much." Vivien began to tear up.

While this was a nice moment of connection between them, and something I felt Vivien really needed to hear, this single exchange wasn't going to fix this common conflict they were having around parenting responsibilities. I invited Henry to share more about his perspective on this conflict around giving Charlotte a bath. He replied, "I had every intention of giving her a bath, just like I told Vivien I would, but after dinner, Charlotte and I were playing and I lost track of time. By the time I realized how late it was, I figured it was better to put her to bed on time and we could just give her a bath tomorrow."

Vivien jumped in: "Yeah, I could have just given her a bath the next day."

Henry replied, "I can give her a bath, too. I wasn't saying that you had to do it or putting more work on you. (*He paused for a few moments.*) This is so irritating. You want me to step in and be a more involved parent, but when I make parenting decisions, all you do is criticize them."

Vivien was silent for a while. I invited her to share what was coming up for her, and we continued to process her experience of wanting Henry to be more involved with Charlotte and having a hard time letting go of something that she did by herself for so long. I also dug deeper into Vivien's reaction about having to give Charlotte a bath the following day herself and invited the couple into a discussion about division of household and parenting responsibilities. It was clear to me that Vivien was taking on the majority of these responsibilities, and we used time in session to identify the household tasks that Henry could take responsibility for on his own.

INTERMEDIATE PHASE OF THERAPY

By our sixth session together, I had developed a strong alliance with Henry and Vivien, they were deescalated, and we had begun reframing their presenting problems in terms of underlying emotions and attachment needs. Vivien and Henry continued to show up consistently to our biweekly sessions, and I felt heartened by their continued commitment to therapy and working on their relationship. The conflicts they presented in sessions continued to center around parenting and ongoing challenges with navigating the multiple transitions they were experiencing; however, they reported their conflicts were less escalated, and they were able to come back together more quickly to discuss them. Vivien also shared that Henry was taking a more active parenting role with Charlotte, and that they had set aside specific time each week for Henry and Charlotte to spend alone together, which gave Vivien a break. Furthermore, Henry and Vivien said that following discussions we had in therapy, they started prioritizing time together in the evenings and had begun feeling more connected and had sex the previous week. I shared how happy I was for them about this new development.

The question of having more children that seemed so prominent for them at the start of therapy seemed to dissipate; that is, there seemed to be less focus on answering this question and more on addressing the more immediate parenting conflicts. In this phase of therapy, I focused on softening with Vivien; she was still quite critical of Henry at times. With Henry, I focused on reengagement—both with Vivien at home and in our sessions when things became too overwhelming for him. My hope was that each of them could gain some insight and empathy for the other's experience and move toward greater mutual acceptance and more effective co-parenting.

Vivien and Henry came to the eighth session reporting that they had yet another huge fight related to parenting. Vivien immediately exclaimed, "I don't even have to tell you what happened . . . I feel like I'm not important, he feels like he never gets it right . . . blah, blah, blah."

I replied, "You seem really frustrated right now."

She exclaimed, "I am!" I responded, "Can you tell me more about that frustration?"

She replied, "I just feel like we keep having the same fight over and over. I didn't used to feel this way, I used to think we just fought about everything. But now you've mapped our struggles around my pursuit and his withdrawal, and I see our fights in that cycle, and it just feels like *Groundhog Day*."

I reflected, "I see. So, understanding your conflicts within that familiar pattern has made you feel like you're having the same fight over and over again."

She replied, "Right."

I then looked over to Henry, who was staring out the window and not making eye contact with either of us. "Henry, what's coming up for you as you hear Vivien share her frustration?"

He was silent for a minute, then replied, "I guess I feel frustrated, too. Despite not wanting to come to therapy, I feel like I've shown up and I've been trying hard, but we've been coming for months and we're still having the same fights . . . "

Vivien interjected, "And if we continue like this, there's no way we're having more children. I just can't. If we can't figure out how to parent one child together, how will we ever parent multiple children?" And there it was again—the initial impetus for seeking therapy.

In that moment, I felt a bit of frustration myself. I believed that Vivien and Henry were making good progress, but their exchanges in session suggested they were not necessarily seeing it. This made me wonder if my perception of their progress was somehow skewed, and caused me to question my perspective. As a client-centered therapist, I value my clients' perceptions of their own progress in therapy. I also had to remind myself, though, that therapeutic change isn't linear. I shared my perspective with them. "I hear your frustration with having the same fight over and over again, and I can understand how that feels like you're not making progress. I want you to know, I've seen a lot of growth in our work together, but I also want the two of you to feel like your relationship is moving in the direction you want it to. I believe understanding your conflict patterns is the first step to changing your cycle of interaction, and I think you both have a good understanding of the pattern, and that's a big step toward change."

Vivien and Henry were both quiet for a few minutes. Vivien said, "Okay, well I'm glad at least you think we're making progress. It's helpful to hear that, because I don't think I always see the progress, or it feels like we should be improving more quickly." I normalized her statement by saying that change can be slow, and validated that it can be difficult to see the progress when you're fighting about the same things over and over again. I also commended the couple for their continued commitment to therapy—consistently arranging child care, so that they could come every other week—and working hard to improve their relationship. They seemed slightly more hopeful at the conclusion of this session. However, Henry was more quiet than usual throughout this session, and I worried that he was becoming more disengaged in the therapeutic process. Given that we were at the end of time for the session, I decided not to pursue his lack of engagement and to address it at the start of the next session instead. I wanted to have enough time to process with him without feeling rushed.

I began the next session by checking to see how they felt during the last session, and what discussions, if any, they had after our session. Henry quickly responded, "I think talking about it in here helped. This is my first time in therapy, so I didn't know what to expect other than for things to get better. It just seems like it's taking us a long time."

I replied, "I could see your frustration during our last session, but I also see growth. Identifying your pursue–withdraw pattern and seeing your conflicts in that cycle are positive steps toward change."

I then checked in with them on the past 2 weeks, and Vivien jumped in right away. "Well, not surprisingly, we had a fight over the weekend. But it wasn't about parenting, so I guess that's progress? As you know, we've been having financial difficulties since Henry started his new job—we just aren't making ends meet like we used to. Anyway, he told me that his job was offering overtime, and I was immediately of the mind-set 'you should take it,' but he feels like working more will take time away from our family, which seems to be one of our biggest problems—so that I feel like I am doing this parenting thing all on my own."

Vivien paused and looked at Henry. I turned to him and said, "Can you tell me about your fear of spending more time away from your family?"

He replied, "Well, I feel like that's one of the biggest parts of our problem—me not being involved enough in parenting—so if I'm spending even more time away from home, that's only going to get worse."

Vivien turned to Henry and said, "But we have to consider our financial situation. I've been really stressed about it, and this seems like an opportunity to make it a little bit better."

Henry looked at me and said, "I didn't know that."

I replied, "Which part?"

Henry explained, "That she's so stressed about our finances. I thought the finances were my thing to worry about."

We processed Henry's feelings about the finances being solely his responsibility and I then asked him, "Can you turn to Vivien and tell her that you didn't know she was stressed about finances?"

Henry looked at Vivien. "I didn't know you were stressed about money. You didn't tell me that before."

Tears began to fall from Vivien's eyes, and in a shaky voice she replied, "No, I didn't. I guess I just assumed you knew." Henry was silent.

I looked at Vivien, "It sounds like it was difficult for you to tell Henry that you were stressed about money. Why do you think that is?"

Still in a shaky voice Vivien replied, "I guess I've never been good about sharing when I'm stressed or letting people know what I need. I just always 'figure it out' on my own. Like I did when Charlotte was born—I just figured it out."

I responded, "Could you tell him that?"

Vivien turned, "I've never been good at letting others know when I feel stressed."

Henry replied, "I'm not your parents . . . "

I interjected, "Henry, I'm going to pause you for a moment; tell me a little bit more about what you mean by 'I'm not your parents'."

He replied, "I just mean that just because she didn't feel like she could share that growing up doesn't mean that she can't share that now with me."

I responded, "So you want Vivien to know she can tell you when she's stressed, and you want to be there for her."

Henry replied, "Right"—and without prompting, he turned to Vivien, "I want you to tell me when you're stressed. I want to be there for you. We're in this together." Vivien started to cry. I handed a tissue box to Henry; he gave one to Vivien and grabbed her hand.

This was a beautiful moment—Vivien was able to let her guard down and share how stressed she'd been and, with just a little bit of coaching, Henry was able to respond in a supportive way. This is a common conflict I see with couples when only one partner works outside of the home, which is often the case for couples with young children. The balance of work and household responsibilities is difficult to navigate, and many couples report a sense of strain around having fewer financial resources. In many cases with different-sex couples, the man is working outside of the home, and the lack of time or energy to put toward parenting is a common source of stress.

I wanted to build on the connection I had witnessed, so I began the next session by inviting brief reflections on the previous session. Henry began: "It was like a lightbulb went off. I understood why she was pushing so hard for me to work overtime. Before, it seemed so contradictory to what I thought she was most worried about—me being more involved in taking care of Charlotte—that I couldn't understand it. I felt frustrated, and it took me back to that space of 'I never get it right' and so I just go away."

I replied, "You feel like you can never get it right. Tell me more about what you mean by 'I just go away.' "

Henry explained: "I get quiet. Like when Vivien and I are arguing about something and I feel like I'm wrong, I just get quiet. It's like, I'm not saying what she wants to hear anyways, so why bother. And I know that makes her mad, and probably just makes things worse. Like we learned at the start of therapy, Vivien gets louder because she's trying to get my attention. And the louder she gets the quieter I get, or sometimes I just leave altogether."

I replied, "I want to go back to something you said a few moments ago: 'It's like I'm not saying what she wants to hear, so why bother'—can you tell me more about that?"

Henry continued, "I feel like I can't get it right. That same feeling I had growing up—Henry is wrong again. I felt that a lot growing up, especially with my dad, I never got it right in his eyes."

I replied, "Ah, I see, so this feeling that you had so often as a child comes up for you again in these interactions with Vivien."

Henry nodded, "Especially around taking care of Charlotte."

I continued, "How do you feel in that moment when you can't get it right?"

Henry paused and said, "I feel sad, I feel disappointed. I want to get it right for her, for Charlotte, I really do, but it's like no matter how hard I try, I just can't do it."

I replied, "So you feel sad, you feel disappointed in yourself in those moments." Again, Henry nodded in agreement. I continued, "Can you turn to Vivien and share that sadness with her?"

Henry looked at Vivien and said, "I feel sad in those moments, I feel like I'm letting you down, and that makes me feel bad about myself. I feel like a failure."

Vivien grabbed Henry's hand: "You're not a failure." Henry was quiet.

I gently said, "How does it feel to hear her say that?"

He replied, "It feels good." Then Henry looked at Vivien and smirked, "Can you say it again?"

Vivien chuckled, "You're not a failure." Henry smiled at Vivien with tears in his eyes—the first time I witnessed tears from him.

This was another moment of connection. The following sessions continued in a similar way, building on the work they had done and integrating new conflicts as they arose in the context of their transition to parenthood and how these new challenges were playing into their long-standing pursue–withdraw pattern. They seemed more connected in the therapy room, and less focused on parenting as the primary point of conflict as they consolidated reinterpretation of those conflicts in the context of their separate vulnerabilities and needs for secure attachment.

Toward the end of our 13th session, Vivien said, "I know we're almost out of time, but I want to make sure we talk about something before we leave. Henry and I had a conversation last night about continuing therapy, and I just don't think we're on the same page."

I replied, "Okay, tell me more."

Vivien continued, "Henry thinks we should stop therapy, but I disagree. Just because we're seeing progress doesn't mean we should stop."

I responded, "You're worried that if you don't keep coming to therapy, the progress that you've made will just slip away."

Vivien nodded, "Yes. I mean, we still haven't decided if we're going to have more kids or not. That was originally why we came here."

I replied, "You set an indicator of how you would know when you were done with therapy, and you haven't reached that yet." Vivien nodded. I continued, "I want to come back to something we were talking about a few minutes ago regarding your fear of what might happen if you stop therapy. Can you tell me more about that fear?"

Vivien explained, "I guess I just finally feel like we're doing a bit better, I feel more connected to Henry now than I have in the last 18 months, and I'm not sure we can keep this up on our own."

I responded, "So I hear you saying 'I feel connected to you' (*gesturing over to Henry*), 'I feel more connected to you than I have in a long time, and I don't want to lose that.'" Vivien nodded.

I wanted to bring Henry into this exchange. "Henry, how does it feel to hear Vivien say that?"

Henry replied, "I mean, I agree with her. That's why I suggested we consider ending therapy. We're doing much better."

I reflected, "So you both believe your relationship is stronger and in a better place than it was before." They both nodded in agreement. I continued, "And Henry, you believe that will continue even without therapy, but Vivien, you're worried that without therapy, you'll lose the connection you have now." Vivien nodded, while Henry had a blank stare on his face. I gently prompted, "Henry, what's coming up for you right now?"

He replied, "Well I guess I don't know for sure that we can continue to feel connected without therapy, and I really don't want to get this wrong, but I think we should at least try."

I continued, "Can you turn to Vivien and tell her that?"

Henry turned to Vivien. "We've been coming to therapy for a while, and I think we're in a good place."

Vivien replied, "And what if we're not? What if we stop therapy and then everything falls apart, what then?"

Henry responded, "Well, I guess we could always come back to therapy," and he turned and looked at me.

I nodded. "Of course, my door is always open if you decide you want to return. I work with many couples who suspend therapy and then weeks, months, or even years later, reach out to do more work." I encouraged them to continue this conversation in between sessions and we could check in on this at the start of our next session.

I was surprised by the couple's disclosure of their discussions about termination. I, too, witnessed significant progress in their relationship and was hoping to have more time to consolidate their new patterns. I also really enjoyed working with them and felt a personal sadness about the possibility of termination. Despite my professional and personal desires for them to continue, I decided in that moment not to share this, but instead to help them process their ambivalence and encourage them to continue the conversation on their own. If I thought that discontinuing services would have been detrimental, I likely would have made a different decision, but I could see the progress that Henry and Vivien had made, and wanted to support any desire they might have to continue to work on their relationship on their own.

CONCLUDING PHASE OF THERAPY

I checked in with them at the start of the next session about termination. They were both silent at first, then Vivien said that she and Henry had discussed it more since our last session and wanted to do one more session and then wrap up. Henry agreed with this. I shared my support of their decision and asked, "How would you like to use our time together today?"

Vivien replied, "We had a parenting issue come up this week. I was worried we aren't ready to terminate, but Henry and I talked about it, and while it was an issue, we handled it better than we would've in the past."

I responded, "That's great."

Vivien continued, "But we still wanted to process it in here with you."

I replied, "Of course." We spent much of the remaining time processing this event and consolidating their new patterns of interaction.

Toward the end of this session, I checked in with them on co-creating a plan for our final session together. They were both initially quiet, so I continued, "It's okay if you don't have specific ideas of how we can use that time together." There was more silence, "If you'd like, I can share some thoughts that I have for our final session together." They both nodded.

"I like to use the time for reflection—you on your experience, and me on the progress I've seen. There are many ways we can do this. We can also use the time any other ways you would like."

There was more silence, then Vivien said, "Can we think about it?"

I replied, "Absolutely."

I approached our final session flexibly, on the one hand creating space for anything they wanted to bring in, and on the other having a general plan for this time in case they were looking for more guidance from me. When they sat down, I noticed Vivien had a stack of papers, and I asked her if she would share them with me. Vivien began, "We decided to make a list of all the things we've accomplished in therapy. We wanted to bring it in and share it with you."

I reflected, "That's great that you all had some time to reflect on the work you've done in here, and I appreciate you sharing it with me." Vivien started to read through each item on this list, and at times I would ask her to pause, then ask them both to reflect further on the ways they experienced a particular item from the list. We continued processing until we reached the end of the list. Then Vivien reached out and handed the papers to me, "This is a copy—we have our own at home—but we wanted you to have this."

I flipped over to the second page and there was a heartfelt note sharing their appreciation for their time in therapy. I was truly touched by this gesture. I expressed this, and asked them whether it was all right to provide some reflections of my own on our work together. They both nodded. I shared the many strengths that I believe they have, and reflected on the hard work they did in therapy, and the progress they made. I also shared my own sadness for our time ending and, at the same time, the excitement I felt for them in taking this next step. Vivien then shared that they had also talked about some of things they were worried about with regard to stopping treatment. We spent the remaining time processing their concerns (e.g., not having a place to process fights), and I reminded them that my door was always open should they want to return. We then said good-bye.

I felt hopeful for Henry and Vivien when they left my office that day. Their concerns around termination were understandable, and I believed they had gained the skills and new patterns of interaction to successfully navigate future challenges. While I had hoped to have some more time to work on consolidating these new patterns, I appreciated having two sessions to do some of this work and to wrap up. I also appreciated them bringing their concerns about termination to the final session, giving us a chance to process these. Although I reminded them that they could return to treatment at any time, I never heard from them again, though I do think of them from time to time.

FURTHER REFLECTIONS AND IMPLICATIONS

I enjoyed working with Vivien and Henry so much. Despite many months of feeling disconnected as they navigated the challenges of becoming parents, their commitment to therapy and to strengthening their relationship was very clear. I believe Henry's deployment, their decision to relocate, and the ongoing financial stress they experienced contributed to unique exacerbating challenges for this couple during this time of transition. What I admired most was their resilience despite the many transitions they experienced simultaneously. Henry and Vivien both wanted to be closer to their families and support system, but becoming parents actually increased the strain on their relationship. While this surprised them, even positive events such as having a baby frequently cause increases in relationship strain. Although Vivien believed Henry was not as invested in their relationship or their family as she was, early on in therapy, Henry was able to share with her how much she and Charlotte meant to him. Throughout the course of therapy, I witnessed Henry and Vivien slowly develop new patterns of interaction and regain connection in their relationship. This was truly beautiful and emotionally impactful for me to witness. Even though they weren't seeing the change as it occurred in the moment, I could see progress and for that I felt hopeful for them.

Having biweekly sessions was one challenge that I experienced in working with Henry and Vivien. When I reflect back, I think the biweekly sessions made our work together move a bit slower and, at times, I think, contributed to their frustration about the change (or the lack thereof) they were seeing. I also believe that these constraints were a contributing factor to their decision to terminate when they did.

When reflecting on my work with Henry and Vivien, there are a couple of important take-home messages for those who may be new to working with couples as they transition to becoming parents. The first is more general: *Meet couples where they are at the time.* I can't stress enough how important this is. Every couple we work with has contextual circumstances—some may be more openly discussed than others—and understanding what these are and how these influence the ways in which the couple presents is essential. I like to believe the way I responded to Henry and Vivien's scheduling constraints contributed to a stronger therapeutic alliance and ultimately created a safer space for them to show up every other week and work on their relationship. The second take-home point is *understand the immense challenges that couples experience during this time, and normalize this.* While having a new baby is often a joyous occasion, it's also a stressful one in ways that are too often minimized or unrecognized in our society. As couples struggle with the inherent challenges of a new infant, there's too little attention paid to the couple's own relationship. It is often difficult for couples to acknowledge the relationship challenges they experience during this time and to feel that their relationship is something they can and should prioritize. It is important for therapists working with couples becoming parents to understand this broadly and to examine how these challenges play out more specifically for each couple.

As a new parent myself, I could identify with many of Henry and Vivien's experiences—renegotiating roles and responsibilities, the lack of time to focus on the couple relationship, and the difficulties in making this transition while being far away from one's support system. Despite being proactive in preparing ourselves, our relationship, and our household for this transition, these changes were still challenging for us at times. For me, becoming a new parent simultaneously brought joy and excitement, and stress and fear—an experience, I think, that resonates with many new parents. My own transition to parenthood also occurred during the COVID-19 pandemic, which added to the stress and many logistical challenges (child care, spending time with family and friends) we had to navigate. Tapping into my own experiences and possibly self-disclosing could facilitate joining with couples coming to therapy during this transition. However, some of my own experiences of becoming a new parent didn't mirror other unique characteristics of this couple (e.g., one partner deployed, financial stressors), and it's important to be aware of this and not overidentify with couples' experiences. For therapists who haven't experienced this transition themselves, being informed about the challenges and common experiences of new parents can help validate and normalize this for your couple and facilitate empathic joining. Reading the literature and talking to new parents are excellent ways to gather this information—especially as it relates specifically to the couple relationship. Therapists can offer a safe space for couples to share about the struggles in their relationship and receive support in navigating these and strengthening their connection.

REFERENCES

Doss, B. D., Rhoades, G. K., Stanley, S. M., & Markman, H. J. (2009). The effect of the transition to parenthood on relationship quality: An 8-year prospective study. *Journal of Personality and Social Psychology, 96*, 601–619.

Epifanio, M. S., Genna, V., De Luca, C., Roccella, M., & La Grutta, S. (2015). Paternal and maternal transition to parenthood: The risk of postpartum depression and parenting stress. *Pediatric Reports, 7*, 38–44.

Faisal-Cury, A., Tabb, K., & Matijasevich, A. (2021). Partner relationship quality predicts later postpartum depression independently of the chronicity of depressive symptoms. *Brazilian Journal of Psychiatry, 43*, 12–21.

Funk, J. L., & Rogge, R. D. (2007). Testing the Ruler with Item Response Theory: Increasing Precision of Measurement for Relationship Satisfaction with the Couples Satisfaction Index. *Journal of Family Psychology, 21*, 572–583.

Johnson, S. M., Wiebe, S. A., & Allan, R. (2023). Emotionally focused couple therapy. In J. L. Lebow & D. K. Snyder (Eds.), *Clinical handbook of couple therapy* (6th ed., pp. 127–150). New York: Guilford Press.

Kan, M. L., & Feinberg, M. E. (2011). Measurement and correlates of intimate partner violence among expectant first-time parents. *Violence and Victims, 25*, 319–331.

Rauch-Anderegg, V., Kuhn, R., Milek, A., Halford, W. K., & Bodenmann, G. (2020). Relationship behaviors across the transition to parenthood. *Journal of Family Issues, 41*, 483–506.

CHAPTER 15

Integrative Behavioral Couple Therapy with Military and Veteran Couples

BARBARA M. DAUSCH
SHIRLEY M. GLYNN
ANDREW CHRISTENSEN

Editors' Comments

Barbara Dausch, Shirley Glynn, and Andrew Christensen provide a perfect example of how to adapt a major model of couple therapy to a specific population. Integrative behavioral couple therapy (IBCT) numbers among the strongest empirically supported and widely practiced couple therapies. As Dausch and colleagues so clearly communicate in their chapter, IBCT is a manualized therapy that presents therapists with the advantage of a clear integrative road map about when to do what in treatment.

The authors present a state-of-the-art example of this approach, adapted to a couple treated within the health care system of the U.S. Department of Veterans Affairs (VA), which offers IBCT as a major treatment option. The chapter captures the efficient way IBCT uses a four-session assessment protocol to develop a case formulation and treatment plan, then shares that formulation and treatment plan with partners in a collaborative feedback session. This case narrative also points to how far IBCT has moved from its original point of origin in behavior therapy to emphasizing partners' affective experience and developmental histories in helping the couple arrive at unified detachment and mutual acceptance. Dausch's skillfulness and wisdom in delivering this treatment are remarkable, as she draws from a wide array of techniques tailored to the therapeutic process at any given moment. She also does a remarkable job of orienting the reader along the way as to where she is in the decisional process within the IBCT framework, and sharing in a deeply personal way what she's experiencing as she works with this couple.

This chapter also focuses specific attention on critical work with military and Veteran couples. One special aspect of this case study is that even though one partner has deployment-related posttraumatic stress disorder (PTSD), the couple therapy targets partners' concerns and challenges that extend well beyond that issue. Even when PTSD is not the specific focus of the therapy, its shadow often traverses multiple aspects of a couple's daily experiences. Fortunately, efforts such as dissemination of IBCT within the VA health care system, as well as specific couple therapies for PTSD, have advanced effective interventions for comorbid trauma history and intimate relationship distress.

My (BMD) love of clinical work with Veteran couples stems largely from growing up with strong ties to the military and parents who struggled as first-generation Americans in the New York City melting pot. My father and grandfather proudly served, and their military experiences shaped our family and influenced my values and life choices. Themes of family separation, loss, trauma, transition, and grit are part of the Veteran experience, as they are the story of my own family. I was taught to be persistent, value education, appreciate privilege, and serve those in need. In carving my own path, I gravitated toward clinical approaches that appreciate the values of self-determination and cultivate resilience in the face of challenge. I feel fortunate to have collaborated with Andrew Christensen and Shirley Glynn in their initiative to provide IBCT to military Veteran couples, and their expertise is reflected in my clinical practice.

Service members and Veterans represent a broad array of experiences and characteristics such as age, ethnicity, service era, service-connected mental health disorders, combat experiences, deployments, and gender (with women as the fastest growing demographic). Because most service members and Veterans are married and have children, family members are impacted when they are deployed, suffer service-related mental health and medical injuries, and face reintegration back to civilian life (for reviews, see Snyder & Monson, 2012; Sayers, 2014). The VA, charged with providing lifelong health care services to Veterans, provides a breadth of specialized services when compared with non-VA facilities to address Veterans' inherent medical and mental health comorbidities and situational complexities. In a recent study of Veterans receiving couple and family treatment within the VA, over one-third of Veterans had combat exposure and nearly two-thirds had a service-connected mental health diagnosis, with PTSD as the most predominant diagnosis (McKee, McDonald, Karmarkar, & Ghatas, 2023).

Relationship difficulties are common among Veterans, and the VA provides couple and family therapy to address these. IBCT (Christensen, Doss, & Jacobson, 2020) was chosen for national dissemination throughout the VA because of not only its robust evidence-base but also its ability to address the multitude and complex issues of Veteran couples, its grounding in both cognitive-behavioral and third-wave acceptance-based approaches, its time-limited nature, and the willingness of its primary developer (Christensen) to work with the VA to adapt it for a Veteran population. IBCT effectively improves relationship satisfaction in couples as it helps them to navigate a host of issues, including low-level intimate partner violence and affairs (see Christensen, Dimidjian, Martell, & Doss, 2023, for an overview). Evaluation data from the implementation of IBCT in the VA from trainees learning IBCT have shown similar benefits as the initial clinical trials (Christensen & Glynn, 2019).

IBCT emphasizes dyadic processes over individual processes; considers causal factors across each partner's lifespan; highlights understanding internal motivations and emotional sensitivities to facilitate emotional connection, as well as behavior change; and capitalizes on contingency-based or spontaneous change versus rule-governed learning (Christensen et al., 2020). In short, IBCT empowers partners to understand both their own and their partner's emotional experience as it relates to their interactions. As a result, interventions prompt partners to express hidden vulnerable emotions related to unmet needs, desires, or hope for change. Understanding or acceptance of a partner's true emotional experience enables a shift away from reactivity toward curiosity and focuses on conditions for change. In this shift from "I'm so angry . . ." to "I feel hurt . . . ," there is an invitation to connect.

There are four phases of IBCT: assessment, feedback, intervention, and termination. The assessment phase comprises an initial conjoint session and individual sessions with each partner to understand the presenting problem and each partner's social learning history, along with assessment of safety concerns such as intimate partner violence. The feedback session integrates this information to offer a conceptual formulation called the DEEP analysis, which serves as an explanatory framework for why a couple struggles and serves as an alternative to the couple's usual fault-based explanation. DEEP stands for the *Differences* between partners, their *Emotional* sensitivities, and *External* circumstances that may magnify the differences, and their *Pattern* of interaction as they encounter problems created by their differences, emotional sensitivities, and external circumstances.

Treatment begins with two primary interventions: empathic joining and unified detachment. Empathic joining gently exposes the hidden, softer emotions and authentic motivation underneath challenging interactions, allowing vulnerability to surface. Unified detachment enables partners to understand how their differences and sensitivities lead them to engage in problematic patterns of interaction. These two interventions set the stage for change-oriented interventions (communication strategies, problem solving) in which practical discussions and spontaneous solutions occur. The final phase of treatment is termination, where progress is highlighted, and sessions are spaced out until the couple is ready to end therapy.

As an IBCT therapist, I appreciate the emphasis on integrating individual stories of struggle and triumph into a shared conceptualization (i.e., mutual understanding), which encourages empathy. When I invite couples to engage in a narrative emphasizing understanding, I'm reminded of my grandmother's advice when I would have a conflict with a friend as a child. She would tell me to "walk in their shoes." Because my grandfather was deployed on a Navy ship during most of my father's youth, she ran a household alone with strength and compassion. Her sage advice is useful as I remind myself to first understand each partner's experience and then encourage each to understand and appreciate the other's perspective.

INITIAL ASSESSMENT AND CASE FORMULATION

I received a referral for Ben and Alisia, a Hispanic couple in their mid-30s, from Alisia's individual therapist, indicating the couple had issues with trust and parenting, and recently had separated and reunited. Alisia served as an Army medic deployed to Afghanistan, where she witnessed frequent injury and death. As a VA clinician, I routinely review the Veteran's medical chart to assess for appropriateness for treatment including safety concerns (e.g., intimate partner violence, acute substance use, or acute suicidality). In doing so, I learn that Alisia is engaged in cognitive processing therapy (Resick, Monson, & Chard, 2016) for PTSD, a trauma-focused treatment in which Veterans examine and challenge upsetting thoughts and beliefs stemming from their trauma.

Initial Session

During the initial session, I discover that Ben and Alisia met online after she separated from the military while she went through a divorce, and have been married 7 years. They have two daughters, one from Alisia's prior marriage. They went through fertility treatments to get pregnant with their own daughter, who has special needs. During a brief separation 3 months ago, Ben moved out and had a few girlfriends during that time. The couple reconciled when both realized they loved one another and decided to try couple therapy.

During the initial session, I ask about what brings them to therapy. Ben jumps in first. "We argue about everything from the kids to the laundry."

Alisia reacts assertively. "Ben is selfish and is always looking out for himself."

Ben rolls his eyes. "Alisia always needs to have the upper hand."

Alisia nods and says, "I make more of the decisions, but I wish I could be a priority to Ben. Our lives have become transactional, and this is what I don't like. I know he had a different experience growing up and didn't have a sense of family like I did, and then he struggled with drinking."

Ben looks down, shakes his head, and says, "Alisia acts like she's still in the military, commander of this relationship. Yes, we have struggles, but I've come a long way with my own sobriety, and I'm invested in the children and in her."

Like many couples, Ben and Alisia present with a litany of issues but are engaged in this discussion. I note they're already making connections between their past experiences and current conflict, although they look to past events to support their critical perspectives.

When I ask about their goals, Ben and Alisia state they want to trust one another again and communicate "like we're on the same team," particularly around parenting. They also want more affection and physical intimacy between them. Ben describes a typical conflict in which he helps a neighbor with a computer issue and when he returns, Alisia accuses him of spending too much time away. He "blows up and leaves" because he doesn't want to fight. Alisia describes how Ben was gone for hours when she needed him at home to go over the kids' schedules for the week. I find myself empathizing with both perspectives. As I reflect on my compassion for each of them, I recognize the culprit for their problems in their reactive interactional pattern.

I ask them to tell me about their initial attractions, being fully aware that I'm moving against their natural tendency to tell me about their challenges. While this may feel abrupt, it provides vital information. What attracts couples are often the very traits over which couples experience conflict. Ben was initially attracted to Alisia's strength, ambition, and caring nature as a mother and military medic. Alisia was attracted to Ben because he was "a rock," valued connection, and his methodical nature made her feel safe and respected. I feel relief as I watch how they smile at each other and can tap into these emotions. As a couple therapist, I find it's easy to become overly focused on couples' challenges or to overaccentuate strengths. Couples need to feel heard and recognized for both their struggles

Individual Sessions

I meet with Ben and Alisia individually to gather information about their histories. Both were raised in tight-knit, Hispanic families. As the oldest of six children, Alisia took charge of her younger siblings amid the chaos. She reports facing prejudice as a Hispanic female and fighting against feeling invisible or insignificant. Alisia reports she got pregnant early in life and joined the military to create stability for her child. Her military experience, however, was full of trauma. Autonomy and decisiveness were vital to success. I admire her resilience and understand how Ben offers the respect, safety, and validation she seeks.

Ben reports that he witnessed his parents' fights leading to their divorce when he was 10. He felt abandoned and ignored after his parents' divorce and craved attention and connection. Both parents were occupied with new partners, and he went through several family transitions. Ben states that his ability to focus and organize helped him navigate the chaos. He engaged in drinking earlier in his life to deal with his loneliness. I can understand Ben's need for belonging, his fear of abandonment, and how Alisia's caring helps him to feel connected.

Feedback Session

The feedback session is my favorite part of IBCT. In this session, I create an experience in which partners can shift their focus from seeing conflict rooted in each other to understanding that their differences and sensitivities generate the reactivity that fuels conflict. I empathize with each partner and convey that all behavior is understandable when put into the larger context of our lives. In the spirit of collaboration, I invite them to agree, disagree, or add anything that I missed. I reflect on how each partner's background contributes to their struggle using a delicate balance of honest compassion and compassionate honesty. It's like holding up a mirror and gently identifying the images that make up the reflection.

I start with what brings Alisia and Ben into therapy, and remark on challenges they've faced in their lives that have left them feeling less than satisfied with their relationship. I remark on their high level of commitment to the relationship and their strengths as a couple, reinforcing their decision to enter therapy. Alisia and Ben smile and state that they've always felt they "had each other's backs." I highlight their resilience and struggle with starting a family together, their similar values and cultural background, their devotion to their children, and common passion for sports. Alisia and Ben look at one another and smile softly. Accentuating couple strengths and seeing their reaction often adds energy and infuses optimism into the process; however, I'm also aware of how it's important to make sure the strengths outlined are authentic and not an exercise in cheerleading.

Why are the issues of trust, parenting, and intimacy a problem for Alisia and Ben? This is where the DEEP formulation helps to demystify the issues in their relationship. Both Alisia and Ben sit up attentively in their chairs.

I start with differences. While most couples have differences, these often serve as forces of attraction. I look at Alisia and relay that she's decisive and "tuned into the big picture." She cherishes time to sit and think, but then creates a plan and acts. She cares deeply, and her military service enabled her to develop her nursing career, but she never anticipated the trauma she experienced. What she witnessed makes her cling to the things that are important even more now. Alisia appears intensely focused and nods her head in agreement.

I turn to Ben. I describe that he's someone who likes to think and talk things through methodically and analyze a situation before acting, which fits with his career in information technology. He recharges his batteries by spending time with others and seeks connection. Ultimately, his natural tendency is to approach matters in an organized, methodical way, which helped him manage the transitions of his youth. Ben nods in agreement.

Ben and Alisia's emotional sensitivities reflect their upbringing, culture, life experiences and history of relationships. I explain that sensitivities operate like a trigger and create a reaction when activated. I lean in as I review Alisia's history and identify her sensitivity as a need for autonomy that has kept her safe and in control. Uncertainty in her youth and military trauma combine to strengthen her impulse to take charge. I pause and make eye contact with Alisia, and she nods and states that it's hard for her to depend on others at times. As I recognize that Alisia is thinking about what may be behind her reactions, I wonder whether Ben is empathizing with her struggle.

I turn to Ben. I review his history and note that he feels safe when connected to others and may become triggered when he feels alone or abandoned. I connect this to past experiences in which he found safety in being methodical and seeking out social interactions when his family was chaotic. Ben nods slowly and agrees that it's difficult for him to feel lonely. At this point, I wonder whether Alisia can grasp Ben's struggle for validation and connection.

After reviewing Ben's and Alisia's external stressors (parenting young children, recent separation, PTSD treatment) and describing how they amplify interactions, I turn to how these three elements feed into their pattern of interaction. It goes something like this: When an issue arises, Alisia acts decisively in contrast to Ben's methodical approach. Feeling minimized or alone, Ben retreats and Alisia approaches to obtain resolution. This creates a secondary problem in which Alisia feels that Ben does not care and Ben experiences Alisia needing to control the issue. I reflect on the reality that during stress, we tend to do more of what we know how to do (push or retreat), and it can leave couples polarized. Alisia and Ben agree that their arguments are less about the issue and more about how the other is reacting.

While I don't present Alisia's military service and her PTSD as a primary issue, I highlight the impact of trauma in her sensitivities, external stressors, and pattern of interacting with Ben. I am careful to follow the lead of what couples present as their core issues and know that Alisia or Ben will bring this into therapy when they are ready to address it. Therapy invites difficult and necessary conversations.

BEGINNING PHASE OF THERAPY

In IBCT, treatment sessions involve discussing specific positive and challenging events that occur throughout the week. To guide content, participants complete a weekly questionnaire independently before each session. This tool provides information on relationship satisfaction, destructiveness, problematic substance use, or major events. It also identifies the most salient positive and challenging interactions from the week and important upcoming events. In using the structure of reviewing each partner's questionnaire to collaboratively set the agenda, I enable each partner to have an equal voice and provide their perspective on the issues. Furthermore, this structure sets the stage for the primary IBCT interventions: empathic joining (uncovering salient emotional experiences), unified detachment (observing and identifying potent dyadic processes), and last, direct change interventions (inviting direct or intentional change). While this structure provides a frame, I need to suggest the framework for reviewing these incidents and issues (the DEEP conceptualization). I anticipate that couples will attempt to "air grievances," even if they understand new ways to see their relationship. As this occurs, I model curiosity, understanding, compassion, and empathy with both partners to establish this as a norm. Couples observe how I solicit emotion and inquire curiously about perspectives, and I hope they can adopt this stance.

Alisia and Ben come to the first session with a challenging interaction in which Ben wants to attend a baseball game with a group of work friends, including a female friend of his who was never a girlfriend but someone whom Alisia perceives as a threat. I ask the couple to describe the conflict blow by blow. Alisia starts. "This is where our trust goes off the rails. He wants to go off and do these things and has no idea how this impacts me! Plus, there's a woman he works with that I don't trust, and Ben doesn't see it."

In order to structure this discussion, I state, "This seems like a great topic that represents the issue of trust in the relationship. I'd like to begin by having each of you talk through the incident when this issue came up and go over what each of you said. Go back and forth, sharing your emotions, perspectives, and reactions." In the beginning stages of therapy, couples want to litigate the wrongs in their relationship and to grandstand to make sure their perspective is heard. Providing structure can shape this desire into productive dialogue.

Alisia asks, "So you want us to go over our fight?"

I reply, "Yes, I'd like for each of you to start with where you think it started."

Ben states, "I brought up going out last Monday, and I know this is a touchy subject. I know Alisia was tired after a shift, but I had to let her know." I ask Ben to talk about his underlying emotions. He notes that he felt like he was "walking on eggshells" and felt fearful of Alisia's reaction, while at the same time feeling as if he should be able to go out independently with work colleagues.

Alisia responds with anger, "Ben just announced this, as if I didn't have a say in this decision at all. I was fuming because of what we've been through in the last year! He also expects me to pick up the slack with the kids all the time and I'm exhausted." While the affect is escalating, I feel assured by the fact that this issue is about taking risks and is an opportunity for them to build trust.

I reflect Alisia's angry response. "Alisia, I hear a lot of anger and some fatigue. I'm just curious to hear you talk more about other emotions you felt when Ben approached you."

Alisia responds. "I just don't know that trust is there yet, even if this seems innocent to him. It hurts me to know that this is the way he wants to spend his time." Rather than focus on her anger, I jump on the opportunity to highlight Alisia's hurt and feelings of not being prioritized and ask Ben what he's thinking—particularly about Alisia's hurt.

Ben replies, "I didn't know this hurt you, I just thought you want me to have a strict routine with the girls. I know you're worried about that woman, and there is nothing there! We work together. I know you're also afraid I'll drink, and I get that, but it's been years and I haven't even come close to wanting a drink."

Alisia responds, "Of course, I feel hurt, and I am concerned about your drinking and anything else that may happen. But we were recently separated, and I need to feel like you want to be with me too . . ."

I jump in to slow down the interaction and focus on a critical piece. I hold up my hands to signal. "I want to highlight something important that you just said, Alisia. You said you 'need to feel like Ben wants to be with you.' Can you say more about this and what this would entail?"

Alisia smiles. "Yes, I need to know Ben wants to spend time with me, and I want his attention to be focused on me."

I ask, "What does this feel like when Ben's attention is focused on you?"

Alisia replies, "It feels like it did when we first met. We spent hours talking about all the details of our lives. I felt appreciated, cared for and loved, which is what I do for everyone else in my life." At this juncture, it's important that I reinforce and direct the expression of needs, particularly when they're aligned with a couple's desires for closeness and connection.

I turn to Ben, "What feelings come up when you hear that?"

Ben replies, "I want that too . . . I guess I feel sad but hopeful that I want that too."

I say, "Sounds like you're both thirsting for that feeling of being cared for and attended to. How can we apply this back to what we started talking about?" Silence. I'm grateful that Ben has heard Alisia and I can summarize their mutual desire for connection in what started as a difficult interaction; however, I want Alisia and Ben to connect the dots, and I give them the time to do so.

Alisia replies, "I want to feel like we're a couple, and it's difficult when you make plans with others, and we don't have any plans."

Ben acknowledges Alisia's perspective, "I'd love to go out together . . . this just came up at work."

Alisia states, "If you go to the baseball game, I'd like to be in on what's going on, like knowing when you get there, what the score is, highlights of the game. Like if you text me a few times during the evening."

Ben replies, "I could do that . . . it would be fun. I could also send you a picture . . ." It makes sense to me that Alisia comes up with a solution, based on her decisive nature. It also makes sense to me that Ben agrees on a solution that enables him to have the social connection he craves.

As I wrap up this session, I highlight aspects of their interaction that reflect choices they made to move toward one another, such as sharing feelings of hurt and the real issue: their mutual longing for connection. I feel hopeful for Alisia and Ben primarily because they're able to navigate a way to connect despite strong reactions. I remind myself to be careful not to reinforce their spontaneous problem solving as the "way out" of conflict (e.g., that now we have a texting solution to their trust issue), but make sure to reinforce their bid for connection and understanding of each other's needs.

During the next session, Alisia and Ben note in their weekly questionnaire under the positive interactions that Ben attended the baseball game. I chose to ask Alisia first to describe what happened. I start with Alisia because when there's perceived or real infidelity, the person on the receiving end often takes longer to recover and is understandably sensitive when similar situations occur. Alisia replies, "Ben went out and I was nervous at first, knowing he was in the company of a woman who I believe wants to hook up with him. I think it went well; he texted me when he got there and sent me a picture. I was also scared that he would drink and come home late, but he didn't, and I was glad to get his texts about the game. I think the best part for me was when he came home—we talked at the kitchen table and he told me everything that happened."

I turn to Ben and ask him to relay his perspective. "It went as planned . . . as I thought it would. There was no drinking—these are the folks I work with, and we enjoyed the game. It really wasn't a big deal to text her. At first it felt a bit annoying, only because it was like 'reporting in,' but I get it. After I sent her the picture of the group, I enjoyed texting her the highlights of the game and was excited to get home and fill her in on the evening."

I use this opportunity to comment on the risks they both took and outline how their actions were consistent with their goal of building trust and fostering connection. Additionally, I begin to introduce unified detachment as I comment on their ability to act on the problem with a nod to their sensitivities (need for autonomy, need for social connection) and pattern of interaction (Alisia pursues and Ben retreats). "Because the two of you engaged in a different pattern of interaction around Ben attending the game, you were able to use this event to get what you both want in the relationship. Instead of giving in to feeling resentful and angry, which pushes Ben away, Alisia, you let him know the issue was that you wanted to be with him. That brought him closer and enabled you to be decisive around creating an opportunity. Ben, you didn't run, but approached the request and then moved closer at the invitation to do so."

During the beginning stages of treatment, both empathic joining and unified detachment are used. The initial focus is on empathic joining—prompting couples' underlying softer emotions, the hurt, the sadness, and the fear. These emotions are more difficult to identify and share initially as couples are primed to respond with defensiveness, anger, and frustration. While I provide the opportunity for the softer underlying emotions (hurt) to emerge, I'm careful not to devalue the harder surface emotions (anger). As couples become less fused with their emotional reactions, they begin to recognize the impact of their behavior and typical patterns that are a natural extension of their differences and sensitivities. As a therapist, I see one of my most potent tools as my ability to hold a light in the darkness and chaos of a couple's distress and point it in the direction of their authentic experiences and ultimate goals.

When I was a beginning therapist, I believed that a successful session involved problem solving, skills training or psychoeducation, ending with a plan for homework. Somehow, I felt like I needed to leave each session with neat resolution. Now, I realize that raw emotional experiences that represent vulnerability give couples a new experience of their relationship, which is powerful. Honoring vulnerability opens opportunities for connection. I've had couples quietly leave sessions after expressing sadness or hurt for the first time, and by the time they got to their car, one spontaneously reached for the other's hand, and the relationship shifted. The beginning stages of therapy are ideal for shaping expectations around therapy and empowering couples to be mindful and take emotional risks.

INTERMEDIATE PHASE OF THERAPY

Alisia and Ben continue to work through interactions that represent what they begin to label as their "toxic pattern." This labeling is one example of unified detachment, in which couples look at their interactions with analytic distance. While both the early and intermediate phases of IBCT are dominated by empathic joining and unified detachment, these interventions begin to work hand in hand as couples begin to express vulnerability and become mindful of their patterns of interaction. In short, I am asking Alisia and Ben to identify key turning points in the interactions they target on the weekly questionnaire and to detach from the struggle of thinking the problem is within each other. When detached, they can see their patterns in a unified way and may spontaneously change certain problematic pieces of their patterns. The following represents excerpts from several progressive sessions that represent the intermediate phase of treatment.

In one session, Alisia and Ben discuss a tense interaction around parenting. Ben starts, "So Alisia comes in from work today and announces plans to visit her parents in New Mexico for our daughter's sixth birthday. She made this decision without even asking me! I didn't know what to say. I was surprised and resentful that this was thrown at me, and it led to a fight." I wonder about the hurt underneath Ben's outrage and how to structure a compassionate discussion around this. I start by validating his surface emotion (anger, surprise) and switch to Alisia to engage her.

I inquire, "Alisia, can you tell me a little bit about how you saw the interaction?"

Alisia adds details of how she mentioned briefly to Ben that there was an invitation from her parents who are hosting a family celebration. "It's a great opportunity for our daughters to be with family. I know we didn't have a big discussion, but I know that family is important, so why would you disagree? I just had to say yes or no to them and start organizing my schedule."

At this point, I engage in empathic joining to help Alisia and Ben explore what was underneath their reactions. "Ben, tell me what came up for you emotionally, besides anger, when Alisia mentioned this to you." I purposely direct him back to their conversation to focus on the interaction rather than the larger issue.

Ben replies, "Well, I feel broadsided by the comment and invisible, like talking to me about it doesn't matter, even if I agree." This reminds me of Ben's chaotic family, in which he felt ignored after his parent's divorce. I notice that Ben is openly connecting emotions to past issues, in part due to his dedication to sobriety and work in recovery.

I ask, "Can you say more about feeling invisible?"

Ben looks down. "What is there to say? It's like I'm worthless as a father and reminds me of my own father." He pauses. "I feel guilty and tend to go along with Alisia, because I don't want to let my daughter down and I don't want to show her the fighting I saw between my parents, and I don't want Alisia to leave me. I just go along to get along, and it becomes transactional."

Alisia responds to Ben, "You're not invisible, our lives are so busy, and I really think I did mention it and you know how my family is . . . "

At this point I remind them of their sensitivities: Ben's fear of abandonment and Alisia need for autonomy. I bring the couple back to the interaction to ask Alisia to talk about what she was feeling at the time this occurred. She responds, "Well, if I don't plan these things, then I get anxious and I feel worried that we're not doing the right thing by our daughters. I see now how this affects you. I've always thought it helped you not to have to think about things like this, but I get it."

In this session, I use both empathic joining and unified detachment to help Alisia and Ben tune into their underlying emotions and to notice their pattern of interaction. They're beginning to see how they both value their children but are responding to their own wishes and worries as they care for them. This leads to pushing each other away inadvertently.

I ask, "How does it feel to have started the discussion on this issue?"

Ben jumps in. "It was good to express what it's like for me when I get handed a decision. I'd like to spend the time to talk through these things in the future."

Alisia responds, "It's not my intention to exclude you, we're just busy . . . I don't think you've ever shared how this brings up your childhood experience and I just had no idea . . ."

I'm reminded that as I slow down the interaction, Alisia and Ben can fully appreciate the depth of emotions as they reflect on the impact of their reactions.

Parenting comes up again in a later treatment session. Initially, Alisia describes herself as a "strict parent," claiming Ben "coddles" the kids. They differ in how they view parenting. Alisia believes that a parent's primary role is to provide boundaries and structure, whereas Ben believes parents should have a close relationship with their children. In one session, Alisia brings up an incident with their daughters when Ben takes them to visit his uncle an hour away and upon returning, they fight.

Ben starts. "I took the kids to visit my uncle, and when I got home that night, I was met with a criticism of how I should bring them home before their bedtime. It's like she's in the military all over again and I'm assigned to her unit! At first, I cringed and thought, 'Here it comes!' Then she stops and recognizes what I'd done and expresses appreciation."

Alisia replies, "Yes, I've been trying to give him more space, and I recognize that he isn't going to do things the way I do. I know that it helps if I don't lead with what I don't like. I was worried because they came home later then he said they would."

"So, you started to pursue Ben for information, but something held you back, Alisia?"

She replies, "Yes, I think we've both been working on taking more time to think about how we approach one another. If I jump in there with telling him something I don't like, it all goes downhill. And, in the end, I do appreciate that he's a good father and thinks about things like our kids getting to spend time with relatives." Ben smiles.

I don't want something positive between them to go unnoticed, so I comment, "Ben, I see you smiling. And I also believe I heard a compliment? Ben, what are you feeling?"

Ben looks at Alisia and says, "It feels good to hear you say I'm a good father and mean it. I know you get afraid when things aren't exactly as you expect, particularly around the kids. I know this comes from a safety perspective and partly from what you saw over there" [referring to her military experience].

In instances when there are positive exchanges, I want to accentuate the exchange between the partners rather than be the one to reinforce the positive. This approach reflects my actions when a partner is crying and needs a tissue. I offer it to the other partner and signal for them to give the tissue to the partner in need. I appreciate the shifts Alisia and Ben make around pulling back from their "toxic pattern" and use questioning to highlight further how they've done so. I ask them both to explain how their interaction didn't turn into a typical fight. They both agree that they take time to reflect on their initial reaction when they notice their emotion rising and imagine the impact of the reaction (e.g., pushing the other away). During this time, they think about their partner's perspective (differences or sensitivities) and their own underlying feelings and experiences, and try to listen before they talk.

I ask, "How is this new way working between the two of you?"

Alisia immediately replies, "It's hard at first, but makes me feel closer to him, like some of the trust is coming back . . . not that I trust him completely, but it's getting better."

As Ben and Alisia progress through treatment sessions, we explore several different interactions where one or the other responded with defensiveness, typically Alisia, whereas Ben would avoid conflict. At this point, relationship satisfaction has increased slightly, with Ben's increasing more than Alisia's.

Following the IBCT structure in the VA, after every fourth treatment session is a recommitment session in which we collaboratively review progress and goals, and determine whether to recommit to four more sessions. This was implemented to enhance therapeutic engagement. I start this by providing information on the couple's progress and goals. It sounds something like this:

> "We've had eight treatment sessions since our feedback session, and I want to talk to you about how couple therapy is going and whether you'd like to continue. You both report increases in relationship satisfaction from our weekly questionnaire and seem to be working through challenging interactions to identify the pattern that gets you in trouble. That's the 'toxic pattern' where Alisia pursues and confronts you, Ben, when she feels anxious or upset, and you first defend yourself and then withdraw from resolving the issue. As a result, Alisia feels like she can't depend on you—and Ben, you feel like Alisia wants to control you. You both seem aware of the impact this old pattern has had on your relationship and are making efforts to stop yourself when reacting. You're thinking about what you really want to communicate and are aware of each other's perspectives."

Ben and Alisia nod their heads.

Ben starts, "Yes, I feel like Alisia is less demanding, and when she is, she seems to back off, and sometimes she even apologizes when things don't come off as she wants."

Alisia adds, "I know I can be demanding, but that's who I am, and I realize that I need to pull back a bit. I'm learning to trust him more . . . and he's stepping it up. To use his 'IT' language, he's like 'Ben 2.0' these days." Alisia smiles at Ben and he smiles back. She continues. "I know I get triggered by things with the kids, work, and starting my individual treatment where I'm being asked to focus on trauma and think about things that are upsetting. But even with this, I know things are moving in the right direction."

I ask about the metaphor presented. "How is Ben 2.0 different from Ben 1.0, and what prompted this upgrade?" The use of metaphor indicates a dyadic mindfulness that provides opportunities for unified detachment as Alisia and Ben step out of their struggle to see the bigger picture.

At the end of this session, Alisia and Ben commit to the next four sessions. I think about how this process of recommitment provides the opportunity to review progress and harness energy to reinvigorate a couple's efforts toward their goals. When I first began to implement recommitment sessions, I thought having this type of discussion with a couple would be distracting or take time away from salient issues and might slow the progress. Instead, I am convinced that it does the opposite. Like many things about IBCT, it feels paradoxical. Slowing things down to understand and explore emotional content related to day-to-day interaction often speeds up progress.

A few sessions later, Ben and Alisia list physical intimacy as a challenging interaction for the first time on their weekly questionnaire. As we set the agenda, I think to myself that this makes sense, as they're both trusting one another more and may be ready to take on this issue that is connected to their separation. We prioritize this issue, and I invite them to start.

Alisia says, "I'll start. I always feel pressure from Ben to have sex. He's always wanted more sex than I do. I feel pressure to have sex and then it becomes transactional, where I'm doing it because he wants it. It came up this past weekend when we put the kids to bed, watched a movie, and cuddled. To him, this meant sex. For me, I just wanted to cuddle, because I don't feel like I'm there yet. When I said 'no,' he acted like I had injured him or something . . ."

I reflect Alisia's desire for caution around physical intimacy and ask her to share how she felt during this interaction. She responds, "I felt guilty, and I don't want to, because I really do want to have sex, but I want to feel like it's my choice, too."

I turn to Ben. "Tell me about what happened from your perspective." Ben shared that he really enjoyed the cuddling "and I thought we were at a point where we could enjoy sex again. It's hard for me—I love being with you (*looking at Alisia*) and I get so much out of it when we're together. I just thought we might be there."

I ask Ben to share what he's feeling as he talks about this issue. "I feel disappointed and confused. . . . It's difficult to feel rejected, although this is nothing new. I feel as if she's punishing me for being with other women when we split."

Alisia reacts. "Really? Well, I see how you think that. It was a big deal for me and makes me feel small to think I could be replaced so quickly—you were so eager to leave me behind after we split."

At this point, I wonder if Ben and Alisia needed to talk more about what the period of separation meant, so I ask if they feel there is unfinished business around that. Alisia replies, "I don't know. It was hard for me to think that he could just take up easily with other women, and I feel disappointed in myself that I failed marriage twice. It was hard for me, because I feel like Ben and I were meant to be . . . my first marriage was when I was much younger and felt as if I was just doing what I should do."

Ben jumps in. "I really thought it was over, and yes, I was with other women, but that's when I realized that they didn't have what we have and that I really love you." Alisia is looking at Ben softly. I ask her to share what she heard Ben say.

She reflects it back. "It just makes me feel like I'm not good enough for you when it comes to sex, because we have differences in our sexual desires. I'm not sure how to do this."

Ben replies, "I'm not sure either, because it's a way I feel close to you . . . whenever I try to be affectionate or kiss you, you shrink or pull away. It hurts, and I feel lonely and rejected. When I wait for you to initiate, it never happens, and I feel ignored. I need you to stop moving the goalpost, so I know where to aim the ball. . . ."

Alisia responds, "I don't know what to say—I'm not sure of the rules of the game sometimes, and you just have to be patient."

After a silence, I summarize: "A lot has been expressed here. There's desire, love, attraction, hurt, rejection, loneliness . . . and finally confusion." Despite the soft emotions expressed, I note the impasse as it dominates the interaction between Alisia and Ben. There's awkward silence and tension. This is where I want to jump in, to remind them of the connection they have built in other domains of their relationship. I stop and ask myself if this is about my own discomfort or about their process. Because it is about their process, I hold my breath and stay silent to let them experience the emotions they are having. After what seems like an hour, but it is only a minute, I reflect their stated desire for connection, and their disappointment around not having a clear path.

I notice the silence out loud and join with their hopelessness—reflecting it and having faith in the process that their path through it will emerge. "This is a difficult space and one that it makes sense you've avoided, with good reason—there's pain and there's uncertainty. There seems to be no easy answer, but as you share your experience and stay in the moment with each other, you can see what may emerge. As we wrap up today, I'm wondering what you're experiencing as we leave?"

Ben leans forward and states, "I know I'm wrapped up in my own expectations, and if they aren't met, I get defensive . . . I need to let go of all this."

Alisia looks at Ben and says, "I need to let go of things, too . . . but I know what I do is try to control when I don't feel safe or understood. I want to be more in the moment."

Alisia and Ben arrive in subsequent sessions having taken time to talk about sex and expectations, as well as experiencing some disappointments. They share that they've been on their own journey of understanding their own needs, conveying these to one another without defensiveness, and slowly moving toward sex that feels mutually satisfying.

In IBCT, we focus on issues that the couple brings up, often on the weekly questionnaire. Issues often don't come up in a linear or predictable fashion. At some point during treatment, I anticipated that issues related to Alisia's military service would emerge. It happens during a session in which Ben describes an interaction in which the couple was on a phone call with Alisia's ex-husband discussing school issues with his and Alisia's daughter. After the call, Alisia and Ben fight about how Ben "talked more than he should" and she feels as if Ben and her ex-husband were making "all the decisions" and leaving her out. Alisia expresses frustration and feeling invisible, alone, and helpless in this situation. Then she proceeds to break down and cry and begins to gasp for air.

Ben reacts by grabbing her hand and apologizing. I hand him a tissue to give to Alisia. Alisia takes a breath and motions that she's okay. "I'm so sorry . . . there's a lot that's coming up for me, and this just triggered me." Ben looks clearly confused.

Alisia continues to cry. "I spent yesterday's appointment at the VA with my PTSD therapist talking about my stuck points with my trauma. I went through the horrible things that happened over there . . . it brings up the same experience—I can't help, people die and it's my fault! (*still crying*) And it's my daughter, so that makes it worse."

Ben starts to talk about how Alisia's ex-husband needs to "get a handle on his own life before he can possibly help his own child." He states that he's angry that her ex-husband is so disrespectful of Alisia, which is why he injected himself into their conversation.

I refocus attention on the affect in the room. "I need to interrupt here to focus on something that's really important, and I want to make sure that we pay attention to it. I'm hearing that Alisia experienced some strong emotions in the incident you described, which resonated with her work on her trauma from deployment."

Alisia sniffles. "I'm okay. It just reminded me of the deep sadness, helplessness, and responsibility I feel for what happened over there. I sometimes feel shame around what happened, and dealing with my ex-husband brings up these feelings. When Ben gets in there and I get pushed out of the conversation, it's just like I'm in Afghanistan all over again. Should I have spoken up? Pushed harder? Done something different? The stakes were always so high, and now with him and my girls, I feel the same."

I affirm her emotion and bravery for leaning into the pain of the trauma and noticing how it shows up in her relationship. I ask Ben what it's like to hear Alisia talk about her pain.

He nods his head, looking at Alisia. "I don't know what that's like for you and you don't talk about what happened over there. I feel like I want to protect you from all of that, and when I see it coming up between you and your ex, I want to step in and protect you . . . "

Alisia interrupts, "You can't protect me from it . . . when you step in, I feel even more like I can't protect myself and my daughters . . . (*getting teary*). I know I don't talk about it, but that's because I'm just beginning to face some of the things that scare me."

Ben asks, "How can I help? I feel like I need to do something."

Alisia replies, "I don't know . . . but I think just being there for me and trusting me to do what I need to do."

Ben looks down as if exasperated. I ask him what it brings up for him. Ben shakes his head. "It brings back all the craziness of my childhood. When I see her cry, I think of my mother, and it makes me feel panicky, as things were always changing and I got left out."

I assure Ben, "So that's important to note. When you feel really strong emotions coming up here for Alisia, it brings you back to a time in your life of instability and loneliness—and that makes you want to . . . ?"

Ben jumps in. "It makes me want to hide."

I state that he isn't hiding here but offering support. As I reflect on this interaction, I realize that this event would have brought about high levels of conflict had it occurred in the beginning stages of treatment, when both of them may have reacted defensively. Alisia and Ben look at each other and agree that they feel more open and honest with one another. Ben asks Alisia if there is some way he can learn more about PTSD at the VA without intruding on her individual therapy. I provide information about a VA workshop for partners and family members of Veterans with PTSD, and other resources, including the National Center for PTSD and the "PTSD Family Coach" app. As I do, I think of my own family and how resources at the VA have changed for the better. In part, this is due to advancements that psychological science has made around the treatment of trauma and how trauma impacts Veterans and their loved ones.

Alisia and Ben are making significant progress, and both have been able to share core vulnerable emotions. They've shared parts of their experience that they haven't revealed in the past. Alisia's honesty with Ben about her trauma opened an area of their relationship that hadn't been explored. Alisia shares her work in therapy in subsequent sessions. Alisia's individual therapy progress enhances her ability to understand how her beliefs, perspectives, and experiences feed her behavior in the relationship. Ben is honest with Alisia about how his past experiences prime him to feel alone or excluded when he doesn't feel able to be useful. This is new territory for both and an opportunity to explore deepening their connection through sharing their hurt, longing, fear, shame, and other vulnerable emotions.

CONCLUDING PHASE OF THERAPY

Ben and Alisia have attended 15 sessions of IBCT, including the assessment and feedback sessions. Their scores on the weekly questionnaire reflect increases in relationship satisfaction that are consistent with the couple's report of more positive interactions, including regular times set aside for them as a couple, shared activities such as going out to baseball games, warm moments, compliments, affection, and intimacy. Alisia states that she and Ben enjoy being together doing more mundane things like going shopping, working out at the gym, taking the kids to the park, all with more physical affection. Their sessions have been spaced out gradually from weekly to biweekly and now every 3 weeks. Because of the routine recommitment sessions, we've had the experience of reviewing progress. Although they still have challenging interactions, they address conflict soon after it occurs and talk more about their expectations and their emotions, similar to what we do in session. Ben attends the VA workshop on PTSD and learns how to actively support Alisia in her individual treatment. Alisia shares more about the impact of her traumatic events while in the military, including her experience of prejudice as a Hispanic woman and a woman Veteran.

The concluding phase of therapy isn't usually as emotionally charged, and I experience it as a review of events. As their therapist, I miss working with them weekly and smile when I see their names on my schedule. Despite Alisia and Ben's progress, they continue to work on intimacy and are actively talking about it. When I think about this, I'm aware that successful therapy doesn't mean that the struggles are over, but that the struggles can continue without therapeutic assistance.

During the concluding phase of therapy, Alisia and Ben describe an interaction that triggered them both. Ben starts. "So it was a crazy week with the kids, the holidays, and work. I was off my game because I forgot to do something special for Veterans Day, and I knew Alisia was bothered by this, but she didn't say anything. I realized we hadn't had sex in 2 weeks, and I brought it up like I used to, you know, 'Ben 1.0,' in kind of a demanding, problem-solving, analytic kind of way. The minute it came out of my mouth, I wanted to take it back."

Alisia is squirming in her seat and jumps in. "Yes! It was demanding and his tone immediately put me on the defensive and a switch flipped inside me. I lost control and started crying, then yelled and ignored him for the rest of the day, which is difficult in our house."

I'm curious about how they see this setback fitting in with their overall trajectory. I ask, "How does this remind you of past interactions around sex?"

Alisia replies, "It brought up my issue around feeling guilty, responsible, and shame around not being enough, and then feeling disappointed that I was back to these old thoughts."

Ben jumps in. "I felt bad about what I said and knew it, but there was a part of me that was exhausted and disconnected, and this is the way I connect—physically. It felt like it took a few days to come back around to where we could talk about it, and I apologized. I now realize that this occurred on the anniversary of one of Alisia's traumas—when she was flooded with injured bodies and felt like she had to choose who to save."

I'm impressed with the empathy Alisia and Ben are displaying for one another. "It seems like the two of you have opened up to each other about many new things, and this also makes your old reactions seem more devastating. I'm curious about how the two of you came back from this."

Alisia looks at Ben and says, "After stewing, I realized that there was more going on with me and it wasn't fair to Ben. We talked and apologized to each other (*Ben nods*), and it's taken me a few weeks to shake this off. I knew the ball was in my court, and we were on the same team after all, so I took it upon myself to put myself out there and initiate sex, and the weird thing was that he was hesitant . . . "

Ben interrupts. "I felt bad about how things went down and didn't want her to feel like she was initiating to make up for things. I wanted to make sure she actually wanted to have sex and wasn't taking care of me or her guilt. I stopped her, and we talked about how to be on the same team."

In an effort to reinforce joining, I ask, "So what does it mean to be on the same team?"

Ben replies, "It's just more about letting each other know what's going on inside, being patient with each other and checking on our assumptions—like having a 'game plan' that works."

Alisia builds on Ben's comment. "Yes, I'd add that it's also taking care of ourselves if we need time or space or something else."

I ask, "So the interaction you had was an example of stepping back into 'old patterns' and you were both able to pull yourself out of that. What did that entail?"

Alisia replies, "I know we'll make mistakes—relationships are work for sure . . . I know now we need to try to understand each other when this happens and know that it's not intentional. To give each other the benefit of the doubt and then talk about it."

At this point in treatment, Ben and Alisia are navigating their conflict and have changed the narrative within their relationship. They're now teammates and exhibit unified detachment by recognizing an old interaction pattern arising when facing a challenge, but they don't stay stuck in the pattern. They engage in communicating in ways that are effective and don't provoke conflict. While I haven't formally introduced any direct change interventions (e.g., problem-solving skills), I've witnessed them summoning existing strategies when they felt safe to do so. I schedule a termination session, which represents their graduation from treatment. I let them know that they can also schedule check-in booster sessions.

During the final session, I review their progress, including the DEEP formulation, accentuating the very things they've told me about how they approach conflict. I commend their efforts and courage to grow together with empathy and compassion for one another. I also tend to share with couples how they've impacted me, and what I've taken from my work with them. In this instance, I feel honored to have witnessed their growing self-awareness and courage in restoring their relationship from a place where they had separated. I admire how they navigated the trauma of Alisia's military service and understand its impact on their relationship and family. Finally, I commend Alisia for her service and express gratitude for being a part of their journey.

FURTHER REFLECTIONS AND IMPLICATIONS

Over the past two decades, I've had the honor of serving a wide variety of Veteran couples. It's difficult to reflect on a single Veteran couple that captured the wide variety of couples with whom I've worked. Because of this, I cherish the opportunity to understand the larger context of each partner's life experiences to see how those experiences come together to challenge their relationship. In essence, this affords me the opportunity to know each partner through a personal lens. I feel honored to have been able to help Veterans understand themselves and their partners, and find their way through struggle. In reflecting on my own family's experience, military service lends the gift of resilient attitudes that get passed through generations. It also asks Veterans to face the unthinkable, and their loved ones to accept and flex around losses, separations, or trauma.

As a couple therapist, I witness this change. Couples enter with their own meanings around what's wrong in their relationship that tend to be fault-based, blame-focused, and limiting. They may believe "my partner is crazy, uncaring, inadequate or isn't attracted to me." With validation of each partner's perspectives while appreciating the larger context of their lives, I invite them to view their relationship in a way that inspires them to find the fulfillment they desire.

Couples often thank me for "all the skills" I taught them. I smile when they say this. For the most part, I haven't taught them skills, but rather have helped them to create an environment to use the skills they already have. Soft emotions invite closeness and compassion, and these set the stage for change. This is the difference between a "bottom-up" and "top-down" approach. A bottom-up approach doesn't assume a specific outcome but it creates opportunity to move toward any number of outcomes. It cultivates a safe emotional climate where vulnerability can exist. Once it does, this safety invites emotional disclosure and creative problem solving. This approach fits nicely with both a diverse Veteran population and the complexities, comorbidities, and trauma that many Veterans experience.

If I were to give advice to myself decades ago as a couple therapist newly employed at the VA, I would offer these thoughts. I remember being overwhelmed with the complexities of Veterans' lives and feeling as if I needed to "give" them something to quell their pain or enhance their joy. In my efforts to do so, I missed key therapeutic opportunities in the room—whether a soft look, a tear, a scowl, or a suggestive glance. My advice to myself would be to notice and lean into emotion, to stay with it and explore it. The gift is in acknowledging these vulnerable emotions. I had to learn to catch my breath and count to 10 so that I didn't try to teach, instruct, facilitate, solve, or educate. I try to reflect accurately, hold the space, extend empathy, and point the couple in the direction of their stated goal. What was most unique at the time I received training in IBCT was the therapist's stance. I was taught that my role as therapist is less directive and more suggestive. In doing so, I allow the couple to be the ones to explore pain, express vulnerability, discover hope, and find their way together.

When I think about why I cherish my work with Veteran couples, I realize that it forces me to open myself up to connect with those who dare to take the risk to show up. It's difficult not to be authentically present when asking others to do so. It offers me the opportunity to tap into my own struggles with trauma, transition, loss, and separation. The struggles of Veteran couples offer an opportunity for transformation. A quote from Ernest Hemingway highlights this process: "The world breaks everyone, and afterward, many are strong at the broken places." Veterans often see themselves as "broken" or changed by war. What they don't see is the prospect of creating something from their experiences. I see it as my job as therapist to ask the questions no one wants to ask, to lean into what feels uncomfortable, and to notice success. As I conclude my work with each couple, I like to reflect on their progress, what I'll remember, and how they've made a difference in my life.

REFERENCES

Christensen, A., Dimidjian, S., Martell, C. R., & Doss, B. D. (2023). Integrative behavioral couple therapy. In J. L. Lebow & D. K. Snyder (Eds.), *Clinical handbook of couple therapy* (6th ed., pp. 79–103). New York: Guilford Press.

Christensen, A., Doss, B. D., & Jacobson, N. S. (2020). *Integrative behavioral couple therapy: A therapist's guide to creating acceptance and change*. New York: Norton.

Christensen, A., & Glynn, S. M. (2019). Integrative behavioral couple therapy. In B. H. Fiese (Ed.), *Handbook of contemporary family psychology: Vol. 3. Family therapy and training* (pp. 275–290). Washington, DC: American Psychological Association.

McKee, G. B., McDonald, S. D., Karmarkar, A., & Ghatas, M. P. (2023). Demographic characteristics, mental health conditions, and psychotherapy use of Veterans in couples and family therapy. *Couple and Family Therapy: Research and Practice, 12*, 11–23.

Resick, P. A., Monson, C. M., & Chard, K. M. (2016). *Cognitive processing therapy for PTSD: A comprehensive manual*. New York: Guilford Press.

Sayers, S. L. (2014). *Coming back together: A guide to successful reintegration after your partner returns from military deployment*. Oakland, CA: New Harbinger.

Snyder, D. K., & Monson, C. M. (2012). *Couple-based interventions for military and veteran families: A practitioner's guide*. New York: Guilford Press.

CHAPTER 16

Couple Therapy and Sexuality
Promoting Intimacy and Connection

TAMMY NELSON

Editors' Comments

In this exposition of couple therapy for issues of sexuality, Tammy Nelson highlights how the pathways to sexual challenges in a couple's relationship vary as powerfully as the pathways to more general relationship distress. Understanding and assessing the diverse patterns and potential sources of sexual issues underlie effective interventions with couples presenting with these concerns. Nelson articulates a clear, overarching model for addressing sexual difficulties—progressing from creating a safe context for discussing sex to providing information and promoting specific exercises to reduce avoidance and facilitate emotional and physical connection and then, when appropriate, exploring prior family or relationship experiences serving as barriers to sexual comfort and pleasure. Similar to some models described in other chapters in this *Casebook*, Nelson's approach is systematic, sequential, and inherently integrative.

Notice in this case narrative how sensitively Nelson blends interventions specific to the couple's sexual relationship with attention to more general relationship concerns and the partners' individual dynamics. For this couple, anxieties about their own sexual adequacies commingle with empathic caring for each other and commitment to improving their sexual relationship. Nelson harnesses the couple's strengths to engage in a 6-week structured erotic-recovery protocol, using intermediate outcomes to identify and address individual dynamics contributing to their distress. Along the way, Nelson describes emerging findings informing her clinical decision making about which issues to address specifically and which ones to allow to evolve on their own.

Nelson distinguishes among various forms that difficulties in embracing sexual pleasure can take, including denial, avoidance, resistance, and rejection—each requiring specific interventions. Because general relationship distress and specific sexual difficulties so frequently co-occur, all couple therapists will benefit from the detailed explication and rich clinical narrative that Nelson offers here. And, more broadly, Nelson orients all of us as couple therapists to the central importance of sex and sexuality in relationships—topics that often are difficult but crucial to explore.

Couple therapy for issues of sexuality is a distinct form of psychotherapy that helps both individuals and couples overcome sexual issues and challenges. Sexual issues that present can be relational and focused on the couple, or the narrative around sex can be about an individual dysfunction. The sexual issue may be procreational as it relates to issues, such as fertility or menopause, or it may relate to the more recreational aspect of sex, such as desire issues or pleasure disorders.

In therapy for issues of sexuality, the work takes place within the context of the relationship—whether in a couple session or in individual therapy—focusing on the sexual dilemma as it relates to sexual identity, as well as partners' attachment to one another. Couple therapy for issues of sexuality takes an integrative approach, one that explores the emotional, psychological, and physical factors that may contribute to the sexual challenges. It approaches each case systemically, focusing on what the partners present and collaborating with their own inner wisdom, acknowledging the interconnectedness of sexual and emotional intimacy without ignoring the innate erotic desires that are essential to the experience of being human.

In couple therapy for sexual issues, the therapist creates a safe and nonjudgmental space where both partners can feel comfortable expressing their thoughts and feelings about their sexual relationship. It then provides education, suggestions, homework, guidance, insight, and intensive therapy to promote healing. The therapist also collaborates with medical providers and other practitioners to create a systemic process that brings a holistic approach to the goals of treatment.

I've been a therapist for over 35 years. I'm certified as a sex therapist by the American Association of Sexuality Educators, Counselors, and Therapists (AASECT), a sex therapist supervisor, and an Imago relationship therapist. I'm also a clinical sexologist. I founded the Integrative Sex Therapy Institute, where I train and certify sex therapists.

As a clinical sexologist, my focus when a couple comes to my office is to ask immediately, "When was the last time you had sex, and how was it?" This creates a space in the session in which both partners know that talking about sex is okay, and not something that has to be tiptoed into after hours of introductory material or extended intake. Most clients respond favorably to the immediacy of this question. Beyond the casual nature of conversation about sex, it lightens the tension of why the couple has come to the session. This question also conveys that I'm comfortable talking about sex and that it's acceptable to bring their most personal problems or questions to the session. My role is to create a comfort level by providing education and guidance around discussing sexual health and wellness, as well as leading the couple in communication and conflict resolution skills that can help them navigate their challenges and build intimacy. Whereas some couples come to the session in high conflict, others simply need permission to discuss their issues.

I follow the PLISSIT model (Permission, Limited Information, Specific Suggestions, and Intensive Therapy) developed by Annon (1976). I also adhere to best-practice models supported by systematic reviews of the literature (e.g., Tuncer & Oskay, 2022). The PLISSIT model posits a sequencing of interventions. First, most couples simply want permission to discuss challenges that are impacting their sexual relationship. While we can explore their current issues, we may not have to dig too deep in order for them to find relief in expressing their concerns in a facilitated discussion. The second most common intervention is for couples who just need limited information about sex, such as education around sex and the barriers to sexual performance, or information regarding arousal and desire, such as the ways women reach orgasm. Many couples are unsure about female orgasm and simply need to know that the majority of women need direct clitoral stimulation in order to reach orgasm, whether alone or with a partner. This limited information is sometimes enough to reduce anxiety about performance and can send a couple happily on their way. Other limited information may include details about the average length of intercourse prior to ejaculation (4 minutes) or what constitutes a low-sex relationship (operationalized as sex fewer than 14 times a year). This information can help shift partners past beliefs and attitudes about sex that may be negatively impacting their relationship.

Other couples need more specific suggestions. For example, a therapist can address any emotional or psychological barriers to sexual connection by discussing the difference between arousal and desire—arousal being the physical experience necessary for performance, and desire being the internal emotional and psychological experience that one may identify as being "ready" for sex. When couples believe they're ready for at-home assignments, specific suggestions might include sensate focus experiences—techniques designed to help them achieve intimacy that aren't goal-oriented but instead help them connect on a sensual level, focusing on mindful touching over time. These mindfulness-based interventions can both build a deeper level of personal understanding and help the couple develop tools and skills they need for sexual satisfaction.

A far fewer number of couples need intensive therapy; these are the couples who may benefit the most from ongoing sex and couple therapy. Cognitive-behavioral therapy and a psychodynamic approach (as well as other theoretical approaches) can help partners explore their narrative or meaning that they each assign to the sexual problem, and then explore a deeper understanding of their childhood and family history around sex and relationships to promote insight into what they each bring to their current relationship. We learn what it means to be in a relationship in our earliest attachments. But it is later, in the separation and individuation stage of development, that we learn to be sexual in our erotic relationships. Both within ourselves and with others, we learn how to be separate and to be wanted, to be desired and to long for, to be attracted to another and have enough distance to find one another again. This coming together and separating is what keeps a long-term sexual relationship exciting and dynamic. The challenges of a committed relationship in which companionship needs have been put first can strain a sexual relationship. The needs of a family, children, home, and negotiations around these responsibilities can lead to conflict, and couples may not be able to keep their sexual relationship a priority. Intensive therapy can help partners explore gender roles and the history of what led them to each other, and develop the interpersonal tools and skills to connect sexually in new and unique ways even when overall relational satisfaction is a challenge.

INITIAL ASSESSMENT AND CASE FORMULATION

Laurie and Todd, a mixed-race, different-sex couple in their mid-50s, came to sex therapy for problems with "intimacy." In the first session, I asked them what they meant by intimacy, because "intimacy" can not only be a code word for "sex" but can also refer to communication issues, or one partner having an affair, or a host of other difficulties that may not be revealed for several sessions. I don't let couples use "intimacy" to refer to sex in sessions. They both answered shyly that, "yes," they were there to talk about sex as well as intimacy and that, for them, intimacy meant emotional closeness, and they missed that as well. From the very outset, I guide couples in their language, educating them on how to talk about sex with me and with each other. I balance an emphasis on using explicit terms with encouraging them to express their desire for sex and discuss sexual fantasies in their own language.

Laurie said she was perimenopausal and was experiencing night sweats, vaginal dryness, and pain during intercourse, which she said had led to a decrease in sex. She said that Todd had withdrawn both emotionally and sexually, and she wondered if he was having an affair. I asked her how she felt about her relationship to Todd. She replied, "I feel disconnected, and I've pulled back. I've stopped initiating sex and I'm . . . well . . . I'm embarrassed about the changes in my body."

I asked Todd to share how he felt about what Laurie had said and he responded, "I love her body, but I can understand. I'd hate to have those night sweats."

I noticed he didn't respond to the question about whether he was having an affair. It was too soon to open up this topic, so I asked him to describe the last time they had sex and how he thought it went. He said, "I thought it was okay, but I'm worried that Laurie didn't like it. When she doesn't like it, I get nervous, I can tell she's not happy. I feel like she's judging me and then, to make matters worse, I orgasm too soon. And then she's really unhappy, and then we just kind of lie there staring at the ceiling. We never talk about it. Never."

Now we have a narrative about their sex life. Laurie feels disconnected from Todd, and Todd has withdrawn from her. She feels insecure about her physical changes since entering menopause, a developmental change in her sexuality. Todd has noticed her shift and emotional changes and has taken it personally, as if Laurie's blaming him for the shift in their relationship and he gets anxious. This affects his sexual performance, and that makes him more anxious and he withdraws, feels bad, and is unable to communicate his feelings to her. They're both shut down and disconnected from the intimacy they crave.

I asked Laurie, "If you were to answer that question—'When was the last time you had sex and how was it?'—how would you answer that?"

She replied, "I think we last had sex maybe 6 months ago. I don't remember, it's been so long. I think we tried to have intercourse but I didn't have an orgasm first, we didn't use lube, and Todd wanted to just do it and get it over with. I think he sees my face and that it hurts, and then he feels guilty."

From the limited information they're sharing about their bodies and their needs, it's apparent that things have shifted in their sex life. They have new needs and desires. She'll most likely need more arousal prior to penis-in-vagina intercourse or any insertion in her vagina. Arousal creates more natural lubrication and also more engorgement, and allows the vaginal tissues to respond more pleasurably to contact. They'll also most likely need to use a water-based lubricant to make insertion more pleasant. His guilt about hurting her makes sense. In fact, research suggests that men's number one desire during sex is to please their partner. Guilt can often lead to anxiety, which can interfere with sexual function. Anxiety can cause erectile dysfunction or premature ejaculation.

I gave them some initial sex education about lubricants, as this seemed to be the most important information they needed in the limited time we had during our first session. I recommended that if they were going to try having sex again anytime soon, to use a lubricant, and that she should be aroused first. However, I added that perhaps they should take the goal of sex off the table for the next 6 weeks. Removing the goal of intercourse can reduce anxiety and decrease performance pressure and it seemed relevant, considering they hadn't had sex for 6 months or longer. I said that if we continued to work together, I'd give them assignments to bring them back to emotional and sexual intimacy. I told them that I have a 6-week erotic recovery protocol they could follow if they were willing to work in therapy for the next few months.

The only requirement was that they had to be willing to close their "exits" for a period of time and give the therapy a real try, focusing on making their intimate life a priority. I explained that "closing an exit" meant that anything that was taking their focus out of the relationship or distracting them from their conflict or their closeness should be put on hold until the end of that time. They could decide for themselves how long that period of time would be, but I would recommend 3 months of meeting weekly for 60 minutes, or every other week for 90 minutes, with home assignments weekly.

I didn't ask either of them if they were having an affair, nor would I have asked them to end their affair if one had been disclosed. As a therapist who has worked extensively with infidelity recovery, I'm very clear that just because I ask someone to close down their affair doesn't mean they will. What will happen, however, is that if they choose to continue their outside relationship, they'll lie about that not only to their partner but also to me. Therefore, both partners have to decide for themselves what closing their exits might look like.

The trust issues that are triggered as a result of infidelity are a unique problem following an affair. If one partner suspects the betrayal has occurred, there can be a natural closing down of the intimate connection as a protection mechanism, and pleasure avoidance can be used as a way to control the emotional balance in the relationship. Opening up to the potential for hurt can start with the vulnerability of physical intimacy, which may cause confusion and misunderstanding. Some couples have more desire for one another after an affair, while others shut down completely. If there has been infidelity, more in-depth treatment has to focus on the crisis stage of disclosure, with more focus in therapy on the meaning and narrative of the betrayal. Erotic recovery may take longer and be more complex for couples who have experienced nonconsensual nonmonogamy.

I do give them examples such as the following:

> "An exit could be compulsively working, or being on the computer all the time, or overfocusing on the kids, or drinking or eating too much, or doing drugs, or shopping or playing video games compulsively, or playing golf all weekend . . . or having an affair. Maybe you decide you still play golf, but only one morning a week. Maybe you don't end an affair, but you stop sleeping together, or maybe you just stop texting. I can't tell you what to do, only you know what your exits are. But if you have an addiction or compulsion of any sort and don't believe you can stop, let's work on that first."

Laurie and Todd decided to come back for the next 4 weeks and committed to closing their exits. I didn't ask them what those exits were. I let them each decide on their own. They had a trip planned to South America in 4 weeks to see her parents, and we agreed to decide at that time how the therapy would continue.

BEGINNING PHASE OF THERAPY

In the second session, Todd said he was getting frustrated with the lack of sex and felt rejected by Laurie's lack of interest in him. They had tried to talk about our first session after we met but found themselves stuck in a cycle of mutual blame and defensiveness. Todd asserted, "It's not about menopause. Laurie has always been like this. She always has an excuse. She won't ever let me touch her."

I asked Laurie to tell me about her past experiences around sex in their relationship. I noticed that she talked about sex in a detached way—sounding almost robotic and describing their history with little or no emotional expression. She said in a flat voice, "I thought we had a good sex life in the beginning. Todd was always gentle and loving. And sometimes we did kinky things. I liked that. Then, when we had the kids, it really dropped off. He didn't want to touch me after our daughter was born."

Todd jumped in. "That's not true. You were breast-feeding. I didn't want to hurt you." As their conversation developed and I continued to encourage them to use dialogue to mirror each other's concerns, a pattern in their relationship began to emerge. Laurie would express emotional or physical vulnerability or pain, and Todd would withdraw to protect her from what he perceived as his dangerous or toxic sexual needs.

I began to hypothesize that the two of them had not only developed coping mechanisms over time to protect themselves from the pain of their unresolved hurt and a pattern of coping in their relationship had developed that they couldn't resolve, but also that there were deeper issues here, possibly brought into the relationship from their childhoods. I wondered what Todd thought his role was supposed to be. Was he was supposed to protect and serve, to comfort and make her life easy, to keep her from being hurt, to shelter her from harm?

I asked him about this pattern that I had begun to notice. "Todd, it's interesting that you seem to always be protecting Laurie. Are you trying to protect her, to keep her from harm or pain?"

And he replied, "Funny, my father was a cop. He always directed me to 'protect and serve' my mother, to take care of her especially after he was gone. He got sick and died when I was 19. He wanted me to make sure she was always 'safe from harm,' so it's funny that you would say that. I guess I learned that, yeah. That's what you do, you keep your woman safe, and if she's hurting, it's my job, I have to help her."

I asked Laurie how she felt about that, and did it apply to their sex life? "Yes, it's true," she replied. "We used to do some light S&M (sadomasochistic) stuff, and I liked that. He would spank me and stuff, and now he doesn't do that; he feels guilty. He said that he can't hurt me. And now that I think about it, after the kids were born, I was in a lot of pain. Breast-feeding was painful, everything was painful. I had a C-section (cesarean delivery), and that hurt. So it makes sense he didn't want to have sex with me."

I turned to Todd, "Were you afraid to hurt her? Did you worry that sex would somehow injure her, maybe even break her?" He started to cry in the session. "I'm still afraid to break her."

While Todd was afraid to hurt Laurie, Laurie also had a preconceived notion of what sex should be. As much as she had begun to experiment with her erotic profile—her map of sexual desire and fantasy—she had just begun to dip her toes in. She felt that Todd had shut down their fantasy life when he decided spanking and light BDSM (bondage or discipline, dominance and submission) were too much for him. As a result, she had closed up her fantasy life, keeping it secret from him. She felt shame about her desire for more impactful play and for a power exchange dynamic in their sex life in which he might "hurt" her during sex, just a little at a time. Laurie wanted to reconnect, but she was afraid that their sex life would be too bland (some people call the opposite of kink "vanilla") and as much as she wanted a sexual connection and sexual intimacy, she admitted she also had not been turned on by their sex life in a long time.

As our work continued, I gave Laurie and Todd specific suggestions, including creation of a sex date once a week. I introduced them to my 6-week erotic recovery protocol that systematically works toward the goal of being sexual and, in their case, retrieving the intimate connection they had felt at the start of their relationship, a little at a time.

INTERMEDIATE PHASE OF THERAPY: A 6-WEEK PROTOCOL

A sex date weekly can be important when a couple has been through a crisis or betrayal in their relationship. A crisis may include an illness, the loss of a job, or an affair. Planning a sex date once a week enables the therapist to suggest specific interventions for each week to create reconnection and slow sexual gains after the intensity of the crisis, titrated in a safe and manageable way. It can also be important for couples like Laurie and Todd who haven't been sexual for a long time and who want to build back up slowly. They needed a plan. They couldn't jump back into sex without some conscious awareness and healing. I assured them that just because we called it a "sex" date, there would be no sex for at least 6 weeks. Taking sex off the agenda would be an important part of the assignment.

I asked Laurie and Todd to review their shared schedules to identify when they could meet at the same time and day every week. Regardless of the children or their jobs, or how they were feeling toward each other or their relationship, they needed to commit to showing up for the date. The date wouldn't be about going out for a meal or to the movies, they could have a separate date night for that need, but this was purely a sensual date. It would be important that they avoided eating heavily or drinking too much alcohol prior to the date, because those could interfere with their capacity to be engaged in the date and the sensations that they were each going to experience.

While I did not share this with Todd and Laurie, I knew that planning a regular date at the same time each week could create what I call "erotic anticipation," similar to the feelings when having an affair. Erotic anticipation is designed into this protocol specifically to create tension that might mimic infidelity, which, for this couple, could trigger feelings for Todd, if he indeed were having an affair. Todd's potential feelings about any outside relationship hadn't been discussed, but it was possible that he was experiencing the relationship energy of an affair. If so, I knew that most people in affairs don't end their outside relationship without first feeling that their current relationship is worth coming back into, and will avoid reentering fully until they feel they can trust the potential of a new beginning. We would have to create a new relationship between Laurie and Todd before any outside relationships would end for good.

What I did share with them was that a date night is a sacred commitment that they were making to one another. I compared the date night practice to meditation or yoga. The date night was a sacred time when they were both pledging to the practice of their relationship. The rest of the week, they could show up for their companionship, the errands of their daily life, the running of their shared world, but this date night was for the erotic side of the relationship. The erotic side of the relationship was the place where they fell in love, where they felt the passion for one another, and where the deficits and longing were showing up currently.

Some couples wonder if planning sex will mean that sex will no longer be spontaneous. My clinical response is always "When has sex ever been spontaneous?" Sex is usually planned at some level by at least one partner. One or both partners know when the sex will happen. Someone is usually the planner and has had sex in mind prior to it happening. Both at some point may have gotten ready, taken showers, gone to bed early—whatever was needed to create the space for sex. Other couples may avoid planning sex dates altogether and find many excuses to reasonably explain why they can't make it happen. Therapists would be wise to confront this as resistance and explore why staying in the same pattern of a sexless or low-sex relationship might in fact be working for them. Is there a secondary gain or benefit to being in this relationship as it stands? Does changing the relationship mean changing a standing role for one or both of them that is actually on some level serving a purpose? Therapists can only make suggestions for home assignments; they can't make a major change in the partners' lives if they're not ready, or if there are other issues that need to be worked through before a date night can be scheduled.

Scheduling sex may not feel sexy or erotic, but sex dates may need to be planned explicitly if the partners are busy, if they haven't had sex for a while and it doesn't seem to be falling into place in their schedules, or if they've been consciously or unconsciously avoiding it. Many couples prioritize their daily activities before their sex life, yet still imagine that sex will somehow fall into place. A sexual life can feel unimportant and therefore make a partner feel unimportant. It's essential, then, to plan regular sex dates to prevent those feelings of disconnection or resentment.

After introducing my specific 6-week proposal, I gave Laurie and Todd directions on how they would slowly reconnect during each weekly date. I assured them that they would not jump into sex, but by following these steps, they could begin the healing process. It would be an adjunct to our work together in our sessions and an important step toward reconnecting in a sexual way.

Introducing the Erotic Recovery Protocol

Each week of the erotic recovery protocol takes the couple slowly from exercise to exercise, beginning with assignments that lead from gentle touch to more sensual touch. I asked Todd and Laurie if they had ever given each other a massage and if they were comfortable with that level of intimate touch. Both had received and given massages to each other; therefore, we could start Week 1 with massage. For couples who have not ever touched sensually or used massage in their relationship, or if they are currently in crisis, the directions can be modified and dialed back to decrease the amount of physical intimacy and reduce the touching exercises.

The erotic recovery protocol is designed to allow partners to approach each other in a personal, sensual way—using mindfulness and cognitive-behavioral techniques, along with touch and somatic therapy. It's important to provide couples with a description and rationale for this protocol. The following narrative summarizes the essential elements of how I introduce the recovery protocol. In actual practice, this narrative would be paced and partitioned into smaller units to facilitate comments or queries by the couple along the way. I shared with Laurie and Todd:

> "The erotic date isn't about having intercourse, although it may lead to that by the end of these 6 weeks. Each week is designed for you to have a sensual experience.

Some weeks you may feel disappointed or let down, but don't let that stop you. The first date night is a time for you to be together without distraction in order to focus on your erotic relationship. Your erotic life together is the one place where you're not just roommates and friends or co-parents—you're lovers. Take it slow and follow the directions to the best of your ability.

"On Week 1, take some time to create an atmosphere in your bedroom. Remember, you're creating a sacred, sensual space for you to practice eroticism together. Light some candles, put fresh flowers by the bed, and lay down sheets and blankets on the bed that you don't mind getting massage oil on, as well as a heater to keep the room warm. Make an extra effort to pick out music you think your partner might appreciate.

"Every date will start with massage. Choose who will be the sender and who will be the receiver. This week there will be no sex, and no touching in or around the genital areas. If the receiver wants to keep their underwear on, great. If they want to be fully naked, that's fine, too. Keep in mind the boundaries are the same. Imagine your partner is wearing a bathing suit or bikini. No touching in those areas. This week only the receiver will get a massage. Set a clock for 15 minutes to keep you both less focused on how long the massage lasts and more focused on giving and receiving pleasurable touch.

"In these beginning dates, the focus is on massage and sensual touch, with limited erotic contact. There are many ways to experience erotic connection, including lying naked together, soft touch, massage, touching your partner in a sensual way, or pleasuring your own body while your partner watches. There is no wrong way to have an erotic date night. However, don't push the sexual contact right now. We're going to take that pressure off of both of you for now and start with just massage.

"If you're the sender, have the room ready before the receiver enters, then ask your partner to get comfortable in order to receive a massage. When you're both comfortable and ready, use massage oil or cream and slowly start rubbing their back gently. Remember to breathe. Try not to talk or use words unless it's to check in with your partner. Spend some time remembering your partner's body. What does their skin feel like? What does it feel like to touch? How can you make yourself more comfortable? Can you take deep breaths? What are the thoughts in your mind? Can you notice them and let them go?

"If you're the receiver, try to relax and breathe. Notice what the touch feels like. Let go of any thoughts, positive or negative, and allow yourself to simply experience the sensations without judgment. Are you thinking about yourself and your body? Are you thinking about your partner and their touch? What's happening in your body? Can you identify any physical feelings? Can you notice any emotions coming up for you?

"At the end of the 15 minutes, allow the receiver to simply rest or fall asleep. This removes the pressure for either of you to process the experience or to have sex after the massage. When we remove the pressure from the *performance* of sex, we can get back to the *experience* of sex. Sex as pure experience means we have the time and space to allow our bodies to have pleasure. Try not to impose any specific expectations on this experience for now. This date will be successful if it makes you feel connected to your partner."

The Pressure of Pleasure

The first 2 weeks of an erotic recovery date night exercise are good experiments in determining how couples handle pleasure. I call this the "pressure of pleasure." Although we like to think we can all handle pleasure and welcome it without stress, for many, pleasure *denial* can be a way of controlling the experience of pleasure, which is really about controlling the self and the urges and impulses that may be interwoven with guilt and shame from the past. For others, pleasure *avoidance* may be a way to control a relationship, using pleasure or the avoidance of pleasure and sex as transactional currency in order to control one's partner or control the flow of intimacy and connection. This happens when someone actively avoids experiences that could bring them pleasure, often due to feelings of guilt or shame. For example, a person may avoid certain sexual activities because they believe they go against their religious or moral beliefs, or they may feel guilty about their desires. This can lead to a range of sexual problems, including low libido and difficulty experiencing pleasure during sex.

One of the main factors that contributes to relationship issues around sexuality is pleasure *resistance*. This occurs when individuals resist experiencing pleasure due to a range of factors including past traumas, cultural conditioning, and negative experiences with sex. For example, a person who has experienced sexual abuse may develop resistance to pleasure as a way of protecting themselves from further harm. Similarly, societal messages that equate sex with shame and guilt can lead to a resistance to pleasure. With pleasure *resistance*, the experience of pleasure may start out without problems, but the body may resist it. When pleasure is resisted, it could indicate something more serious such as sexual abuse or trauma in the relationship or in one's past.

Pleasure *rejection* is an unconscious and hard-to-control physical reaction. When pleasure is outright rejected as a bodily sensation, it's usually felt as outside of the person's control. Pleasure rejection is an indication that trauma is still stored in physical form and somatic memory, and the individual is looking to rewrite their stored narrative in order to maintain control of their destiny.

When Laurie and Todd came in to discuss their first two date nights, Laurie was upset. "I wanted to enjoy it, I really did," she said. "Todd liked it—he had to go into the bathroom afterward and take care of himself. When it was my turn to be massaged, I lay there stiff as a board and couldn't relax. When I was massaging him, it was nice, but I felt like he wanted more."

I asked her what was pleasurable about the experience—could she remember the feeling of it, the skin-to-skin contact, or did she remember any of her thoughts at the time? She answered, "I had some awareness of my physical sensations, some I remember, I know that it made me uncomfortable. I think maybe I was turned on? I don't even know what that feels like though, so I'm not sure." I asked how she felt emotionally. She replied, "I had some emotional feelings, I guess. I was more trying to figure out what he was feeling. I had a lot of guilt."

I asked her to tell me more about her feelings when she was being massaged. "I had this weird memory," she said. "I felt like I was in my room as a kid. I started feeling anxious and afraid. I was afraid someone would walk in. I was waiting for someone to open the door. But that was weird, because no one was home in real life, at our house with Todd. The kids were gone, the door was locked. But I felt guilt and shame almost, like we were going to be caught."

I was wondering then about Laurie's experience with masturbation and self-pleasuring. Self-pleasure can lead to all types of feelings of shame and guilt, depending on how we're raised to understand masturbation and its role in our sexual development. I wanted to ask Laurie about the negative sexual messages she received about sex in her past and what she might have associated with these feelings, but I didn't want to lead her in any specific direction.

Because of Laurie's resistance to pleasure in their relationship, I also wondered about possible sexual abuse in her childhood. Her memory of her childhood bedroom could be a physical memory of guilt and sensual pleasure accompanied by shame. Her regression to the experience of being a young person could be related to self-pleasure or it could be something more. I asked Laurie if she experienced any pain, vaginal or otherwise, during the massage experiences. "I did, actually, even though he was good, he never touched me there."

I winced when she said that. I felt that identifying Todd as "good" or "bad" was parentifying, and I wanted to avoid that association, as it was at risk of desexualizing an already low-sex couple. "It sounds like Todd followed the directions and that made you feel you could trust him?" I asked.

"Yes," she replied. "I appreciated that."

I asked them both to share what they appreciated about the dates. Sharing appreciation is one major way of changing a couple's sex life. Instead of having them state, "I hated it when you went to the left," I find it much more beneficial to have them each share, "I loved it when you went to the right." Using appreciation can reduce the reactivity and central nervous system response of flight or fight and can open the prefrontal cortex, preparing them both for further conversation about how to make positive changes in their sex life. I also provided psychoeducation on sexual anatomy and function to help normalize Laurie's pain during the massage and reduce shame and guilt. I explained that when the vulva or vagina is engorged during arousal and is inflamed, it's called vulvovaginitis and can be painful with or without intercourse. Atrophic vaginitis is caused by low hormone levels, common in peri- or post menopause, when the vagina is dry and irritated. Both of these can happen without any type of insertion. (If vaginal pain happens during intercourse, it's called "dyspareunia." This may also be caused by low hormone levels, or it could result from relationship issues or even a history of trauma.)

Todd said that he felt guilty because he didn't understand or support Laurie's experience. He thought she was just being resistant to him, not necessarily to sex. He said, "I thought when she said she didn't want sex that she didn't want *me*." Laurie began to cry and said she didn't feel that way. I asked her again about the experience of feeling like she was in her childhood bedroom. She didn't want to talk about it.

For the next two date nights, I gave them the assignment to continue the massages with consent, and only if they were comfortable. Weeks 3 and 4 would be slightly riskier. Now they would massage each other, but they could add in being completely naked, and incorporate massage to the breasts and buttocks. However, I cautioned them, there was to be no vaginal insertion and no orgasm. I also said they could slow things down if they wanted, or speed things up by adding another night. I asked them what they wanted—and Laurie said, "Slow down."

Todd asked, "When do we get to the actual sex?"

Laurie responded, "This *is* sex," but Todd countered, "Not for me." I could tell he was growing impatient. I asked again what he appreciated about the exercise, and he said he liked being close to Laurie and finally felt that she was open to touch, and that he had permission to touch her, without guilt.

Because they were experiencing their progress at different paces, I wondered if they would sabotage their progress at this point in the assignment. Todd wanted things to speed up and wondered if they were at a standstill and were perhaps not moving forward. For Laurie, it seemed intimacy was finally at a place that made her feel comfortable, and she was beginning to trust the exercise, and I wondered if she would begin to back off now and distance herself from him.

When they returned 2 weeks later, we discussed pleasure disorders. I explained.

"Pleasure disorders are coping mechanisms that interfere with your enjoyment of sex. When you have trouble experiencing pleasure or enjoying either giving or receiving it, this may be because you're struggling with pleasure. Let's just call it *that* instead of identifying either of you as having trouble with sexual performance. If you're resistant to pleasure, let's talk about why, or about why this isn't feeling pleasurable.

"Pleasure disorders can manifest in different ways, including low libido or lack of desire, difficulty reaching orgasm, pain during intercourse, or sexual aversion. All of these can be a sign that you want more control over your own urges for pleasure, or that you're finding it hard to climb over the pile of resentment in the middle of the bed to share pleasure with your partner. Or that you enjoy pleasure, but your body is giving you the message that it's not safe, and that you can't trust the experience of pleasure. This type of pleasure problem could be related to past trauma, either in your current relationship or from something in your past."

This caught Laurie's attention. "Could it be from my childhood?"

I replied, "Sure. Is there a reason you're wondering?"

She continued, "Well, we did the exercises for Weeks 3 and 4 and we were fine at first, but then I flipped over onto my back when I was the receiver and he started rubbing me, and I freaked out. I had to stop."

I asked, "Were you in pain? Or was it uncomfortable? Were you able to ask him to change the way he was touching you?" We had practiced ways to let each other know what was liked and what each of them wanted more of, or how to use a safe word to let their partner know they needed to stop the massage immediately.

"No," she said, "it didn't hurt. Actually, it felt really good, too good, and suddenly I was frozen, and I started feeling like I was little. Like a little girl. I had this memory of my mother coming into the room and yelling at me. I can't remember what she was yelling about, but I was scared—and suddenly in the room with Todd, I felt guilt and I wanted to cover up. I felt ashamed, and we had to stop. I started crying."

I asked her, "Were you able to let Todd know that it wasn't about him at the time? At that moment? That you were having a traumatic memory?" I purposely inserted the word "traumatic" into my question to gently begin a conversation that could open up the difficult topic of sexual trauma.

Todd jumped in. "I could tell she wasn't in the room with me, that her head was somewhere else, and I don't know if I did the right thing, but I just hugged her. She was crying and at first, I thought I did something to hurt her, you know her breasts sometimes hurt since the kids and the breast-feeding, but she said 'no' that wasn't it, so I just held her."

"Was that helpful?" I asked Laurie.

"Yes," she replied. "I think so. I don't remember it much."

I continued, "How do you feel right now, talking about it? How do you feel in your body? What do you feel in your body?" I asked these questions slowly, so Laurie could adjust to what she was feeling in the moment and be mindful of her body sensations. If what she had experienced during the massage was a dissociative experience in which she remembered a past trauma, I wanted her to know that she could control the experience now, in this moment of being in her body, and recognize what she felt and be present in the room at the same time. I told her that she could still talk to us and that we were here to listen. I asked what she needed from Todd at this moment.

It's important in couple therapy to create a collaborative experience between the partners, as the experience of triangulation is inherent in working with couples. It's likely that the therapist will align with the victim or the perpetrator at some point in the therapy and try to stay in the rescuer position, yet this trauma triangle is destined to shift around unless the therapist can remove themselves from the enactment and remain a witness—stepping out of the superior role and not allowing either partner to be inferior to the other. Each serves a purpose in the healing of the system.

I said to Laurie, "A person who has experienced abuse, especially sexual abuse, may develop a resistance to pleasure as a way of protecting themselves from further harm. Similarly, societal messages that equate sex with shame and guilt can lead to a resistance to pleasure. Either way, we know that something happened when you were young that you now connect in your unconscious with a resistance to pleasure. There's shame and guilt there—your words—and it feels like it's connected in your body as well. Can you tell us more about what happens in your body when you feel pleasure?"

Laurie held Todd's hand as she replied, "There's a sinking feeling in my stomach, and then it feels like something heavy is weighing me down, and then that someone is—well, this is awful—but they're punching me between my legs." She started crying again, and Todd caringly held her.

Laurie and Todd decided then to delay their trip to see Laurie's family. Until Laurie was comfortable knowing what had happened in her childhood bedroom when she was young, she wasn't comfortable visiting her family or bringing her young adolescent children to her parents' home.

We continued our sessions over the next couple of weeks. Laurie and Todd continued their sensual date nights, keeping their massages at this stage, only switching on and off every other week and keeping the touch to body, breasts, and buttocks only, no genitals. Slowly Laurie worked through her intense reactions. She was able to extend the massage, tolerating more pleasure, and with her consent added in some kissing at the beginning and end of the massage. After a month or so, she then became the initiator of the date nights. If Todd was late, she didn't cancel the date but instead encouraged him to come to their bedroom. She was now invested in the date night and looked forward to it. She bought the flowers and candles and started wearing sexier clothes to the bedroom.

They reported that in between the sex date nights, they began going to the movies one night a week in addition to the sex date. They then purchased my books, *Getting the Sex You Want* (Nelson, 2012), as well as *The New Monogamy* (Nelson, 2013). Both books have dialogues about fantasy and how to add in riskier discussions about what each partner desires in their sex life. We never discussed whether Todd had engaged in an affair, but *The New Monogamy* addresses redefining a relationship after infidelity. Todd was the one who purchased the book and even brought it into the session for me to sign it.

Because this couple didn't present with infidelity as their major issue, it seemed intrusive and perhaps disruptive to create more conflict by pursuing the affair narrative in therapy. It may be that they needed more trust in the therapeutic process and in me as their therapist in order to bring up their affair history, or they may have been worried that their current issues were too intense as presented, and the past would be a distraction. More likely, Todd was avoiding the topic and Laurie was colluding with the avoidance. That said, I wasn't inclined to force them to discuss something they would rather avoid unless I felt it directly interfered with the treatment. If they continued therapy and they each had individual sessions as part of the couple treatment, there may have been more details revealed. Considering their current progress in creating emotional and sexual intimacy, the possible history of infidelity did not seem a pressing issue for the moment.

CONCLUDING PHASE OF THERAPY

Over the next few sessions, Laurie was able to identify a past trauma related to sexual abuse that she thought might be contributing to her pain during sex. We talked about a memory she had of someone sexually penetrating her. We didn't identify who the perpetrator was, but she did experience the feeling in her vagina as she talked. I referred her to a pelvic floor therapist for more work in that area. A pelvic floor therapist could do physical therapy with the muscles and internal organs in and around her vagina and genitals, working on her sexual pain and healing any ongoing issues in those areas. Todd worked on his guilt over his initial lack of understanding and support for Laurie's memories.

We worked on their sharing feelings with each other, a new and vulnerable experience. They began to rebuild trust in their relationship and deepen their emotional connection. We talked about the importance of continued work on their sexual relationship even while Laurie was confronting this memory, and they both agreed they trusted each other more than they ever had and wanted to stay close to one another. Laurie declared, "I want to own my vagina again."

Pleasure disorders are a common and complex set of conditions that can have a significant impact on a couple's relationship and sex. I encouraged Laurie and Todd to use "I" statements to express their needs and feelings, and to avoid blaming or criticizing each other. We practiced active listening skills and provided feedback using dialogues with empathy and validation to help them understand each other's perspectives. Todd was able to express his needs for physical touch and affection, and Laurie felt more comfortable sharing her boundaries and her desires.

As our therapy progressed, Todd and Laurie were able to slowly rekindle their sexual connection. In their sex dates, they experimented with different types of sensual touch and activities that were comfortable for Laurie. I suggested that they move forward into Weeks 5 and 6, exercises that included sensual massage and genital massage, but with no penetration. This meant they would each explore ways to incorporate pleasure and even orgasm into their sexual experiences outside of intercourse.

I gave them additional information about basic anatomy and about how women orgasm, and referred them to websites like *OMGyes.com*, an interactive website designed to teach people the many ways women orgasm. We also reviewed the ways that Todd liked to be touched, and once they were over their embarrassment talking directly about how they both liked to experience pleasure, they reported feeling more connected and satisfied with their sexual relationship than ever before just by communicating in this intimate way. When they actually practiced the massage to orgasm, they went very slowly, each of them talking to the other about how they felt, with Laurie using her safe word if she needed to stop.

FURTHER REFLECTIONS AND IMPLICATIONS

The 6-week erotic recovery protocol for working with pleasure disorders can help couples rediscover pleasure but must be accompanied by improved communication as well. Through my work with Todd and Laurie, I developed several clinical hypotheses that contributed to the therapeutic process. I hypothesized that they had developed coping mechanisms to protect themselves from the pain of their unresolved sexual and emotional issues, leading to detachment and disconnection. By creating a safe and nonjudgmental space for them to explore their experiences, they were able to lower their defenses and become more vulnerable with each other. Being in a low-sex or no-sex relationship can be caused by a multitude of factors, including sexual pain, erectile dysfunction, premature ejaculation, anxiety, depression, illness, childbirth, lack of communication, infidelity, or a history of sexual trauma.

Less than 40% of couples have sex weekly, and Americans today are less likely to have sex than in past generations. Therefore, normalizing a low-sex relationship—particularly at the developmental stage of Todd's and Laurie's relationship—was important. Letting couples know that stress and ongoing pressures of monogamy and cohabitation are common causes of low desire, and normalizing the phases of low desire and the gap in desire between partners, can help remove the pathologizing and shame from the experience. Most people have waves of high and low desire throughout their lives, and our expectation of consistent attraction isn't natural in domestic partnerships.

Comorbid issues such as depression and anxiety also affect sexual issues, as well as substance and alcohol use. Further exploration in this area for Todd and Laurie, as well as ongoing follow-up would be important, as anxiety is the number one influence on sexual function and arousal. Anxiety can be a vasoconstrictor that prevents blood flow, thereby inhibiting erectile tissue in both men and women. And anxiety around sexual behavior and arousal can create more anxiety. This anxiety spiral is common in erectile dysfunction and orgasmic dysfunction.

The decline in Laurie's and Todd's sex life was due to a variety of factors. I hypothesized that past trauma related to possible sexual abuse was contributing to Laurie's pain during intercourse, along with perimenopause symptoms and low hormones. By addressing this trauma and providing psychoeducation around symptoms, and by including Todd in the conversation, we were able to reduce her shame and guilt, and increase her comfort with sexual activity. Additionally, I hypothesized that their communication style was contributing to their cycle of blame and defensiveness. By teaching them active listening skills, validation and empathy, and use of "I" statements, we were able to improve their communication and deepen their emotional connection.

Couple therapy for issues of sexuality can be a powerful tool for helping couples navigate issues related to intimacy, trauma, and emotional connection. The PLISSIT model emphasizing permission, limited information, specific suggestions, and intensive therapy provides a foundation for integrating specific interventions across a spectrum of theoretical approaches (e.g., cognitive-behavioral, emotion-focused, and psychodynamic) to optimize their synergistic impact.

REFERENCES

Annon, J. S. (1976). The PLISSIT model: A proposed conceptual scheme for the behavioral treatment of sexual problems. *Journal of Sex Education and Therapy, 2,* 1–15.

Nelson, T. (2012). *Getting the sex you want: Shed your inhibitions and reach new heights of passion together.* Rockport, MA: Quarto Publishing, Quiver Books.

Nelson, T. (2013). *The new monogamy: Redefining your relationship after infidelity.* Oakland, CA: New Harbinger.

Tuncer, M., & Oskay, U. Y. (2022). Sexual counseling with the PLISSIT model: A systematic review. *Journal of Sex and Marital Therapy, 48,* 309–318.

CHAPTER 17

Couple Therapy and Spirituality
Finding Faith in Love

JAMES L. FURROW

Editors' Comments

As Jim Furrow notes in this splendid explication of couple therapy, issues of spirituality are often foundational in how partners create connection, manage conflict, and envision their future. Matters of spirituality, religion, and faith may serve to foster intimacy and sustain couples through challenging times—or they may function as sources of conflict, separation, or disillusionment. The field of couple therapy has been slow to develop clinical practices that specifically address the unique role of religion and spirituality in individual and relational well-being.

    Observe in this case narrative how skillfully Furrow integrates his approach to couple therapy from an emotionally focused perspective with a specific framework for addressing the dynamics of spirituality across phases of relationship formation, maintenance, and transformation. Listen as he describes his decisional processes regarding when and how to interpret recurring negative patterns in the context of partners' enduring attachment insecurities. Notice how intentional Furrow is in creating a safe place for both partners to access their deepest vulnerabilities, to risk sharing these aloud with the other, and to offer corrective experiences of compassion and comfort. Attend also to how deftly Furrow promotes partners' understandings of self and other by linking their vulnerabilities to both historical and contemporary influences—their respective families of origin and communities of faith—that at times have hindered their capacity to sustain intimate connection or explore their respective faith lives to construct and claim these as their own. And consider the cultural humility and multidirectional partiality required to enter partners' spiritual worlds and help them process any differences that may threaten their relationship.

    Furrow exhorts us to engage with couples around their own experiences of spirituality—harnessing their strengths and addressing their complexities—as a means of fostering deeper connection and discovering the transcendent. The shared journey can be mutually enriching.

I grew up in a small Midwest community in the United States, where family and faith could often be found in the same sentence. Not that everyone shared similar beliefs or valued spirituality in the same way, but there was a common awareness and some level of acceptance that spirituality mattered to many folks. This was most obvious at weddings and funerals, where futures were promised and loved ones grieved. These were often sacred occasions that brought community and family together, finding a language to express deeply felt affection and ritual to make meaning of life's most grand and fragile moments. This was brought home in the sudden death of my father at an age too early for both of us, and the ways that a family and community could hold together loss and love with hope and promise.

In my work with couples, I find similar themes of love and loss, and seek to offer a space where partners can find agency, hope, and healing. Finding a language for spirituality and faith in therapy begins with couples as they share their stories and express their ultimate concerns of life. In years of training and practice, I often felt underprepared for the ways my couples' stories and primary concerns might intersect with themes of faith and spirituality. My hope in sharing this case is that you'll find some guidance and perhaps wisdom for engaging couples seeking direction and solace in sacred places.

Periods of unrelenting relational distress often impact a couple's confidence, commitment, and hope for their shared future. Partners' uncertainty may also raise deeper concerns about the nature and promise of romantic love. Spirituality often lies at the intersection of the practical realities of companionship and the ideals partners hold for what could and should be experienced when one is in love or commits to a relationship. Partners' spirituality may prove a significant resource to a couple's efforts to resolve conflicts, deepen intimacy, and gain confidence in their future together. Alternatively, their differences in spiritual perspectives may place their relationship at greater risk for distress.

Both in the literature and in clinical training, themes of spirituality and religiousness are often subsumed in a more general understanding of multicultural assessment focused on cultural attunement and ethnically informed understanding of a couple's unique experience. Consequently, clinicians vary in how they address spirituality as a part of couple therapy. For example, one therapist may share a similar religious tradition with a couple and rely on this shared experience to guide and inform their work around related themes (Hook, Worthington, Ripley, & Davis, 2011). Others may adopt a more intentional approach by employing spiritually integrated approaches that formally incorporate spiritual practices into treatment (e.g., Ripley, Worthington, Kent, Loewer, & Chen, 2022). Still other therapists acknowledge the importance of locating partners' experience in terms of social location and identity, yet the role of spiritual beliefs, practices, and values specific to a couple's relationship remain unaddressed in treatment. Increasingly, greater attention is given to the unique role of religion and spirituality in promoting health and relational well-being and to clinical practices that specifically address these influential aspects of human experience (Koenig, King, & Carson, 2012; Sandage, Rupert, Stavros, & Devor, 2020).

In this chapter, I illustrate a couple's journey as they navigate obstacles that spirituality presents in their efforts to recover a more secure emotional bond and sacred connection. Much of my clinical work draws on the principles and practices of emotionally focused couple therapy (Johnson, 2020; Johnson, Wiebe, & Allan, 2023). I also draw on Mahoney's (2013) multidimensional approach to relational spirituality as a guide to identifying the risks and resources of faith in family life.

"Spirituality" refers to a range of human experiences animated by a search for the sacred or a transcendent reality addressing the ultimate concerns of life (Mahoney, 2013). "Religion" identifies a similar search for significance, but typically within the context of an institution that exists to promote spirituality. Together these terms underscore the role of beliefs, practices, and communities that often purvey ultimate or transcendent meaning into the everyday decisions and values that shape one's life and relationships. Spiritual beliefs, practices, and community may provide important sources of positive coping, personal meaning, prosocial behaviors, and relational intimacy (Mahoney, Chinn, & McGraw, 2023). However, issues of spirituality or religion may also present challenges when differences in background, affiliation, or expression promote conflict or division between partners.

Key decisions in a couple's relationship often draw on individuals' respective spiritual or religious belief systems as they decide to partner or move on, marry or divorce, have children or not, and prioritize other life decisions that impact the trajectory of their relationship. Spirituality's influence may be felt at personal, relational, and communal levels as partners navigate an understanding of self, other, and the divine. As a couple, partners may ascribe a sacred significance or "sanctification" to their bond and join in various religious rituals (e.g., worship or intercessory prayer). They may be affiliated with religious communities whose values and practices provide support to couples seeking to integrate their life of family and faith.

However, spiritual practices and beliefs may also present a risk to a couple's wellbeing. Partners may struggle to reconcile differences in sacred beliefs or values with their shared commitments or visions for their relationship. One partner may turn toward God for divine comfort, solace, and support—and turn away from the other as a form of emotional distancing. Religious rules for a life properly lived, spiritual reasoning, and coping may become justifications for position-taking and power differentials between partners. Or one partner may "one-up" the other through the exercise of spiritual superiority. The impact of these spiritual struggles becomes evident when there's a threat of loss to that which is sacred (e.g., the sanctity of a relationship) or a perceived loss of faithfulness (e.g., unbelief).

Similarly, religious communities may either provide a vital source of support or contribute to increased distress between partners. One partner may find others who support their cause or justify their side of a relationship transgression. Or a partner's beliefs or actions may create reason to withdraw from a shared faith community, precluding the partners' ability to find social support together in this way.

The case narrative I offer here highlights the unfolding attachment drama of a couple as they struggle to break free from a negative interactional pattern that has taken a vicious hold on their relationship—leaving the partners locked in a growing distance, at odds with the purpose and promise of their sacred bond.

INITIAL ASSESSMENT AND CASE FORMULATION

Ayla and Trent have been together 10 years, and married for 7, when they contact me. Ayla's request for couple therapy captures a malaise that set in after years of navigating dual careers and young children. The recent demands of remote work and pandemic stress have put this couple over the edge. She describes growing emotional distance that is quickly reaching a point of no return and has considered leaving the relationship. The slow grind of distress has become not only a marital crisis but also a crisis of faith. "We need help. We can't do this on our own anymore and finding someone to help us with some deep-seated issues has been a challenge. We believe God can heal our relationship, and we're committed to doing this, but we need someone to guide us—someone we can trust with our relationship and our faith."

I've learned that expectations vary widely when faith intermingles with a presenting problem. Some couples seek a form of religious counseling that includes advice and spiritual direction. Others seek a safe environment in which their faith is valued and understood as a life priority. For others, spirituality is in their background and integral to their context but not primary to their everyday experience. In my initial consultation, I seek to establish and clarify my role and therapeutic approach.

I explain to Ayla and Trent that I don't offer "religious counseling" per se, then share how I interact with couples from a breadth of faith beliefs—seeking to recognize the importance of partners' values, practices, and world views in shaping the commitments and experiences that impact their life as a couple. Clarifying expectations is essential to building a working alliance, and I want to be as clear as possible about what they can anticipate in our work together. I can take their beliefs seriously and the impact they have on their relationship, yet I need to be clear about my focus and the direction of our work. Accepting their experience doesn't mean I share their beliefs, or their assumptions about how a relationship "should be." They appreciate that I've acknowledged the significance of their faith to their current challenges and reaffirm their wish to work with me.

We then explore the hopes they each have for our work together. Trent frames the issues diplomatically, seeking guidance in making decisions together, especially given their differing assumptions and expectations about work and parenting. Although clear about his intentions, Trent appears cautious in answering questions that hint at his own uncertainties and personal disappointments. Ayla is strikingly more direct: "Our relationship is an emotional minefield. Anything I say can set off a bomb! Then there's no discussion, we don't talk, everything shuts down, no words, even for days." Tears well up in her eyes. "It's hollow, a relationship with no soul." The pain between the two is palpable. They're exhausted physically and emotionally, and their past patterns of "gutting it out" are failing.

For years, Ayla has walled off her frustration and hurt, presuming that their situational demands would dissipate over time and they'd regain ground together. After the death of a close friend and participating in grief therapy, Ayla recognized how disconnected she has become from her own needs and emotional experience. She's tired of fighting for something better, trying to make it work alone, and has retreated to a place of contemptuous discontent. "I'm done with words and excuses. Actions and follow-through matter." Trent frames their disconnect in terms of differences in personality and approaches to problem solving. She pushes for action, whereas he pulls away into abstraction and avoidance. His protracted silences in this initial session foreshadow the paralysis he often feels given the increasing gap between their hopes and the distance in their everyday world as a couple.

Following our initial conjoint session, I spend time with each partner separately to further our therapeutic alliance, to assess for contraindications of conjoint treatment, and to survey their relationship history. I seek to identify key attachment experiences and whom each partner turns to in times of uncertainty or trouble. I follow the CARE framework (context, attachment, relationship, and emotion)—a recent development in an emotionally focused approach to assessment and therapy (Johnson & Campbell, 2022).

Through the lens of context, I seek to understand how current and historical influences have shaped the trajectory of the partners' lives personally and relationally. Ayla and Trent identify as a mixed-race, cisgender couple living in a middle-class, urban neighborhood. As parents of three young children, they now find their lives defined by traditional roles. Trent focuses on his demanding but financially lucrative career, whereas Ayla has taken a leave from her career to focus on her children prior to elementary school. Ayla often feels invisible in the rush of external demands that feel soul crushing, and Trent carries his own frustrations regarding the unrelenting expectations of a profession he believes is defining him and eroding joy in life.

Tensions in their relationship are fueled by a growing divide in their spiritual lives. Ayla describes faith as the glue for their relationship and homelife. Her positive childhood experiences in a highly religious household reinforced hope that a similar approach would bring a deeper peace to the couple's growing discontent. Trent struggles to fit into Ayla's religious family story. Although aligned in their religious tradition and a core value to their relationship, Trent struggles with doubts about his own beliefs. These differences are suppressed to keep the peace and avoid further aggravation of Ayla's eroding trust in him. Ayla holds onto her faith as the one sure resource she can rely on, whereas Trent questions his own beliefs privately. He feels caught between his own renewed spiritual searching and Ayla's doubling down on the stability of a faith commitment in their marriage.

I then pursue a deeper understanding of Trent and Ayla's attachment histories and how those shape how they see themselves in their relational world. Ayla's earliest memories are of a warm and responsive family. Although her family, shortly after immigrating, moved often and she had to adjust to new schools and neighborhoods, her family provided a stable foundation amid the change. Religious commitment and community were strong aspects of her family's identity, and she found comfort, strength, and belonging in her faith. She describes having experienced comfort in the rituals of bedtime prayers and the soft reassuring touch of her mother's care and singing.

Trent grew up in a working-class family that valued hard work and independence. He'd been a daydreamer and was often teased by his siblings. His family viewed vulnerability as weakness, and hurt feelings were to be expected and gotten over. Trent, raised under the shadow of rejection, believed he had to perform to be seen. Although he achieved accolades in both sports and academics, his family seldom acknowledged these. Trent had been drawn to Ayla because of her belief in him and her admiration for his efforts and ability. However, by this time, as I meet them, Trent is exhausted from the performance demands and believes Ayla doesn't appreciate his efforts or successes, even while he understands that those achievements have come at a personal cost both to her and to their relationship. Ayla is put off by Trent's constant introspection, as in her mind he's self-obsessed. Her reactions now mirror the themes of rejection and distance that Trent experienced in his family.

I keep my primary focus on their goals for their marriage while fostering a sense of safety and felt understanding in their relationship with me. Trent expresses reservations about therapy and questions whether they really need counseling. He sees therapy as an expensive addition to a growing list of what is "expected" and another prospect to disappoint Ayla. Nevertheless, he relents, agreeing to proceed given Ayla's urgency and despair.

Ayla's wish for couple therapy follows her own growing awareness that her efforts to cope and contain the negativity in their relationship have led to her own loss of self. This perpetuates a lifelong pattern of relying on a pragmatic and disconnected approach to getting things done for others at a personal cost to her own interests and passions. I'm struck by how Ayla's confidence and Trent's doubt about therapy parallel their respective religious experiences. My appreciation and acceptance of these differences are pivotal to a strong alliance through active acceptance and validation of unique experience.

The couple's pattern of sharing and managing their emotional responses is initially more difficult for me to discern. Ayla's pragmatic approach protects her from layers of mistrust that have grown between them. She no longer confides in Trent, as he seems distracted by work or lost in his own thoughts. Trent quickly defends his position in arguments through intellectualizing and reinforcing his position with reason. The couple's disagreements have become emotionally detached, cautious, and unproductive. The growing distance and cold is broken by Ayla's declarations that change is non-negotiable and she isn't willing to continue in the marriage as it is.

BEGINNING PHASE OF THERAPY

In our initial sessions, my focus is on deepening my alliance with each partner and expanding our understanding of the negative interaction patterns that increasingly define their relationship. The sessions often follow a dispute or difficulty from the week that offers a window into the felt experience of each partner's distress and the predictable strategies they use to influence each other and protect themselves. I work to identify a predictable pattern of behavior (e.g., their demand–withdraw cycle) and make explicit the underlying or disowned emotions that are shaped and confirmed in these difficult moments. For many religious couples, these cycles also embody perceptions and beliefs that justify expectations of how their relationship or partner "should be." Adding to the relationship drama, these expectations can promote a moral position or ideal that can be seen as a "spiritually superior position" in the interaction. Balancing a focus on the emotional experience partners share and how that is reflected and informed by their spiritual experience has attachment significance, particularly when that experience is of a transcendent nature. This is a delicate balance, and at times I've been too easily pulled into a couple's reactive cycle, often around charged emotions and polarized beliefs.

The recurring periods of high demand and low support in Ayla and Trent's relationship erode their capacity to trust each other's availability. The strains from parenting and Trent's work have taken a toll on their marriage. They had envisioned a heathier and more satisfying life balance once Trent had settled into his career. Instead, his career demands, coupled with the birth of three children in 5 years, have created an unexpected path into more traditional gender roles. Ayla often feels lost within these situational constraints, and her own professional interests have been postponed. Furthermore, their daughter's recently identified learning disability requires additional support, primarily from Ayla. Chronic stress has left both parents questioning whether their lifestyle is sustainable and whether they fit the lives they've made for themselves.

It's painful for me to witness how quickly the couple's arguments can escalate and cast partners into well-honed defensive positions. Ayla complains that Trent's responses are evasive and he lacks commitment to confronting the practical issues that the family faces. Trent takes issue with her tone and tendency to frame her complaints in terms of his deficient character and lack of judgment.

AYLA: (*irritated*) Trent complains about the responsibilities and burdens he carries around his office, and I know it's difficult now with his workload, but when I want to make a decision about our children's school, our budget, or other issues—much less our future—he's nowhere to be found. He avoids the issue . . .

TRENT: (*interrupting*) We often have a difference of opinion in how we decide things, and she's looking for a decision, whereas I'm looking to understand the problem. I focus on the "big picture," while she wants the decision now. It's a lot of pressure between us in that moment.

AYLA: (*countering*) It's avoidance. You give long explanations that never get to a decision. You don't want the responsibility. You push it back on me or just go away. It's not right.

Trent turns away, and Ayla continues to describe her frustration with this dynamic and how her irritability shows up in arguments and tensions in their parenting. Her tears begin to fall as she recalls her own experiences as a child and the ways her home was a place of peace. Her parents held their home as a "sacred space," where it was important to shelter those under their care. She then shares, "I wish Trent saw us this way. You know . . . we have a responsibility to each other and to our children, and ultimately to God. I doubt that this matters to him, not like it does to me. And as much as I try to help him see, he doesn't get it or doesn't want to."

As I hear the sincerity and frustration of Ayla's longing, I'm struck by two underlying themes. First, Ayla expresses the impact of Trent's doubts and the ways his uncertainty shakes her confidence around their "sacred" bond. The gravity of this concern is rooted in her early family experiences and her identification with her faith community. Second, I discern ways in which the couple's conflicts are shaped by feared differences in their essential commitments to being a family. Although Trent has expressed similar beliefs and values, Ayla questions whether he truly understands her concerns and needs. I validate Ayla's values and the importance of her faith, often using her words and language to reflect the felt significance of her faith, even as I explore the underlying distance between them. Both are important to her experience.

As an emotionally focused couple therapist, I follow a sequence of interventions intended to access, process, and engage experience at increasingly deeper levels of vulnerability and connection. These interventions, referred to as the "EFT tango" (Johnson, 2020), provide a focus for helping Ayla and Trent move beyond the rigid pattern of pursuit and withdrawal that typically defines moments when one or the other has a need or seeks to engage the other.

AYLA: (*tearing up*) I feel like we're growing apart and can't find our way back. It's gotten harder and harder as parenting and work take over. (*Trent looks away as he hears her voice break with emotion, and Ayla reacts to this.*) See how he just goes away!

ME (JLF): This is such a hard place. Ayla, you begin sharing the ways you feel, how you're drifting apart, both of you divided by outside demands. Tears come to your eyes in this moment as you feel the distance and disconnection from Trent, especially as he looks away. Trent, you look down and away, like there's nothing to say here that would answer her concern or reassure her. It's like you're failing again. It's like the gap between the two of you is growing, even right here, right now.

Reflecting their emotional dance with empathy and validation maintains a focus on the partners' insecurity and how it has taken hold in organizing their responses to the threat of distress and distance. I want to help each partner see and be seen in their pattern and to focus on the emotional music in the moment by mirroring the present process. As the moment unfolds, I comment to make this pattern explicit.

> ME (JLF): In these moments, you both get caught and lose touch. The differences between you get bigger, and the conversation gets harder and harder. Like many couples, you find yourself further and further apart when this pattern takes hold—where you reach for each other and there's little response, or you try to respond and it's not what's wanted. This is so difficult when you're focused on what matters most—your family, each other, and your faith.

When addressing spiritual themes with couples, balancing a focus on the context versus the content is helpful in processing the emotional impact of the difference that partners experience, especially when insecurity arises in the interaction. Ayla's "sanctified" expectations for family life can lead to a one-sided conversation about the couple's shared devotion. Her experience, highlighted by her family of origin, increases the imbalance of her conviction and Trent's doubts and reservation. The threat of failing Ayla grows in Trent's experience, as he doesn't have reassuring answers for Ayla's convictions and feels pushed into expectations that he won't be able to meet. For Ayla, the conversations are confusing, because their common faith commitment is central to their story as a couple and she can't help but see Trent's doubts as a loss of faith—not just in God, but in their bond.

Reaching for a shared religious narrative only heightens the insecurity that is organizing this couple's negative pattern. Ayla frames her sense of security in the ways her family organized life around religious rules and sentiment. Trent's reluctance to accept her language and story creates fear for their future, all the while missing the way that Trent's doubts reflect his own struggle to redefine the importance of faith in his own story. Following Mahoney's (2013) framework, Ayla is "maintaining" and Trent is "exploring" within their spiritual experience. Faith is simultaneously both a resource and a risk for this couple. From an attachment lens, God is a source of security for Ayla and, for Trent, religious uncertainty has clouded his confidence in Ayla's conviction. It's important for me to hold space for Trent's doubt as a form of protest or review rather than join Ayala's fear of doubt as disbelief.

I look to use both context and patterns of insecurity as a frame for looking deeper into the individual experiences of each partner and the attachment longings and needs that are blocked by fears and uncertainty. I focus on the emotions that accompany these moments and work to assemble and deepen the experience of each partner around these blocks. In assembling Ayla's experience, I work to delineate and regulate her underlying fear of losing Trent, while holding on to her faith. I ask Ayla to focus on her own physical responses as Trent turns his body away.

AYLA: I tense up. There's a flash of anger, and it's hot. I have to manage my response.

ME (JLF): Yes, there's a flash of anger, you hold back, tense up . . . and you're feeling this now? What's this like on the inside?

AYLA: It's overwhelming. I don't know what's happening and why he closes off like this.

ME (JLF): It's like the alarm sounds. He's looking away, you're in tears, and he's gone . . . yes? And what do you say to yourself?

AYLA: (*choking back tears*) He doesn't care . . . I'm on my own . . . I'm too much.

ME (JLF): And when this happens—and it is now—what do you do? How do you respond?

AYLA: I get harsh—question his commitment to me, to our family, to God. "Man up, Trent!"

ME (JLF): (*emphatically*) Right! You let him know and call him back. "Don't you see? Don't you see us? See me?" [Then I reflect more softly.] This matters, and it feels like it could all slip away.

AYLA: (*her voice breaking with emotion*) If we don't have our faith and we don't have each other, what do we have? It's gone.

ME (JLF): Yes, it's so hard in these moments. You're reaching for Trent, and when he turns away or doesn't respond to all this, that matters so much. The alarm rings, the anger comes, your body reacts. You push for a response, and he goes further away—leaving you alone and afraid it could all slip away. [Then, focusing on her emerging fear, I take another step toward the leading edge of her experience.] And so it makes sense that when you hear his uncertainty or doubts, you look to the comfort of your faith in God—but you're holding that alone. All alone, calling him back, and he turns away. "Our foundation is crumbling, and I'm so afraid." [I then seek to create a new encounter in which Ayla can engage her fear and share it more effectively as an expression of the desperation that drives her anger and critical attack.] So, could you let Trent into a bit of this fear that happens in these moments? The arguments between the two of you can quickly become defensive and angry, but these are also times when you're so afraid. Can you share how scary this is for you?

Ayla shares her fears about the distance she feels, and how these moments take her to scary conclusions about the future of their relationship. She begins to recognize and can articulate that when she pushes Trent on questions about his faith, she's actually seeking reassurance. When she doubts his commitment, she holds tightly to the one thing that gives her hope—her faith. Trent responds to Ayla's softened disclosure by admitting that when he turns away from her anger and disappointment, it's because he often feels that his attempts to answer and reassure her only make their conflicts worse.

I validate Trent's intention to end the escalation, even if it often backfires in those moments. I ask whether he heard Ayla naming her own doubts, and what that was like for him. Trent turns to Ayla and says, "Yeah, that surprises me. I know that you're trusting me when you say that. This isn't easy for either of us." As the partners share their vulnerabilities, a softer conversation emerges. Trent discloses how he's often felt like his doubts were a disappointment to Ayla, and he's failing as a husband and father, particularly when compared to her family. Along the way, his own questions about faith increasingly became a private matter, safe from the scrutiny of shortcomings.

I use the opportunity to illuminate this moment when the couple can see something together about their distress and underlying fears. I feel the ways their doubts and fears have intertwined, and shame, silence, and protest block the couple from meeting in the midst of their uncertainties. Their block is influenced by different experiences but is charged by the fear that divides. Focusing on faith without addressing their fears would only recirculate their reactive pattern.

I contrast this new exchange with their past patterns of interaction. As fears are named and concerns expressed, Ayla and Trent are better able to maintain their emotional balance and put into context the ways that doubt and fear play different roles in their conflict. They begin to recognize that new ways of relating require more than simply agreeing on religious views and practices. Instead, they each must rise to a new level of emotional accessibility, responsiveness, and engagement to face the fears, hurts, and vulnerabilities that have divided them.

Through these interactions, the couple develops greater clarity about their pattern of approach and retreat and its impact. Ayla empathizes with Trent's reluctance and tendency to downplay differences for fear of increasing the distress between them. Trent now hears Ayla's fears and despair underlying her attempts to fight for something new between them. Trent expresses a new appreciation for Ayla's religious coping and her need to express hope in the promise of her faith. Ayla expresses more understanding for the ways that Trent's doubts speak to an uncertainty about himself, not just about God. Yet caution remains given the vulnerability of confiding their fears and needs to each other. In Ayla's words, "We're closer and kinder to each other, but I'm not sure we risk all that much. We're better at staying out of the deep end of the pool—you know, the hard things."

INTERMEDIATE PHASE OF THERAPY

As we enter the next phase of our work together, I continue to promote both partners' deepened understanding of their shared vulnerability and encourage them to risk sharing their attachment needs and making clear bids for reassurance, comfort, and care. Trent assumes more initiative and expresses appreciation for Ayla's efforts to be more positive and less harsh in her comments about him. Ayla shows appreciation for Trent's attention and affirmation, but it remains difficult for her to always trust that he means it. Over time, there is more emotional safety in our sessions and the pace of conversation becomes more reflective.

The issues of faith and doubt are less radioactive, although conversations about trust and vulnerability still fuel the uncertainty that Ayla and Trent feel but are hesitant to engage. Ayla now understands how her pragmatic approach in pushing for solutions reinforces their "spiritual divide" and creates more distance from Trent. Her new, less strident approach to issues of faith has also led to an unexpected struggle with feeling alone and at times abandoned—not just by Trent, but more often by God. She longs to reexperience the deep "peace" she once felt in her own family and offer the same to her children.

This shift in her understanding of her faith moves Ayla toward reorientation: Questions arise, and her anger becomes focused toward God. In its own way, this draws Ayla and Trent closer together as they meet in a shared struggle to work out their faith. The couple's lack of religious community also impacts their sense of isolation from others who know their story, and could hold and validate what they describe as a "wilderness" experience. Their common search for direction and hope creates a sense of togetherness in this spiritual struggle. However, Trent also feels a sense of shame and responsibility for the uncertainty that now defines their lives. I appreciate again how issues of spirituality and family life are multidimensional, as beliefs, practices, and experiences are often shared in faith communities that may simultaneously both nurture and impede relationships. Couple therapy can provide a "third place" where partners can disentangle the emotional and relational dynamics that may be obscured in certain social and religious settings.

Key elements of our work together focus on supporting Trent's efforts to reengage with Ayla following conflicts and resist his impulse to withdraw, and strengthening Ayla's capacity for softening in her pursuit of Trent to facilitate a safe space where they could come together.

Withdrawer Reengagement

As I encourage Trent to share more of his struggle with feeling lost and overwhelmed by the competing demands of work and concerns, he describes feeling "hollowed out" by juggling the expectations of others and his own internal sense that his best efforts aren't enough. Trent often tries harder, pushing himself. Over time, his efforts leave him in a cynical and ambivalent place, further amplified by Ayla's stories from her family upbringing. I want to help him confront his fears of trusting others and loosen the grip of self-reliance that often block him from turning toward Ayla. His uncertainty in career and life are amplified by his own ambivalence around a sense of purpose and his faith. He avoids sharing these struggles with Ayla, as he fears she will see this as a loss of faith and a risk to the foundation of their relationship.

The process of withdrawer reengagement is often two steps forward and one step back. This gradual, iterative process provides an expanding platform of trust in which a more withdrawn partner can move more deeply into their core emotions and attachment-related experience. Trent reflects increasingly on the tension he carries as his "cross to bear." He recognizes that his feelings of uncertainty ultimately leak out in fights with Ayla when the "dam breaks" and his fears foment into an angry rage. Ayla, however, continues to carry her own fears about Trent's doubts. Recognizing that he often keeps these doubts "bottled up," she has stayed away from these topics, anticipating that if she gets too close, he'll withdraw into solitary silence.

In a key session, Trent reacts to Ayla's complaint that he has "checked out," and that her attempts to show understanding and care were rebuffed. Trent pushes back, offering excuses for his distraction and redirecting his frustration to Ayla's lack of understanding and critical tone. He protests, "No, I was there. I was involved. Yes, I was distracted by a text from work, but I was engaged. You don't give me the benefit of the doubt." I reflect the overriding pressure he feels when the message he hears is that he's failing others' expectations—particularly when Ayla is the one he's disappointing. I seize this moment to deepen Trent's understanding of these attachment-related fears and promote an opportunity for engagement rather than withdrawal.

> TRENT: I used to go for a long bike ride when I felt this way—just work it out of my system. But I don't do that lately and I think it shows. She picks up on my tension

and tries to understand, but that doesn't work so well when I'm trying to bottle up those feelings.

ME (JLF): Right, she's checking in on you and you're trying to manage all this—not burden her with your uncertainty and fear—and you know that frustrates her. So you tense up and your chest tightens. Can you feel this now?

TRENT: It's uncomfortable. It's intense and I feel it all over—like I can almost taste the stress of it all.

ME (JLF): So, if you tuned into that tightness, that feeling you have right now in your chest, what's it like? What's happening as you focus on this tension?

TRENT: I don't know, it's difficult to put words to. It's overwhelming, like my heart is racing.

ME (JLF): Your heart races and it's hard to find words to describe it—just overwhelming.

TRENT: Yeah, I get lost in the uncertainty, it's like a fog. The more I push to get somewhere, the more lost I am. (*He pauses and sighs deeply.*)

ME (JLF): And you're alone in it all. It's up to you to figure it all out on your own.

TRENT: (*looking down*) I'm failing. [I transition to focus on Trent's emerging sadness—the softer core emotion underlying his secondary reactive anger—as we reflect together on this lonely place of defeat. I gently ask Trent to consider what it would be like to share with Ayla about this lost, lonely place of failure.] Would you ever turn to her in a moment like this to let her in on this dreadful place? [I'm asking Trent to experientially imagine confiding his underlying vulnerability with Ayla. This brings to the surface his fear and shame in response.]

TRENT: I think she knows already. But no, I don't think I would. I'm not sure she would want to hear it—not about these things. They're too big, too uncertain. She has no patience with me this way.

ME (JLF): So, there's concern here. She may not take this well or really see you in this place. There's some fear that she's going to react badly or reject this. Reject you, maybe?

TRENT: Yeah, exactly. This isn't what she wants. I don't want her to lose faith in me, this side of me.

ME (JLF): Right. There's fear, and there's shame here, too. Fear that she might think less of you and this core feeling you have of not being good enough, not being who she wants, a failure in her eyes. Maybe in your own, too?

TRENT: It's tough. I mean, I know she's hearing all this, and she's always pushing to go deeper. But it's hard to be this open. I don't like this feeling, much less talking about it. [The conversation weaves back and forth between staying present with his fear and shame and his struggle to share his experience. Ayla attempts to reassure Trent, but inadvertently ends up dismissing his concern.]

AYLA: You know I wouldn't see you that way. This is a tough time for you and it's confusing, but I see you trying. I wouldn't judge you for this. [I decide to honor Ayla's effort to support Trent in this difficult moment but then refocus on Trent's emerging efforts to share his fear and uncertainty.]

ME (JLF): It makes sense that you need to know this is going to be okay, and she's offering some reassurance. Did you hear that? (*Trent looks up making eye contact but shakes his head.*) It's like you want her to know that at times, it's too much, but you hold back when what you need is to let her into this fearful feeling of confusion and doubt. Like you're saying, "I need you to know that I can be overwhelmed and confused, afraid I'm not going to make it, and that's when I actually need you the most." Can you share that with her in your own words?

TRENT: (*to Ayla*) Yes, that's what I need most in those times—to know that I can turn to you, that my fears and doubts won't drive you away. And I need to know that you're going to be okay, that you're not going to judge or condemn me for that. That would crush me.

ME (JLF): (*turning to Ayla*) What's it like to hear him put this together in this way—to hear and feel his fears that he keeps hidden away? He's not hiding now! He's trusting this moment to share this with you. What's this like for you?

AYLA: (*looking intently at Trent, speaking softly*) Really good. You know, I know this. I know you've been in this dark, hard place alone and that's horrible—and when you share it like this, we're in this together. There's so much to all this and our families are a big part of this struggle, their expectations and pressure to do things right. Life is overwhelming and we all get scared and don't know what to do.

ME (JLF): And do you think less of him for sharing his fears this way? Are you disappointed in him?

AYLA: No, no—this is what I want. We can face this together. We can figure it out, and we usually do. It just hasn't been safe between us to go to this level, because when we'd try to get close, things would go bad between us. This is different. [Trent begins to reflect further on the difference in Ayla's support as she names the pressures from their families and faith community. Her confidence in him makes his doubts less troublesome or threatening. Later in the session, he shares.]

TRENT: (*to Ayla*) You know, in moments like this I wonder if God is working in all of this. It's a chance for me to be more of the person I want to be, more of who I was created to be. Like there's a choice here toward more freedom, more grace, more ease. It's a risk to let go of this part of me that just sees the "never good enough"— but I don't like the person I was becoming, grinding out an existence without joy in those things I value the most. You and the kids have paid the price for that and I'm starting to see I have, too. This is my chance to let go, to trust that I can be enough for you and for me, like a new step of faith—one I don't have to take alone.

Blamer Softening

The process of blamer softening is similar to withdrawer reengagement as core attachment emotions and needs are accessed, deepened experientially, then shared with one's partner. As we continue our work together and Trent grows in confidence that he can express his own needs, he encourages Ayla to do the same. She appreciates Trent's more explicit support but remains cautious about trusting his consistency and true commitment. There have been too many years when she's felt she had to forfeit her interests for the sake of Trent or her family. Ayla's ambivalence also reflects a growing tension with her religious community, where she has felt similarly disregarded. Role assumptions and rituals often place her in an unseen position, and her faith now comes into question—even more so as Trent now sees more freedom and opportunity in his own faith journey than she's ever known.

Trent begins one of our sessions describing positive strides the couple is making and ways he's finding more freedom to assert his needs and stay engaged in more difficult conversations. He expresses remorse for the ways his avoidance has impacted Ayla and appreciation for her fighting to be heard while drowning in the stresses of their family life alone. Ayla tears up, then reacts harshly. "That pattern is long-standing and today it's better, but those times were horrible for me—just trying to keep our family going and support you. I lost myself in that process. All I had was my faith, and we didn't really share that, so it felt devastating to me."

I wanted to honor her feelings of loss and fear before encouraging a softer and more vulnerable response. "It's hard to trust what he's offering you, after going at this alone for so many years. Trent is here now—but what comes up for you is the anger, the loss, the risk of trusting him." As Ayla moves more deeply into her loss, she expresses her abiding fear that she could lose everything precious to her: her family, her marriage, and even her faith. Her emotional survival has required protecting herself from disappointment and not voicing her desires that too often seemed invisible or less important to Trent.

> AYLA: I know he means well and he's trying to be supportive, but I don't think he sees how long and hard this has been, and how difficult it is to just turn the switch and trust that he's there.
>
> ME (JLF): Right. This seems different now—he makes this invitation, but somehow the pain and the history just speak so loud in this moment. It feels like it is too much to imagine turning to him and sharing your fear of trusting his offer—even right now, yes?
>
> AYLA: I feel like I'm damaged, like a part of me in all this was lost and he doesn't see or want to know about that. It will just trigger his shame, or he'll give me reasons to move on, convince me otherwise.
>
> ME (JLF): Yes—if he doesn't see you, then there's no comfort or reassurance that you do matter in his world. To tell him about this forgotten and hidden part—to show that part is a big risk. It's like you're saying, "I can't let you into this, you wouldn't want to see this, it's too hard to share about this broken part of me."
>
> AYLA: I can't, it's too hard. I just don't know anymore. (*Her voice trails off into silence.*)
>
> ME (JLF): (*after a few quiet moments*) And that fear is here, now. It makes so much sense to question . . . to really wonder if he could be here for you. He says, "I'm here. I want to know this part, too," and your fear says, "No, I can't, it's too big of a risk."
>
> AYLA: I know he's sincere, it's just that I can't be that strong person anymore. It broke inside me. What I have now is doubt about me, about my faith. I'm not that person. Maybe I never was.
>
> ME (JLF): It's like you're saying to Trent, "I know you're here for me, but you don't know this part of me . . . the vulnerable part of me that's scared that if you really see me, you would be disappointed, you wouldn't want me." (*Ayla looks away even as Trent reaches toward her, and so I continue.*) Can you tell him? Tell him about this fear right now?

The softening process involves processing fears associated with a partner's negative view of self and negative view of the other. Ayla's endemic struggle reflects years of being an anchor for the family, a source of strength and stability. Others would admire her confidence and strength to carry on through uncertainty and adversity. Trent is chief among them. But her strength has crumbled under the weight of years of caring for others at the expense of her own needs. Her faith community once provided a narrative that gave meaning to this sacrifice, but it has become increasingly hollow and has slowly eroded her identity as a person of strong faith. Her self-reliance has masked a deepening fear impacting her own worth and doubts regarding her own view of faith and God.

After years of studying softening events and their importance in promoting bonding interactions with couples, I'm often humbled by the power of vulnerability to organize new understandings of self and other. I'm also challenged to hold the intensity of these moments without rushing toward resolution. As therapists, we need to trust the power of core emotion as it unfolds and hold with an inner confidence the importance of the present moment. The impact of guiding a couple through their fears to the connection they seek is life changing. As Johnson and Campbell (2022, p. 29) suggest, "The goal is, then, not to simply increase our clients' ability to cope with or understand their problems but to shape a corrective growth experience that fosters development into a more fully functioning person."

In this key moment, Ayla now turns to Trent and describes her fear as a "tangled ball of yarn" and the harder she pulls, the more tangled and stuck the knots become. The role of faith in her family, the expectations she's held for herself as a mother and partner, and the utter sense of failing to find herself have led Ayla to close off her vulnerable side. The reassurances she often found in her faith and "playing by the rules" have become increasingly unsure, especially as she experiences the growing freedom Trent has found in his new pursuits and his efforts to support hers. And in this moment of deep vulnerability, as Ayla softly expresses these things, Trent reaches to hold her as her words turn to tears. The corrective experience emerges as Ayla shares her need for reassurance and discovers that, in this moment, Trent can just be with her—his words of reassurance affirming his care for her, his validation of her struggle, and a hand to hold faith and uncertainty together, not as a lack of faith, but a path toward growth.

CONCLUDING PHASE OF THERAPY

During the last stages of our work together, Ayla and Trent return to common issues that often reignite their pattern. Decisions about work schedules, leisure time, and enduring expectations from their family-of-origin experiences all provide opportunities to revisit the steps each partner has taken to move toward vulnerability and away from their self-protective strategies. Our sessions, now more intermittent, follow a typical pattern. They revisit a conflict or notice how they've avoided their negative pattern, and we walk through their "tango" together—highlighting newfound responses of emotional accessibility, responsiveness, and engagement. At times, these moments are painful and uncertain, but not in the same way as in earlier sessions. There's a growing confidence in their ability to face their challenges together—to disagree and to value differences. This becomes even more important in confronting questions of faith in their relationship.

Often, in my work with highly religious couples, there's a figure–ground relationship between religious belief/practice and relational process. Initially, relational concerns are framed as problems of belief and conviction but, as therapy progresses, themes related to being loved, having worth, and trusting others become more central. For Ayla and Trent, the language of faith had often been an exit from intimacy or a justification for change. Through our work together, they now recognize faith as a bid for a deeper bond—an invitation to a love that, for this couple, has a transcendent value and eternal purpose. Inviting and honoring expression of their deepest convictions has focused more attention on their longing and needs relationally.

In our final sessions, we explore ways Trent and Ayla can invest in the security they have created through the steps of growth each has taken. Ayla shares how the process of working on their relationship has opened a new pathway in her own spiritual journey. She acknowledges that not only has she reclaimed some of her faith tradition but has also found the need to explore her own place in this spiritual narrative. Together, Ayla and Trent begin to revisit their need for a faith community that will hold space to challenge and grow their love for one another and their care for their children and their community.

As our work concludes, Ayla and Trent continue to confront challenges common to a developing family facing the demands of an urban life. Together, they've created an emotional balance that gives them freedom in their expectations of life and their efforts to shape a common purpose for their togetherness. Months after our last session, I'm surprised to receive a note from Trent, who had expressed skepticism toward therapy during our first session.

> "Over the past year, I'm finding a more hopeful and optimistic path for our family, our relationship, and my soul. It's been hard for me to see past the present and grasp a sense of the future—but in our time together, I've gained a sense of promise and faith for our relationship. We've been able to live in the day-to-day with more peace and look to the future with greater hope."

FURTHER REFLECTIONS AND IMPLICATIONS

The role of spirituality in a couple's relationship is by nature a sacred matter and, when the topic enters the therapeutic dialogue, a sacred trust. I've admittedly become more cautious over the years when clients request a religious focus in therapy, particularly when they have a preconceived notion of what a spiritually focused therapy should be. As I met with Ayla and Trent, our alliance was shaped around a common focus on the insecurity each experienced as they sought to shift from rigid, reactive positions to greater confidence and trust in their relationship. Often, these interactions reflected enduring struggles between religious convictions and existential doubts. Separate from such challenges, each partner held hope that they would be seen, accepted, and loved. Our work together followed a path illuminated by guiding principles of emotionally focused therapy, and the couple's experience along the way was also a sacred journey.

The nature of spiritual and religious experience reflects a dynamic balance between stability and change. Ayla and Trent approached therapy with different assumptions about the importance of their faith for working on their relationship. Ayla initially sought to consolidate her current family's experience of spirituality around the traditions of her faith community and her experience of religion growing up. Her convictions often resulted in an emotionally charged triangle wherein Ayla's passions increased the distance and distress between herself and Trent as he struggled with doubts in his own faith. He was moving away from prior religious perspectives to reorient his spirituality—particularly after several disappointments and losses in his religious community. The growth that both Ayla and Trent achieved in their own spiritual journeys reflected the growing security of their own relationship bond and their ability to approach differences in spiritual experiences and expectations with curiosity and support rather than mistrust and suspicion.

Other couples may reach an impasse when differences in religious or spiritual conviction come to define the future of their relationship. The blocks to partnership are impassible as partners face irreconcilable differences. For some partners, this impasse would be determined in the initial phase of assessment, precluding conjoint treatment or further assessment regarding readiness for couple therapy. For other couples, this impasse may be discovered through the process of working toward deescalation. Emotionally focused therapy may help these latter couples identify their negative pattern and its impact on their individual experience. Religious conflict and spiritual superiority may also be used to reinforce power differentials, increasing risk for intimate partner violence. With such couples, further assessment is required in determining possible contraindication for conjoint treatment.

Cultural humility is an essential component of fostering a therapeutic alliance that prizes the lived experience of couples—even more so when faith and cultural experiences uniquely intersect, especially among more marginalized groups. General assumptions about attachment, vulnerability, or spirituality may limit a therapist's understanding of a couple and how to construe the resources and the risks that a religious or spiritual community may bring. An intersectional approach to culture, ethnicity, and spirituality warrants a therapist's attention to the unity and diversity found in spirituality and religious experience.

Partners' spirituality is often foundational to how they sustain intimate and secure connection, manage inevitable tensions and conflicts, regulate emotions, and envision their future together. Spirituality as a personal expression, relational experience, or community engagement is common to the pursuit of love for many partners. Only recently has the field of couple therapy moved toward developing clinical practices that specifically address the unique role of religion and spirituality in individual and relational well-being. Becoming an effective couple therapist requires honing both the skills and attitudes essential to engaging partners around issues of spirituality—harnessing the strengths, addressing the risks, and mining the complexities these may bring. Embracing such work creates both challenge and opportunity for couple and therapist alike. Joining the couple in their journey can be a privileged and sacred experience.

REFERENCES

Hook, J. N., Worthington, E. L., Jr., Ripley, J. S., & Davis, D. E. (2011). Christian approaches for helping couples: Review of empirical research and recommendations for clinicians. *Journal of Psychology and Christianity, 30,* 213–222.

Johnson, S. M. (2020). *The practice of emotionally focused couple therapy: Creating connection* (3rd ed.). New York: Brunner-Routledge.

Johnson, S. M., & Campbell, T. L. (2022). *A primer for emotionally focused individual therapy (EFIT): Cultivating fitness and growth in every client.* New York: Routledge.

Johnson, S. M., Wiebe, S. A., & Allan, R. (2023). Emotionally focused couple therapy. In J. L. Lebow & D. K. Snyder (Eds.), *Clinical handbook of couple therapy* (6th ed., pp. 127–150). New York: Guilford Press.

Koenig, H. G., King, D. E., & Carson, V. B. (2012). *Handbook of religion and health* (2nd ed.). New York: Oxford University Press.

Mahoney, A. (2013). The spirituality of us: Relational spirituality in the context of family relationships. In K. I. Pargament, J. J. Exline, & J. W. Jones (Eds.), *APA handbook of psychology, religion, and spirituality: Vol. 1. Context, theory, and research* (pp. 365–389). Washington, DC: American Psychological Association.

Mahoney, A., Chinn, J. R., & McGraw, J. S. (2023). Positive psychology and religiousness/spirituality in the context of couples and families. In E. B. Davis, E. L. Worthington, Jr., & S. A. Schnitker (Eds.), *Handbook of positive psychology, religion, and spirituality* (pp. 445–459). Cham, Switzerland: Springer.

Ripley, J. S., Worthington, E. L., Jr., Kent, V., Loewer, E., & Chen, J. (2022). Spiritually incorporating couple therapy in practice: Christian-accommodated couple therapy as an illustration. *Psychotherapy, 59,* 382–391.

Sandage, S. J., Rupert, D., Stavros, G., & Devor, N. G. (2020). *Relational spirituality in psychotherapy: Healing suffering and promoting growth.* Washington, DC: American Psychological Association.

CHAPTER 18

Working with Couples Encountering Serious Illness
It's More Than Medical

DONALD H. BAUCOM
DANIELLE M. WEBER

Editors' Comments

Don Baucom and Danielle Weber invite us to enter the world of a couple encountering major illnesses. Unlike many other couples who are in focus in this *Casebook*, this couple doesn't enter therapy with major problems of relationship distress. And unlike late-life couples, the health issues challenging the couple arise mid-life and "out of sync" with what the partners had anticipated.

    The authors describe how a skillful therapist (Baucom) works with such a couple. Although fully grounded in enhanced cognitive-behavioral therapy, observe his focus on generic aspects of couple therapy such as the therapeutic relationship, collaborating with the couple about their process of decision making, and accessing and processing both cognition and emotion. The case provides a great example of merging the very different personal styles of partners around crucial life events and how they process and react to those events.

    Notice as well the adaptation of cognitive-behavioral couple therapy to a longer-term therapy relationship. In that context, the earlier work with Grace and William around William's illness naturally segues into therapy focused on Grace's breast cancer. This reminds us that therapies are often presented in models in more fixed ways (e.g., a plan for 12 sessions) but are adapted in various contexts. Here, Baucom and Weber offer a prime example of providing couple therapy episodically as needed, over a long period of time—a common way that couples seek out therapy. Moreover, separate from the specifics of this case, the authors articulate general principles for working with couples struggling with physical health challenges.

> The juxtaposition of Grace's breast cancer and Baucom's processing similar issues in his own life also offers a superb example of what to do when couple issues overlap with those occurring in the life of the therapist. The case offers an excellent model of how to effectively and empathically use self-closure in therapy to enhance the therapeutic process.

I (DHB) began conducting couple therapy decades ago, when I was a doctoral student. This quickly became a passion for me and, along with numerous outstanding colleagues over this time, I've devoted my professional career to developing the theoretical, research, and clinical base for cognitive-behavioral couple therapy (CBCT). Throughout this time, I've maintained a small clinical practice, because I greatly enjoy working with couples, and most of my research and ideas about clinical innovations come from these direct clinical experiences that I've had with couples.

When I began this work, my focus was primarily on relationship distress, trying to help couples reengage, get back on track, or develop new ways to treat each other with love, kindness, and respect, rather than the hostility and criticism that often dominated our therapy sessions. While trying to understand the intricacies of various interaction patterns that distressed couples exhibit, I also realized that relationships aren't that simple. The couple's interaction patterns and communication patterns are hugely important, yet who each partner is as an individual, and how they're integrated into their environment also are central in relationship well-being. Of course, navigating inevitable differences can be difficult (e.g., partners' differences in preferences for closeness). Yet, there is more. One or both partners may be experiencing a significant health problem when they enter couple therapy, or such problems develop during the course of therapy. The Centers for Disease Control and Prevention (CDC) estimate that approximately 60% of adults in the United States currently have a chronic disease, and 40% have two or more chronic diseases (National Center for Chronic Disease Prevention and Health Promotion, 2022). The majority of deaths in the United States each year have been from chronic diseases. Therefore, if you're in a close relationship and live long enough, one or both of you are likely to experience notable individual difficulties—either psychological, medical, or both—and these become woven into couples' relationships.

So I realized early on that if I were going to be a couple therapist, I needed to understand how health problems play out in couples' relationships and how we might use their relationship to address these individual concerns, whether within the context of a happy or a distressed relationship. Thus, I've spent considerable effort developing interventions for working with couples when one or both partners experience psychological problems such as fear-based or anxiety disorders, depression, eating disorders, and sleep disorders. In the physical health area, I've focused primarily on couples with cancer, with effort also devoted to cardiovascular difficulties, respiratory disorders, and pain disorders.

I've been the therapist for many couples dealing with cancer over the years. I've helped develop some of these treatments, trained therapists to conduct this important work, and supervised therapy sessions ranging from couples experiencing early-stage cancer to couples with late-stage cancer who are preparing to say good-bye to loved ones. It's demanding but valuable work, and I welcome an opportunity to share those therapeutic experiences with other professionals.

Yet it isn't that simple—professional and personal life often intersect. "After all," as the research suggests, "if you live long enough. . . . " I've had close family members, friends, and former students die from cancer in the distant and recent past. And within the past year alone, my wife Linda and two colleagues were diagnosed with breast cancer.[1] In essence, cancer is a part of reality for many people, as it is for me. Sometimes it remains in the background, but it becomes activated when it touches someone close to you, and it doesn't disappear when you enter the therapy room. Can a therapist balance these personal and professional experiences and, if so, how? Learning how to use personal experiences as a resource rather than an intrusion during therapy becomes the challenge, particularly when you care deeply about the people you are seeing clinically. Clients typically are frightened by the uncertainty and unpredictability of cancer, even if the "statistics" say they have a good prognosis. As a therapist, I have to be willing to enter into that world of fear with them. Although I'm not shielded from cancer in my personal life, I can't lose my clinical perspective.

I find it easy to empathize with a couple dealing with cancer, yet the experience varies based on how well I know them and the journey we've been on along the way. In some instances, I know the couple because they're participating in a treatment research study that we're conducting for couples dealing with cancer. In those instances, my work with them is often brief, perhaps six sessions, focused almost exclusively on how the couple can deal with the cancer in their own unique situation. In other instances, the couple has come to see me for relationship distress or other reasons and cancer is part of the initial complicated picture, or it develops during treatment. Sometimes I know these couples well, either due to our current ongoing therapy or because I've seen them in the past and know them and their lives as they've evolved over time. This was Grace and William.

This chapter is first and foremost about helping this couple address Grace's breast cancer, along with addressing William's major medical problems. The chapter also explores how a therapist (in this instance, DHB) integrates professional and personal life when they overlap. That important focus of the chapter required not only self-reflection but also the perspective of my coauthor (DMW); that is, just as a couple benefits from a therapist who knows and cares about them and can see their experiences from an outside perspective, I knew I needed a coauthor who could offer that understanding and external perspective. DMW offered that critical outside perspective. Her expertise in research and clinical work with couples (including couples experiencing a variety of health conditions) and our close working and personal relationship over the years made her essential in thinking through how my experiences with this couple and reflections about this work come through in this chapter.

ASSESSMENT AND EARLY CASE FORMULATION

I knew Grace and William quite well when she received her cancer diagnosis. The diagnosis arrived unexpectedly as a result of a routine screening mammogram, but even before then, William had developed a serious medical diagnosis as well. Yet both of their health

---

[1] We're grateful to "Grace" and "William" for allowing us to tell their story. Identifying information and details of their medical conditions have been altered somewhat to protect their identities and to highlight certain factors of importance in treating breast cancer. We also greatly thank Linda Baucom for allowing us to share her medical condition for the purpose of bringing to life the complex issues when therapists and their loved ones are confronting issues similar to what the therapist is addressing with a couple in therapy.

concerns evolved within the context of our intermittent therapeutic relationship, which began much earlier. I had seen them on and off over a number of years, and they had generally found our therapy to be very valuable. Both are highly skilled, successful professionals who are insightful, and who manage various routine stressors quite well. Yet, at various times over the years, they've encountered challenging, ongoing family developmental issues (e.g., balancing individual, couple, and family needs with limited time). They also have had more than their share of major stressors, with extended family members needing a great deal of time and resources. At such times, they might reach out and ask to see me if they were struggling to resolve complicated issues on their own. They had come to experience me as a helpful resource, a type of primary care, mental health professional who understands and cares about them, knows their history and can quickly help them focus on the issues they were confronting at a particular moment.

Therefore, I wasn't surprised several years ago when I received a message that read, "Can we get together soon?" What concerned me was the next sentence, "This one is big." When we met at my office, they shared with me that William had been experiencing some lingering symptoms over the past year and finally had seen a doctor. After a series of tests, they had learned that William had a rare chronic disease that, over time, typically shows ongoing deterioration. However, the speed of decline is unpredictable, and much of the treatment is experimental. There was no imminent danger of death and William, overall, was feeling well but, as they stated, their lives had "just taken a major turn in a very bad direction."

And none of us was surprised by how they responded upon learning the news. Both William and Grace are outgoing, engaging people who have good friends, love their children, are highly successful in their work, and give a great deal to others. In many ways, they're quite compatible with each other, yet they deal with adversity quite differently. William grew up with a very demanding, critical father who had unrealistically high expectations. Little affection or warmth was displayed either toward William and his siblings or between his parents. The atmosphere vacillated between neutral and negative, and William found a way to deal with it successfully while growing up: "You just learn to let it roll off your back. Put on your raincoat and hood, and keep your head down. Even if it's pouring down on you, don't listen to it, and don't let it get to you. You can't change it, so don't focus on it. Keep moving forward and do your best." And his "best" was impressive; he had succeeded professionally throughout life, felt very fortunate to have Grace as a loving partner, and was devoted to their children. Not surprisingly, when either William or the couple experienced the inevitable adversities that are a part of adult life, his response was to make it better if he could, but otherwise not to focus on it.

Grace's experiences growing up were very different. Her parents were warm and caring, and when bad things happened or people were upset, those feelings were expressed, and the situation was addressed. As we discussed together over the years, Grace has a "rich emotion system" and experiences both positive and negative feelings strongly. When life is good, she experiences it to the fullest. When things go badly, she experiences that as well. Her typical approach when distressed is to reach out and connect with people close to her, both giving and receiving emotional support at tough times, and William is her main person.

Therefore, when the news about William arrived, they both responded in predictable ways. For William, this was to acknowledge the seriousness of his illness, make changes where possible, but not to dwell on it. Grace's response was to reach out to him and be close during this vulnerable time, voice her concern, and express her love for him. Although we met for a session soon after William's diagnosis, they were already struggling with their different approaches to dealing with distress. William was not in denial or withdrawing from Grace, but he didn't need or want to have long conversations about how they were feeling about his disease. Grace felt shut out at a time when she needed to feel closer to William; she also wanted to be able to express her own fears and worries about his well-being. She knew he wasn't attempting to push her away—it was just his way of dealing with distress—but still it didn't fit with her need to feel close and safe at a time of such danger.

We had discussed these differences between them a number of times over the years, but this was the first time within the context of mortality, and the gravity of their situation felt palpable in the room. I needed to help them with this, while also having my own reactions when hearing about William's diagnosis. I'm fond of these two people, both as a couple and as individuals. My own personal way of dealing with distress is closer to Grace's—after all, I'm a therapist. Plus, in Western cultures like the United States, we have a tendency to teach clients that experiencing and expressing emotions is inherently adaptive. Yet people differ in the extent to which expressing emotions is adaptive for them overall, and it also depends on timing and where they are in dealing with the illness. I knew I needed to be thoughtful and not simply encourage William to open up and delve deeply into his feelings, doing it Grace's (and my) way. Yet I needed to be responsive to Grace's needs as well. We know that partners of individuals with chronic diseases often have as strong or stronger emotional responses than the patients themselves, typically with a great deal of anxiety and depression. Also, I had helped them create a couple's perspective on most of what they had confronted over the years: "You each have your roles, but it can be valuable to approach this as a couple, working together as a team and recognizing what will work well for you together as a unit, as well as what you both want or need individually." That principle seems to ring true, but applying it in complex situations can be challenging when the two partners deal with stress in very different ways.

They knew, and I reminded them, that they had to find a way to meet in the middle when deciding how much to talk about William's disease, how much to make it an ongoing focus of daily life, and how to address their feelings. Basically, William needed to "hang in there" at times when Grace wanted to talk about her feelings and wanted to know his feelings as well. This was difficult, because William not only didn't want to experience being distressed about things he couldn't change, but he also knew Grace has strong emotions, and he couldn't see the value in upsetting her. This very common pattern among partners when a health concern is present is called "protective buffering" (Coyne & Smith, 1991), which is attempting to protect or buffer the other person from your own feelings, so that the other person doesn't have even more with which to deal. We had talked previously and discussed once again that, for Grace, such conversations don't add to her stress; for her, sharing her feelings and listening to his feelings actually decrease her stress, even when they're talking about difficult issues. Grace had to remember, when William did engage and open up, not to push him too far or for too long. It didn't have to be an all-or-nothing approach.

We spent several sessions fine-tuning the process, and William acknowledged that at times, it was actually helpful for him to share his own feelings about his health within a broader context of continuing to move forward with life and not dwelling on his condition. Grace felt that they found a good midpoint, where she got enough of a glimpse of what

William was feeling and felt that he was caring in his responses to her disclosures. She also found that it worked to turn to some of her good friends to discuss her worries about his health. They were valuable additions in providing support, but she was clear that they weren't substitutes for William. Many partners make this point: Turning to friends, family, or professionals is helpful, but you can't simply substitute one person for another. There's something unique that comes from turning to the most central person in your life when times are tough, and you often can't transfer that role to someone else. For Grace, that someone was William, and we discussed his centrality in her dealing with her own emotions. After a few sessions, all of us knew that we had done what we needed to do, and they were aware that they needed to remain attentive to avoid falling back into each person's more characteristic approach to dealing with this ongoing stressor in a way that would polarize them. I felt that I'd been helpful to them, and it was gratifying to see that a couple I knew so well had found a way to deal with this unexpected turn in their life journey. I felt privileged to be a part of it.

EARLY PHASE OF ADDRESSING BREAST CANCER INVOLVING MEDICAL DECISIONS

Two years later, I heard from Grace and William again, asking to see me. Grace was frustrated that William had taken on increasing responsibilities at work with a recent promotion, such that he was working very long hours, seemed exhausted much of the time, wasn't sleeping well, and was exercising less. They also seemed to have little time for each other. They agreed that this made no sense—that this wasn't healthy for William or for their relationship, and they needed to get it under control.

We began addressing these issues. But then, less than a month into our sessions, Grace announced at the beginning of our couple session, "This is really too much, but here we go again—round two. I just found out I have breast cancer. I had a routine, annual mammogram; they followed up a suspicious lump and have now confirmed this. They said it looks small, and they think we found it early, but we won't know for sure until surgery and they biopsy some lymph nodes. Of course, those results are crucial, but regardless, I think I'm losing it. We've been living with this cloud over our heads, not knowing how things are going to go with William, and we came back to see you because we haven't been living in a healthy way to protect him and us. And now me. I don't know how to make sense of any of this. So, do I now take center stage when this might turn out to be much more minor than William's disease? That feels selfish, but I'm so scared, and the 'encouraging statistics' I'm being given don't really make much of a dent—I have cancer!"

Then Grace sobbed, and William held her tightly. I was witnessing and being allowed to be part of a very intimate moment: Someone I know and care about was directly confronting having cancer. Simultaneously, I had to be me as a person and as a therapist. Within a moment, I needed to allow myself to experience what I felt and then quickly turn to the therapeutic process. With a tear in my own eye, I sat quietly with them, observing William hold her while I was thinking, "Well done, William. You two have laid the groundwork for dealing with this as a couple. We'll draw on that. This might tax you, but we know the process."

Because what much of therapy is about is process, we can't know or promise a certain outcome. But we can help lead a couple through a healthy process, and the outcome will evolve from that process. It might sound strange given that CBCT involves teaching skills, psychoeducation, and a moderate amount of structure—yet, philosophically, we believe it's somewhat of a self-actualization model. Help create a healthy relationship environment for the couple that often involves building skills, minimizing negative exchanges that disrupt their relationship well-being, providing a conceptualization of how to think about their circumstances, and helping them make the changes that are consistent with their values and life goals. Then the couple will take it where it needs to go and become the couple they want and have the potential to be. Like William and Grace, I was concerned about how their medical conditions might impact all of this, but what we needed to focus on and what we could control was the process of the two of them working together as a team through this difficult time, with me providing a caring yet somewhat outside perspective to assist them during this ill-defined journey.

This might sound good on a broad level, but what does a therapist actually do to help a couple confront a major medical problem with this philosophy and theoretical perspective? My colleagues and I have written about some of the major domains that can be useful in helping couples when addressing medical problems (Baucom, Porter, Kirby, & Hudepohl, 2012), always adapted for the specific disorder and the unique qualities of the couple and their circumstances. These domains include (1) providing psychoeducation about the disorder; (2) sharing thoughts and feeling about the disorder; (3) making decisions focal to the medical disorder; (4) implementing relationship changes that are nonmedical but that result from the disorder (e.g., stepping back and deciding what's really important in life and how to live consistent with those values or life style changes resulting from medical concerns); and (5) addressing relationship functioning unrelated to the disorder (e.g., broader relationship distress). The following narrative describes how Grace, William, and I focused on several of these broad domains. We engaged in psychoeducation about the integration of emotion and logic; we focused on communicating feelings and thoughts, along with making medical decisions, as well as broader life decisions triggered by their illnesses. These issues arise in treatment not because I have a checklist of topics to address, but because medical complications often lead couples into discussions of such issues.

Integrating Emotion and Logic in Making Decisions

Grace and William quickly became quite knowledgeable about the medical literature about breast cancer from the medical staff and the internet. However, learning how to navigate medical problems involves much more, in addition to knowledge about the physical aspects of the disorder. For Grace and William, psychoeducation in our therapy focused on the emotional impact of cancer and the idea that both feelings and thoughts/reason are important components of experience. When Grace expressed worry that she might die and William countered that she wasn't being rational, we discussed that emotions, by definition, aren't rational but are still valid. It was a new idea but helpful for him to consider that telling Grace that she needed to be rational might not be productive; to the contrary, it might actually feel invalidating to her. William didn't need to have the same feelings that Grace had, but just listening and accepting what Grace feels has great value—a fundamental tenet of our work with couples that *acceptance* is not *agreement*.

Helping Grace and William make good medical decisions highlighted the complex association between feelings and logic, and how the two of them integrated these important facets of reality differently, particularly when making decisions. This integration of feelings and thoughts is crucial in almost all approaches to therapy, whether it is called *wise mind* in dialectical behavior therapy or *insight* in many other therapeutic approaches. Different individuals seem to have a general tendency to weigh one factor more than the other in making decisions. For William, logic typically has greater weight than emotions in the decisions he makes individually and what he emphasizes in conversations with Grace. Grace in general gives relatively equal weight to both sets of factors, but when she has strong emotions about something, those emotions take an increased role in decision making. And, of course, the particular issue at hand influences the role that emotions and logic might play in the final decision. There are times when you need to pay primary attention to the facts, no matter how you feel; at other times, the decision might be a matter of personal preference, with emotion weighing heavily in the process.

This integration of information and emotions became tantamount as Grace and William were approaching medical decisions related to her cancer. Grace needed surgery to remove the lump in her breast, and both a lumpectomy and total mastectomy were options. There was no strong medical evidence to indicate one approach over the other, although a lumpectomy was common in cases similar to hers. To William, the answer seemed obvious: "Having a lumpectomy is simpler, the recovery is faster, and if something comes up that indicates a more extensive removal of breast tissue is needed, do it then. Don't start with a more extreme surgery; that makes no sense." Grace knew the facts but, in some ways, felt that she would be calmer and worry less if she went ahead and had her breast removed and was "done with it." When we discussed this together in a session, I reminded William that Grace's feelings were an important part of the decision process, and he listened. And when he listened, and Grace felt understood and cared about, she backed off from her initial decision: "I know I'm having a strong reaction at the moment, and I also know that with time, I often calm down and then I can see things more clearly, particularly when I feel like you've heard and understand me. Like now. So, thank you, William. Can we set up another appointment so we can discuss it further before we make a final decision?"

Medical Decisions—Mine, Yours, or Ours?

At the next session, Grace stated that she was still leaning toward a mastectomy, but she realized there was another important part of the puzzle. How would she feel about her body if she had her breast removed, and equally important to her was how William would feel about her body if she had a mastectomy—would he still find her to be attractive? William caringly assured her that he would love her and find her attractive no matter what she decided, and those concerns shouldn't factor into her decision. But Grace balked at the notion of "her decision." Our therapeutic approach and this couple's mind-set had been to manage issues as a team and to make decisions together, so, for Grace, this felt like a couple decision. This was confusing to William: "Of course, we'll approach this together, but it's your body and you have the cancer, so you should ultimately make your own medical decisions."

This led to an important discussion among the three of us. There are many issues where it seems pretty clear to most couples that the matter is a couple decision: "Do we move in order to be closer to our aging parents? Do we take out a loan to renovate the house?" Likewise, some decisions seem highly personal for one individual: "How am I going to set up my office at work to create a comfortable working environment?" But what about medical decisions when one person has a disease? Does that person unilaterally make the decisions about treatment? At the same time, often medical decisions significantly impact both people, and perhaps others. Some medical decisions might greatly impact both partners' roles in life, for example, if deciding not to pursue a treatment results in one person needing to work only part-time or stop work entirely, or treatment might impact a couple's intimate or sexual relationship. Or in late-stage disease, deciding to decline treatment might mean a shorter but higher quality of life that remains. Such decisions can drastically impact a wide range of people. And what if the person who has the medical condition truly wants it to be a joint decision between the two of them or, alternatively, wants the primary role in the final decision? I shared with Grace and William that there's no inherent right or wrong way to go about making such decisions. What's important is that they be clear on how they want the process to proceed regarding who has what say in medical decisions and then to use that process to arrive at a good decision.

Grace and William both agreed: "We've never been confronted with this before. I don't think we've ever really thought about it, and it seems like we should." They realized that this was about Grace's cancer at present, but they might confront very difficult decisions about William's disease in the future. They had a touching conversation about being responsible to each other and recognizing that not only does each person's behavior impact the other person but also each person's health. For them, it felt like the ultimate "couple commitment" to say, "We're going through this together, and we'll decide together about medical treatments. Maybe the person with the medical problem wins the tie breaker or holds 51% of the voting power if it ever comes to that, but we don't anticipate ever being in that situation. Neither of us would ever try to force our partner with a health issue to make a medical decision about their own body against their will. But basically, these are joint decisions, and we'll make them with love, caring, and full commitment to each other, taking both our own and the children's views into account."

Oh my, they had come a long way from debating emotion versus logic, and who was right and who was wrong! We discussed that whereas their approach seemed to be an excellent decision for them, other couples might decide differently. For example, others might address the disease as a couple and each partner would listen to the other's perspective, but the ultimate medical decision would rest in the hands of the person with the medical issue. I knew in my own marriage that Linda and I might confront similar decisions, and I was grateful to see a couple navigate these issues with such grace and caring. Sometimes, as therapists, we receive from our clients.

Grace had a lumpectomy, and both she and William agreed with the decision. The tumor was small and early stage, with no lymph node involvement, and they were greatly relieved that she had an excellent prognosis for her future. The remaining medical procedures seemed pretty clear and, at least for now, additional medical decisions for Grace wouldn't dominate their lives. Of course, other couples must address ongoing medical decisions when late-stage cancer is involved, such as contemplating bringing life to a close, making sure that one's "affairs are in order," and so on. Regardless, cancer isn't about medical decisions only; it affects life much more broadly in ways that can be helpful to address in therapy.

INTERMEDIATE PHASE OF ADDRESSING BREAST CANCER AND LIFE

The focus for Grace and William, a couple who had always been active, vital, and full of energy, became how to live with both partners having a notable medical problem. And as Grace noted, "Don, with all due respect for all the good things that you bring to us with your seniority, William and I are too young to have our lives dominated by disease. We can't start to see ourselves as victims—but at the same time, we have to deal with all of it. And what about our grown children? I don't think we're on the same page about what to tell them and how to bring them into this altered world we're in now.

We've told them about both of our illnesses, but William keeps low-keying it with them. I think we need to let them know this is really serious, particularly William's problems. Also, at the moment, both of us are feeling fine. I'm worried that we'll continue to keep living as we've been living, which is what brought us back to see you this time. William keeps working all the time, and if this isn't a wake-up call, I don't know what is."

There's a lot in that one statement from Grace and, in many ways, she outlined the next phase of our work together. "Don, with all due respect. . . . " I'm more than a decade older than the couple, and most people would consider it normative if either I or someone else my age developed a major medical problem. I'm fortunate that I have no major medical problem, and I'm conscientious about my lifestyle to optimize my physical and emotional health. Yet so do Grace and William—they're younger than I am, and they've both been facing major medical challenges. I could tell that at times it was a bit awkward for both of them to talk about physical health and feeling cheated by being younger and having to confront such concerns, and they certainly didn't want to suggest in any way that life would be much fairer if it rained down its medical problems on my generation. And, to be honest, at times it hit me the same way; here they both have major medical problems, yet I'm older with no serious medical issues yet. It was clear that we needed to talk about the unfairness of life and make certain that we could talk openly about where they are in their life journey, without holding back in some way because of my being further along that path.

"And what about our children?" Cancer affects not only the individual and their partner—it affects many people, particularly family members who are a part of the couple's lives. Both of their children are adults and no longer living at home. But how much do you bring them into the process? Do you inform them about the facts and be honest but interact with them in a way to encourage them to live their own lives and not be "burdened" by their parents' problems? Or is there a healthy way to make this more of a family experience, still preserving boundaries, while everyone adapts to the reality that the parents' lives have changed, and we all need to respond in a way that works for each of us individually and as a family.

Finally, "I'm worried that we'll continue to keep living as we've been living . . . " Well, should you, or shouldn't you? As Grace had said, she didn't want them to become victims, yet life is different now. For many people, getting bad news about their health is a major wake-up call. For some, these medical experiences precipitate somewhat of an existential crisis in which people step back and reevaluate life, its meaning, and what's important. Even if a major medical complication doesn't create such a reevaluation of the meaning of one's life, as therapists, we've found it useful to help people step back and consider how they're living, what they want to retain in light of new health issues, what aspects to focus on and enrich, and where to decrease or stop engaging. In essence, we're asking them to become more mindful about their lives. At times, this experience has been referred to as "benefit finding," or seeing what is good or what can be learned from difficult circumstances (Affleck & Tennen, 1996) or as "posttraumatic growth," when the experience has been more traumatic and the person has learned about how they and others have handled it well, or strengths they've experienced in the midst of difficult times (Tedeschi & Calhoun, 1996). What seems to be important is not trying to force a positive mind-set when someone is rocked by adversity but rather to allow it to happen at its own pace and then to address it. Alternatively, as the person or couple recovers from the immediate shock and is coping more effectively, we gently ask about what they're learning about themselves or how it might put life in perspective.

Often individuals and couples mindlessly drift into patterns of behavior over time, without ever deciding to do so. It just happens, so it's important to step back and reevaluate how life has evolved and whether they've inadvertently drifted into unrewarding or maladaptive patterns. Conversely, many couples get into trouble because they don't change, even when circumstances have changed. For example, if one partner develops osteoarthritis, they might continue to push with vigorous exercise in order to prove they're still capable, when more regular yet less stressful movement might be indicated.

A number of years ago, a man in his mid-50s set up an initial appointment with me (DHB), and I asked him, "Very briefly, why did you want to see me?"

He humorously responded, "Well, Doc, I think I'm having a Big MAC attack. You know, a Middle-Age Crisis." Very appropriately, he wanted to address whether he preferred to continue with life as he was living it or to make changes. Since that meeting, I've started to think that it might be wise if all of us have a Big MAC attack at least every decade or so. Hop off the treadmill, step back, and see the big picture before continuing. Perhaps it was time for Grace and William to make theirs a Double Big MAC. The table was set for our next phase of treatment.

Our Therapeutic Relationship and Addressing Health and Aging

Given that they had raised the issue of our respective ages and their medical problems, I thought we should take some time to talk about our relationship relative to health, so I initiated that conversation.

> "We've known each other for a long time, and I think we all agree that we've learned to work well together. And in addition to working well, we've all expressed that we respect and value each other, which is why we have this long-term history. You've always felt comfortable sharing openly with me, and I want to be sure we maintain that openness now. We all know that I'm older than you and, by the odds, I should be more likely to experience medical problems than you. So I don't want you to hold back if you feel that life is being unfair to you, that it's the 'older folk' who should be having these problems, or that it's uncaring to raise these issues. So let me know—have there been times or aspects of this situation so far that have made it hard for you to raise issues related to health and aging because I'm your therapist?"

They both appreciated my introducing this issue, and they both said it might be there a little bit, but William laughed and said, "Don, I think we should definitely take your being older into account as most important, and I don't want to burden you with our stuff; so let's not talk about these health issues anymore. (*Then, after a pause and a smile*) No, seriously, I'm good. I know you can handle whatever we throw at you. That's why we keep coming back."

Grace remarked, "I do want to be sensitive to your feelings, and it's so helpful to know that I don't need to back off or monitor what I'm saying. Of course, you can handle it, and from knowing you, I bet you handle this with real grace and depth in your own life. So, I'll say what I think is important and continue to express my feelings, and if I'm ever insensitive, I apologize and let me know."

Then I had a decision to make: How much do I disclose? For the past year, my wife Linda and I had been dealing with cancer in our own lives, the first time either of us has experienced a notable medical problem. Linda had received a diagnosis of early-stage breast cancer, and her health and cancer treatment have been a major focus of our lives. Her long-term prognosis is excellent, and treatment has gone well. But it frightens both of us at times, regardless of the likely long-term picture; we have to hold both the fear and the good at the same time. Linda is extremely well adjusted and has amazing strength, and we have a wonderful marriage of 50+ years. I believe we're handling this very well, and we're extremely grateful to have an excellent long-term prognosis, superb medical care, and a loving family and broad range of caring friends and community. So, what do I say to Grace and William? I decided to tell them. I had just told them they can be open with me, and I can handle it. Yet it seemed disingenuous to suggest that everything was fine on my end, when actually Linda and I were on a similar journey, only a few months further along than they were.

So I continued, "I want to let you know that I really do understand because my wife and I have been going through a very similar experience this past year." I briefly explained her medical situation. "I didn't want to bring it up when you were in the midst of your initial shock; I didn't want to possibly confuse or complicate our time together at that point. But I want you to know. And I want you to continue to be open with me, express the full range of your feelings and thoughts as we continue to talk about your health problems, and know that you don't need to hold back. Plus, it's fine to ask about Linda when you wish, and of course, we want to keep the focus on you. I hope that we can use these common experiences to help as we continue our time together. I know you didn't expect to hear this, so let me know your reactions."

They both expressed concern for Linda and me in a caring way, and I think they felt honored that I would share this with them, without it seeming to cross appropriate therapist–client boundaries. As our sessions continued, they asked about Linda and me, but we always kept the focus on them. I believe they internalized that I understood on multiple levels what they were going through.

You certainly want clients to be aware that you're a human being, at times experiencing or contemplating issues similar to theirs. But that can't become a clinical barrier; clients can be considerate and caring without taking care of you as the therapist. I recognize that some therapists would choose not to disclose as I did. These decisions regarding disclosure are complex, but I believe those decisions involve the same considerations as many other clinical decisions—taking into account the therapist's style, the couple, their relationship, the therapeutic approach, and the implications of the disclosure. Had I not known them well, if the intervention had been brief, or if I thought they would engage in "protective buffering" to take care of me, then I might not have disclosed this information.

So, we dealt with what was in front of us within our therapeutic relationship with openness and caring. We could talk about their experience that it seemed unfair that they were confronting serious health problems at an age when such was not expected, and when they had followed most guidelines for healthy living. And we addressed our common journey through the maze of the cancer experience. I believe we found the sweet spot that worked in our relationship.

Interacting with and Integrating Children into the Couple's Medical Problems

Grace and William's children are grown and live on their own. From the couple's description, they seem to have made the broad transition to being a happy family with adult children. William and Grace together had told the children about William's medical condition, and Grace had agreed to go along with William's approach of being open about the seriousness and unknown aspects of the future, while not emphasizing worry and concern, and remaining upbeat about approaching it thoughtfully. The children were concerned about him, and they asked Grace from time to time about how he was doing, given that he kept working as hard as he typically had and seemed to feel fine. He had given them the message that everyone should continue to live their lives as they were living them and not make a big fuss about something they couldn't predict or control. Grace was concerned that his health concerns were being minimized, and she believed that if the children understood the seriousness of his problems, they would make a special effort to be around more, call more, join the couple on holidays and vacations—all without overdoing it.

Now they had to decide again how to handle health issues with the children given that Grace had breast cancer. Grace's cancer was a real concern, but relative to William's medical problems, it was probably less threatening in the long term. She didn't want to overdo it in discussions with the children, but she was bemoaning that with both of them having notable health complications, "the whole is greater than the sum of its parts." For the first time in their lives, their own health and mortality as a couple had become a reality. She didn't want to frighten the children, but she wanted them to know that this was now a prominent part of life for them, and she didn't want to shield the children from that reality. We had a conversation in which she expressed this concern to William, and he hinted that, in spite of his calm and optimistic outward appearance, there were times when he felt down and believed that his life would be considerably shorter than he had previously anticipated. They subsequently had a discussion with the children in which they explained that their health was now a more central part of life, that they would be stepping back to reevaluate how to spend their energies, and their desire was to keep an open conversation going with the children about how they all might think about this together. Those conversations continue.

Moving Forward: What to Keep, What to Change?

With cancer and with other major chronic medical conditions, life often feels different—it has changed. And the partners have to figure out what that means. This situation has sometimes been referred to as "the new normal." For some people, this concept rings true; for others, it misses the mark, because life feels anything but normal. Some individuals and couples continue living as they did previously, others make minor tweaks in their lives, and still others make more fundamental changes. The magnitude of change does not necessarily relate to their previous quality of life. Some people who haven't been particularly happy prior to the diagnosis continue to live as they did before. Others who felt that life was very meaningful prior to the diagnosis now step back and make notable changes in their lives, recognizing that a meaningful life doesn't just happen and maintaining it requires considerable thought when circumstances change notably.

Although Grace was taking the lead in approaching this issue, William agreed that though it was difficult to think about changing life in any notable ways given how thoughtfully they had been pursuing their life goals, they should take time to step back and think about this next phase of life. They had learned over many conversations that when Grace pushed hard for change and became more emotional, William would push back, and they would become polarized. However, when she expressed these same sentiments in terms of her deep concern for him and for them, he could join with her. Both were value-driven people who were also good planners, fully capable of exploring this next phase of life together. They merely needed to address these important issues in a manner in which they didn't let their old relationship dynamics get in the way.

This consideration would involve some thinking about the "big picture," which eventually would get to specifics and decisions that they might make. Over the years, they had developed not only communication skills but also the trust in each other to address these important and perhaps vulnerable topics. We started big, and after some discussion, they both agreed it really involved reevaluating "how we spend our time as individuals and as a couple, and where we devote our energies—living what is most important to us." Grace had retired from her successful and rewarding full-time career when William became ill, and she continued with part-time consulting, often turning away people who sought her involvement in professional activities. William had continued with his career, going full throttle, as had always been the case. In fact, with his most recent promotion, his responsibilities had increased considerably. He often worked 12+ hours on weekdays and used weekends to catch up on work and do household chores and maintenance. He often was tired, wasn't sleeping well, and had decreased his lifelong commitment to exercise. He had extraordinary stamina, performed at the highest level, and was greatly valued by his professional colleagues. He felt that his work had always been an area where he had contributed to others, and it also had given his life meaning. He was clear that Grace and the children were the most important aspects of his life, yet he acknowledged that he had a tendency to put them on the back burner when the explicit demands at work and deadlines were looming. They had discussed this work pattern over the years, how William would set limits at work that lasted for a while, but then gradually return to his longer work hours.

Grace expressed her perspective:

"I'm concerned that if we don't do something rather drastic or profound, we're going to keep having this pattern where you cut back on work, but then you gradually resume. We don't know what the future holds for us healthwise, but I think we both agree we probably don't have as long as we once thought we would have. And I know you feel like work is a way that you give to the world, and I wouldn't want to try to take that away from you. Still, I suspect no one would think your work habits are healthy for any individual, much less a person with your medical condition. Then there's us—I love you, and I miss you! I want us to become the clear and major focus of both of our lives from here forward."

William shared his dilemma:

"If you ask me what's most important in my life, absolutely, it's you and our family. But you know I have this sense of commitment and responsibility at work. So I don't know if I can cut back at work, either. Do I think that the way I'm working is healthy? Absolutely not. But this seems to be the only way I know to work, so I don't know what to do. We have enough money that I can retire, but I also need to know that I'm contributing to the world. Of course, you and I are of utmost importance, but focusing just on us actually feels selfish, so I'm stuck. But when I get down to reality, I don't think I can sustain this work pattern long term. So, I agree—I think we need to make a plan, but I'm just not sure what that will be. This is what I've done my entire adult life."

My role as therapist is to help them make that plan, taking into account their health, what they want for this next phase of life as a couple, and what each of them wants and needs as an individual in order to live their lives fully. Grace's cancer and William's chronic health problems precipitated this important, multifaceted issue that they now face. However, every couple addresses similar decisions all along the way in their journey together: Do we continue doing what we've been doing? Have changes occurred within our relationship for either or both of us that push us to reevaluate how we're living? Has our environment changed in such a way that we need to adapt? And are we moving into a new phase of life, such that we need to have a Big MAC attack and embrace those changes? These transitions are hard, because they almost always involve giving up something. At the same time, they provide an opportunity for growth, for making tweaks or a more major recalibration of how to reconfigure life. I am passionately committed to helping Grace and William, and couples in similar situations, adopt this approach to recognize that while some aspects of life might go away, or at least become less prominent, now is a time to embrace this opportunity and move forward to create their future together, however they choose that to be within their current situation. That's the process. To rephrase from one of my favorite movies, *Field of Dreams* (Robinson, 1989), "If you build it, [you] will come."

CURRENT PHASE OF THERAPY

At the time of this writing, Grace, William, and I are still working together on their plan for the future. They're trying to decide about William's current position and whether he continues with it. Not surprisingly, we had a conversation similar to the discussion about Grace's treatment for breast cancer: Since it's his work, does he decide what to do—or given that it affects both of them, do they decide together? They appear to have adopted a general operating principle: "If it affects both of us in a notable way, we decide together." This approach will likely work for them, because they respect each other and have ongoing goodwill to make sure to consider each other's needs in important decisions. Grace knows that pushing William to retire before he is ready would likely result in long-term resentment, and that is not how she would want to honor her partner. William is trying to balance his top priority of Grace and the two of them as a couple, while continuing to maintain his professional contributions. I anticipate that as they make that plan and put it into effect, we will have finished our work—at least for now.

At the moment for both of them, things are quiet on the health front. Yet Grace and William both know it's likely that at some point, William's disease will progress, and they might have a new set of issues to address. Grace has finished her cancer treatments and, as many people do, she has a fear of recurrence that is activated when she goes for her routine checkups. She now can talk to William about those fears, and he listens well.

Grace and William are well equipped to address whatever these next years hold for them. They might do this on their own, or at some point I might get a message saying, "Don, can we set up an appointment?" Of course, we can.

FURTHER REFLECTIONS AND IMPLICATIONS

We chose to write about my (DHB) work with Grace and William for several reasons. First, therapy with this couple is atypical, because it has continued intermittently for quite some time. Most of our work with couples involving health concerns is typically time-limited. However, there are exceptions, and we wanted to share one of those instances in which the exception makes sense. In a broad way, when addressing couples and health concerns or psychopathology, we think of ourselves as mental health primary care professionals. For most couples, that means assisting them for a limited time as they're addressing their health concern. We complete our therapy and don't see them again, although we let them know they're welcome to contact us in the future if that would be helpful. However, there are couples such as Grace and William who return at strategic points in their lives. While being highly effective people, they seem to benefit on occasion from brief consultation—in this specific case, because of my professional expertise, and because we connect well as human beings. They've let me know they trust me, and that makes a real difference. I can be that third voice, one who knows them, values them, yet is on the outside, with professional expertise to help them envision the present and the future. We believe this is one important way to conduct therapy, even within a cognitive-behavioral model, which is typically more time-limited.

Second, we wanted to emphasize the importance of the therapeutic relationship in working with couples. I've written extensively about various intervention strategies and techniques in working with couples from a cognitive-behavioral approach. Yet, in our book on working with couples and psychopathology (Baucom, Fischer, Corrie, Worrell, & Boeding, 2020), we included a chapter on the therapeutic relationship before addressing any intervention strategies. We believe that the best couple therapy evolves from the integration of developing a positive, constructive therapeutic relationship in which a couple knows we care about them and are committed to them, along with the use of appropriate therapeutic interventions. In sharing this narrative of Grace and William, I didn't focus on and often didn't label such specific interventions as psychoeducation, communication skills training, behavior change, cognitive restructuring, and the centrality of emotions in couples' lives—although these interventions were woven together in an integrated fashion into what the couple needed to address. We and our colleagues don't follow step-by-step session manuals in our routine clinical work, because life varies too much couple by couple. We know the principles and core interventions, and those guide our work.

Finally, we wanted to address how to conduct meaningful treatment when the issues confronting a couple overlap with experiences in one's own personal life. At times you might opt not to provide the treatment, either because you're not in a good place yourself, or your current experiences might compromise your clinical perspectives. I (DHB) thought about this when the issue of Grace's breast cancer arose. Had it been a different circumstance in which a couple I didn't know contacted me for assistance, I probably wouldn't have taken the case—choosing not to accentuate my involvement with cancer further at that moment. Yet, Grace, William, and I were in the middle of our work when her diagnosis arose. I had a long-term relationship and an ongoing commitment to them, and ending our work in the middle would only have happened if I felt I couldn't give them the best therapy, or if working with them would result in a notable personal cost to me. I had confidence in myself and in them that the three of us could do this work, and that I would share, as appropriate, what Linda and I were confronting. I felt they needed to know where their therapist was, and we dealt with it well and respectfully, and in a manner that actually might have enhanced our sessions.

It might sound trite to say that life is a journey—yet it is. The couple is on a journey—as a therapist you're on your own journey—and these can intersect at times in unexpected ways. We teach couples to embrace that journey and hope that's reflected in our own lives and in our clinical relationships with the couples we seek to help. We teach couples that between the partners there's reciprocity—the more they give to each other, the more they're likely to receive in return. Although the specifics of what is given and received might differ, we've found that when we do our best work, the same is true between a therapist and a couple.

REFERENCES

Affleck, G., & Tennen, H. (1996). Construing benefits from adversity: Adaptational significance and dispositional underpinnings. *Journal of Personality, 64*, 899–922.

Baucom, D. H., Fischer, M. S., Corrie, S., Worrell, M., & Boeding, S. E. (2020). *Treating relationship distress and psychopathology in couples: A cognitive-behavioural approach*. Abingdon, UK: Routledge.

Baucom, D. H., Porter, L. S., Kirby, J. S., & Hudepohl, J. (2012). Couple-based interventions for medical problems. *Behavior Therapy, 43*, 61–76.

Coyne, J. C., & Smith, D. A. (1994). Couples coping with a myocardial infarction: Contextual perspective on patient self-efficacy. *Journal of Family Psychology, 8*, 43–54.

National Center for Chronic Disease Prevention and Health Promotion. (2022). Chronic diseases in America. Available from *www.cdc.gov/chronicdisease/resources/infographic/chronic-diseases.htm*.

Robinson, P. A. (Director). (1989). *Field of dreams* [Film]. Universal City, CA.

Tedeschi, R. G., & Calhoun, L. G. (1996). The Posttraumatic Growth Inventory: Measuring the positive legacy of trauma. *Journal of Traumatic Stress, 9*, 455–471.

Index

Note. *f* or *n* following a page number indicates a figure or a note.

Abandonment fears, 48
Abuse, 33
Active listening. *See* Listening
Adaptation, 81
Adaptive child responses, 198, 204–205
Addiction
    discernment counseling and, 137
    integrative couple therapy and, 35–39, 40, 41–42
Admiration, 70–71, 74
Adolescents, 120
Adult children
    working with couples experiencing illness, 314, 317
    working with Latinx couples, 160, 172
    working with older adult couples, 220, 223–225, 229–230, 232
Adults couples, older. *See* Older adult couples
Adults couples, younger. *See* Young adult couples
Affection, expression of
    Gottman method and, 64
    working with Latinx couples, 64
Affirmative care. *See also* LGBTQIA+ relationships
    beginning phase of therapy, 203–206
    concluding phase of therapy, 210–212
    intermediate phase of therapy, 206–210
    overview, 196–199, 212–214
Agency, 132
Alcohol use, 285. *See also* Addiction
Alliance formation, 12–13. *See also* Therapeutic alliance; Therapeutic relationship

Alzheimer's disease, 226–232
Ambivalence
    integrative psychodynamic couple therapy with personality dysfunction, 47
    working with couples experiencing spirituality issues, 299–300
Anger
    concluding phase of therapy, 115–116
    integrative relational–neurobiological approach and, 91–92
    working with Latinx couples, 165
Anxiety
    initial assessment and case formulation, 308
    integrative psychodynamic couple therapy with personality dysfunction, 53–54, 55
    transition to parenthood (TTP) and, 235
    working with Black couples, 151–152
    working with couples experiencing issues of sexuality, 274–275, 285
    working with multicultural couples, 192
Appreciation
    Gottman method and, 75–76
    working with couples experiencing issues of sexuality, 281
    working with couples experiencing spirituality issues, 296
Approaches, therapeutic, 2, 6
Arousal
    compared to desire, 273
    working with couples experiencing issues of sexuality, 274
Assertiveness, 165

Assessment. *See also* Initial assessment and case formulation; Questionnaires
  common factors approach and, 102
  discernment counseling and, 121
  emotion-focused therapy for couples and, 10–11
  Gottman method and, 64
  integrative behavioral couple therapy (IBCT) and, 254
  working with couples experiencing spirituality issues, 303
Atone–attune–attach approach, 66. *See also* Attunement
Atonement phase, 66, 68–69
Atoning conversation, 66
Atrophic vaginitis, 281
Attachment
  emotion-focused therapy for couples and, 9, 13, 16
  Gottman method and, 75–76
  negative cycle deescalation and, 16
  personality dysfunctions and, 44, 45
  working with couples experiencing spirituality issues, 290–291, 296, 303
Attack strategies, 198
Attentiveness, 202
Attraction, 9
Attunement
  common factors approach and, 102, 105, 117
  working with young adult couples, 240
Attunement phase, 66, 68–69
Authenticity, 9–10
Automaticity, 93
Autopilot, 81–82. *See also* Habits
Avoidance. *See also* Withdrawal
  Gottman method and, 69
  integrative couple therapy and, 37–38
  working with couples experiencing issues of sexuality, 280, 284
  working with couples experiencing spirituality issues, 293, 300
  working with LGBTQIA+ relationships, 203, 209–210
Avoidance of conflict, 38, 41
Avoidant attachment style, 50. *See also* Attachment

B

Beginning phase of therapy
  common factors approach, 105–108
  discernment counseling, 122–129
  emotion-focused therapy for couples, 14–19
  Gottman method, 65–68
  integrative behavioral couple therapy (IBCT), 257–260
  integrative couple therapy, 31–33
  integrative psychodynamic couple therapy with personality dysfunction, 53–54
  integrative relational–neurobiological approach and, 84–88, 85*f*
  transition to parenthood (TTP), 240–244
  working with Black couples, 146–148
  working with couples experiencing illness, 310–313
  working with couples experiencing issues of sexuality, 275–277
  working with couples experiencing spirituality issues, 292–296
  working with Latinx couples, 164–168
  working with LGBTQIA+ relationships, 203–206
  working with military and veteran couples, 257–260
  working with multicultural couples, 181–187, 182*f*, 185*f*
  working with older adult couples, 221–226
  working with young adult couples, 240–244
Behavioral psychoeducation, 50–51
Benefit finding, 315
Betrayal. *See also* Infidelity
  beginning phase of therapy, 65–68
  concluding phase of therapy, 75–76
  initial assessment and case formulation, 64–65
  intermediate phase of therapy, 68–75
BIPOC (Black, Indigenous, and People of Color) couples. *See* Black couples; Cultural factors; Interracial couples; Latinx couples; Multicultural couples; Race
Black couples. *See also* Interracial couples; Minority populations; Race
  beginning phase of therapy, 146–148
  concluding phase of therapy, 152–154
  initial assessment and case formulation, 141–146
  intermediate phase of therapy, 148–152
  overview, 139–141, 154–155
Black feminist critique, 198. *See also* Feminist approaches
Blame
  emotion-focused therapy for couples and, 18–19
  Gottman method and, 70, 71
  integrative couple therapy and, 27

integrative relational–neurobiological approach and, 84–85, 86, 94, 97
LGBTQIA+ relationships and, 205
working with couples experiencing issues of sexuality, 276
working with couples experiencing spirituality issues, 299–301
Bonding, 120
Bottom-up approach, 269
Boundaries
integrative couple therapy and, 34, 35
integrative relational–neurobiological approach and, 81
working with Latinx couples, 165
Breast cancer. *See* Illness, couples experiencing
Breathing exercises, 32–33
Building an alliance, 12–13. *See also* Therapeutic alliance; Therapeutic relationship

C

Calming strategies
integrative couple therapy and, 32–33, 38
integrative relational–neurobiological approach and, 92
Cancer. *See* Illness, couples experiencing
Care
common factors approach and, 112
integrative relational–neurobiological approach and, 81
working with couples experiencing spirituality issues, 296
CARE framework (context, attachment, relationship, and emotion), 290–291
Career factors, 48
Caregiving partners, 230–232
Case formulation. *See* Initial assessment and case formulation
Case narratives overview, 6–7
Change
common factors approach and, 102
discernment counseling and, 125, 131–132, 134–135, 136–137
integrative relational–neurobiological approach and, 81, 87
motivation for, 27, 33, 41
overview, 4
stages of change, 119
working with couples experiencing illness, 317–319
working with LGBTQIA+ relationships, 210
working with young adult couples, 245

Childhood experiences. *See also* Family of origin; Trauma
common factors approach and, 109–111
working with couples experiencing issues of sexuality, 282–283
Children, adult
working with couples experiencing illness, 314, 317
working with Latinx couples, 160, 172
working with older adult couples, 220, 223–225, 229–230, 232
Choice, 28, 93
Circular coercive cycle, 119. *See also* Interactional cycles
Class
working with Black couples, 140
working with Latinx couples, 157, 169–170
Classism, 197–198, 213
Client factors, 101–102
Clinicians, 2, 4
Closing an exit, 275
Cognitive functioning, 218, 226–232
Cognitive techniques, 92
Cognitive-behavioral couple therapy (CBCT). *See also* Cognitive-behavioral therapy
beginning phase of therapy, 310–313
current phase of therapy, 319–320
initial assessment and case formulation, 307–310
intermediate phase of therapy, 314–319
overview, 305–307, 320–321
Cognitive-behavioral therapy. *See also* Cognitive-behavioral couple therapy (CBCT)
common factors approach and, 100
working with couples experiencing issues of sexuality, 273, 278
Collaboration
integrative couple therapy and, 27
integrative relational–neurobiological approach and, 84, 86
Colorism, 169–170, 174. *See also* Race
Commitment
integrative psychodynamic couple therapy with personality dysfunction, 48, 49–50
working with LGBTQIA+ relationships, 199
working with young adult couples, 239–240
Common factors approach
beginning phase of therapy, 105–108
concluding phase of therapy, 114–117
initial assessment and case formulation, 103–105

Common factors approach (*continued*)
  intermediate phase of therapy, 108–114
  overview, 99–103, 117
Communication. *See also* Feedback; Listening; Responding; Summary
  common factors approach and, 105–108, 112, 117
  concluding phase of therapy, 115–116
  Gottman method and, 73–74, 75–76, 77
  integrative relational–neurobiological approach and, 92–93
  working with Black couples, 146, 150
  working with couples experiencing illness, 318
  working with couples experiencing issues of sexuality, 284–285
  working with LGBTQIA+ relationships, 210–211
  working with multicultural couples, 191
  working with young adult couples, 236
Compliance strategies, 198
Compromise, 64
Concluding phase of therapy
  common factors approach, 114–117
  discernment counseling, 135–137
  emotion-focused therapy for couples, 23–25
  Gottman method, 75–76
  integrative behavioral couple therapy (IBCT), 266–268
  integrative couple therapy, 40–41
  integrative psychodynamic couple therapy with personality dysfunction, 58–59
  integrative relational–neurobiological approach, 96–97
  transition to parenthood (TTP), 249–250
  working with Black couples, 152–154
  working with couples experiencing illness, 319–320
  working with couples experiencing issues of sexuality, 284–285
  working with couples experiencing spirituality issues, 301–302
  working with Latinx couples, 170–172
  working with LGBTQIA+ relationships, 210–212
  working with military and veteran couples, 266–268
  working with multicultural couples, 190–191
  working with older adult couples, 230–232
  working with young adult couples, 249–250
Conflict avoidance, 38, 41. *See also* Avoidance
Conflict escalation
  integrative couple therapy and, 33
  integrative psychodynamic couple therapy with personality dysfunction, 56
Connection. *See also* Disconnection; Intimacy
  discernment counseling and, 120
  Gottman method and, 75–76
  integrative relational–neurobiological approach and, 81
  working with couples experiencing issues of sexuality, 273–274, 284
  working with couples experiencing spirituality issues, 303
  working with military and veteran couples, 257, 259, 260
  working with young adult couples, 238–239, 240, 241, 248
Consolidation, 23–25
Construal humility, 84
Contempt
  Gottman method and, 64
  integrative relational–neurobiological approach and, 93
Contextual developmental model, 218
Contextual factors
  discernment counseling and, 137
  working with couples experiencing spirituality issues, 291
  working with older adult couples, 233
  working with young adult couples, 250
Contextual therapy, 80
Control, 280
Co-parenting. *See* Parenting
Coping ability
  personality dysfunctions and, 46
  working with couples experiencing issues of sexuality, 285
Corrective experiences, 45
Countertransference
  integrative psychodynamic couple therapy with personality dysfunction, 49, 60
  personality dysfunctions and, 46
Couple Therapy 1.0, 44
Critical consciousness, 155
Criticism
  Gottman method and, 64, 65, 69–70, 71, 72–73, 76
  integrative psychodynamic couple therapy with personality dysfunction, 55, 56
  integrative relational–neurobiological approach and, 85
  LGBTQIA+ relationships and, 205

Criticize–shut down pattern, 15–16. *See also* Interactional cycles
Cultural factors. *See also* Multicultural couples
  emotion-focused therapy for couples and, 16–18
  integrative psychodynamic couple therapy with personality dysfunction, 47, 53, 54–55
  working with Black couples, 140–141
  working with couples experiencing spirituality issues, 303
  working with Latinx couples, 158, 160–161, 165, 172, 173
  working with LGBTQIA+ relationships, 198, 213
  working with older adult couples, 233
Cultural genogram, 181–184, 182*f*, 186. *See also* Genogram
Cultural humility
  working with Black couples, 155
  working with couples experiencing spirituality issues, 303
  working with multicultural couples, 192
  working with older adult couples, 233
Culturegram, 184–186, 185*f*. *See also* Genogram
Curiosity
  integrative relational–neurobiological approach and, 84–85
  working with multicultural couples, 192, 193
  working with older adult couples, 222
Cycle compass, 10
Cycles, interactional. *See* Interactional cycles

D

Decision making
  discernment counseling and, 120–121
  working with couples experiencing illness, 311–313
  working with older adult couples, 223, 232
DEEP analysis
  integrative behavioral couple therapy (IBCT) and, 254
  working with military and veteran couples, 256–257, 268
Defensiveness
  Gottman method and, 64, 65, 67, 69–70, 72–73, 76
  integrative relational–neurobiological approach and, 93, 96, 97
  LGBTQIA+ relationships and, 205–206
  working with couples experiencing issues of sexuality, 276
  working with military and veteran couples, 265
Demand–withdrawal cycle. *See also* Interactional cycles
  working with couples experiencing spirituality issues, 292–293
  working with young adult couples, 234
Dementia, 226–232. *See also* Cognitive functioning
Demographics
  discernment counseling and, 137
  working with older adult couples, 217
Denial, 280
Depression
  initial assessment and case formulation, 308
  integrative couple therapy and, 35
  transition to parenthood (TTP) and, 235
  working with couples experiencing issues of sexuality, 285
  working with multicultural couples, 192
Desire
  compared to arousal, 273
  pleasure disorders and, 282–283
Detachment, unified
  integrative behavioral couple therapy (IBCT) and, 254
  working with military and veteran couples, 260–262, 268
Difficult dialogues, 198, 203–206
Discernment counseling
  beginning phase of therapy, 122–129
  concluding phase of therapy, 135–137
  initial assessment and case formulation, 122
  intermediate phase of therapy, 129–135
  overview, 119–122, 137
Disconnection. *See also* Connection
  Gottman method and, 65
  working with couples experiencing issues of sexuality, 273–274
  working with couples experiencing spirituality issues, 292
  working with LGBTQIA+ relationships, 204, 207
Discrimination
  emotion-focused therapy for couples and, 17–18
  working with multicultural couples, 193–194
Disease. *See* Illness, couples experiencing
Disengaging in conflict, 33

Division of labor
	integrative relational–neurobiological approach and, 82–83, 89
	working with couples experiencing spirituality issues, 291
	working with older adult couples, 221
	working with young adult couples, 243–244, 251
Doing, 102
Dreams-within-conflict intervention, 73–75, 77
Duration of treatment
	discernment counseling and, 120–121
	Gottman method and, 62, 77–78
	integrative couple therapy and, 41
Dysfunctions of personality. *See* Personality dysfunctions
Dyspareunia, 281

E

Emasculated feelings, 143
Emotion compass, 10
Emotion regulation
	emotion-focused therapy for couples and, 9
	integrative relational–neurobiological approach and, 91–92
	neurobiology of, 87–88
	personality dysfunctions and, 44, 45–46
	working with couples experiencing spirituality issues, 303
Emotional blocks, 11
Emotional generosity, 27
Emotional intimacy, 104. *See also* Connection; Intimacy
Emotionally focused therapy (EFT)
	beginning phase of therapy, 240–244, 292–296
	concluding phase of therapy, 249–250, 301–302
	initial assessment and case formulation, 236–240, 289–292
	intermediate phase of therapy, 244–248, 296–301
	transition to parenthood (TTP) and, 235–236
	working with couples experiencing spirituality issues, 290–291, 293–294
Emotion-focused approaches. *See also* Emotionally focused therapy (EFT); Emotion-focused therapy for couples (EFT-C)
	common factors approach and, 100
	integrative relational–neurobiological approach and, 79

Emotion-focused therapy for couples (EFT-C)
	assessment and interventions and, 10–11
	beginning phase of therapy, 14–19
	concluding phase of therapy, 23–25
	initial assessment and case formulation, 11–14
	intermediate phase of therapy, 19–23
	overview, 8, 9–10, 12, 25
Emotions
	common factors approach and, 111–112
	working with couples experiencing illness, 311–313
Empathic capacity, 44. *See also* Empathy
Empathic conjecture. *See also* Empathy
	emotion-focused therapy for couples and, 14, 19–23
	integrative couple therapy and, 27
Empathic joining. *See also* Empathy
	integrative behavioral couple therapy (IBCT) and, 254
	working with military and veteran couples, 260, 261–262
Empathic listening, 60. *See also* Empathy; Listening
Empathy
	discernment counseling and, 127
	emotion-focused therapy for couples and, 19–23
	Gottman method and, 68
	integrative psychodynamic couple therapy with personality dysfunction, 56
	integrative relational–neurobiological approach and, 84–85, 96
	working with Black couples, 151–152
	working with couples experiencing illness, 307
	working with couples experiencing spirituality issues, 294
	working with Latinx couples, 166
	working with LGBTQIA+ relationships, 202
	working with multicultural couples, 194
	working with older adult couples, 222
Empowerment, 260. *See also* Power
Enactments
	emotion-focused therapy for couples and, 10
	working with young adult couples, 234
Equality
	integrative relational–neurobiological approach and, 82–83
	working with LGBTQIA+ relationships, 214
Erotic recovery protocol, 277–284, 285. *See also* Sex therapy

Escalation of conflicts
  integrative couple therapy and, 33
  integrative psychodynamic couple therapy with personality dysfunction, 56
Ethnicity
  emotion-focused therapy for couples and, 12
  working with Black couples, 140–141
Exiting strategies, 198
Expectancy, 101. *See also* Hope
Expectations, 290
Experiencing, 102
Expressions of affection
  Gottman method and, 64
  working with Latinx couples, 167–168
Extratherapeutic events, 101–102

F

Fairness, 147–148
Faith. *See* Multicultural couples; Spirituality issues
Family differentiation, 100
Family therapy, 34
Family of origin
  initial assessment and case formulation, 308
  integrative relational–neurobiological approach and, 79, 93–96
  working with Black couples, 145, 147–148, 152–153
  working with couples experiencing spirituality issues, 291
  working with Latinx couples, 162, 165–166
  working with LGBTQIA+ relationships, 207, 208
  working with military and veteran couples, 256
  working with multicultural couples, 179, 181–184, 182f, 190–191
  working with older adult couples, 224
Fantasy, 276–277, 283
Fear, 307
Fear of abandonment, 48
Feedback. *See also* Communication
  integrative behavioral couple therapy (IBCT) and, 254, 256–257
  integrative couple therapy and, 30–31
  integrative psychodynamic couple therapy with personality dysfunction, 47, 49
  working with Black couples, 145–146
  working with LGBTQIA+ relationships, 205, 209–210
  working with military and veteran couples, 256–257

Feminist approaches, 198, 203, 205
Fertility issues. *See* In vitro fertilization (IVF) issues
Fight-or-flight
  Gottman method and, 64
  integrative relational–neurobiological approach and, 81, 87
Financial concerns
  integrative psychodynamic couple therapy with personality dysfunction, 48
  integrative relational–neurobiological approach and, 83, 89–90
  working with Black couples, 142–144, 146, 148–153, 154
  working with older adult couples, 218
  working with young adult couples, 245–247
First consciousness responses, 198, 204–205
First-order change, 210. *See also* Change
Flexibility, 5, 102
Flooding, 64, 69, 73, 77. *See also* Physiological arousal
Forgiveness, 147–148
Formulation. *See* Initial assessment and case formulation
Freeze response, 87

G

Gay couples. *See* Emotion-focused therapy for couples (EFT-C)
Gender
  emotion-focused therapy for couples and, 12
  integrative relational–neurobiological approach and, 97
  overview, 139
  working with Black couples, 151–152, 154
  working with couples experiencing issues of sexuality, 273
  working with Latinx couples, 157, 163, 165, 172–173
  working with multicultural couples, 185–186
Gender roles, 125. *See also* Division of labor; Gender
Genogram
  integrative relational–neurobiological approach and, 84
  working with multicultural couples, 181–184, 182f, 186
Gottman method
  beginning phase of therapy, 65–68
  concluding phase of therapy, 75–76
  initial assessment and case formulation, 64–65

Gottman method (*continued*)
    intermediate phase of therapy, 68–75
    overview, 62–64, 76–78
Gottman Relationship Builder, 76
Gridlocked issues, 65, 73, 77–78
Grief
    working with couples experiencing spirituality issues, 290
    working with older adult couples, 231
Guilt
    working with couples experiencing issues of sexuality, 280–281, 284, 285
    working with older adult couples, 231

H

Habits, 81–82, 87, 93
"HDYFAB" question ("How do you feel about being here?"), 142
Health concerns. *See* Illness, couples experiencing
Help, asking for, 57
Heterosexism, 197–198, 213
Homework
    emotion-focused therapy for couples and, 10, 24–25
    integrative psychodynamic couple therapy with personality dysfunction, 57
    working with Black couples, 154
    working with couples experiencing issues of sexuality, 275
    working with military and veteran couples, 260
Honesty, 37–38. *See also* Trust
Hope. *See also* Expectancy
    common factors approach and, 101
    discernment counseling and, 121
    emotion-focused therapy for couples and, 14, 21
    integrative couple therapy and, 41
    integrative psychodynamic couple therapy with personality dysfunction, 46
    overview, 3–4
    working with Black couples, 153
Household labor
    integrative relational–neurobiological approach and, 82–83, 89
    working with couples experiencing spirituality issues, 291
    working with older adult couples, 221
    working with young adult couples, 243–244, 251

Humanistic–experiential tradition, 9. *See also* Emotion-focused therapy for couples (EFT-C)
Humility, 42
Humility, cultural
    working with Black couples, 155
    working with couples experiencing spirituality issues, 303
    working with multicultural couples, 192
    working with older adult couples, 233
Humor
    Gottman method and, 64
    integrative psychodynamic couple therapy with personality dysfunction, 60
Hurtful comments, 38

I

Identifying with one member of the couple, 34–35. *See also* Therapeutic relationship
Identity
    common factors approach and, 103
    discernment counseling and, 137
    emotion-focused therapy for couples and, 9, 13, 16
    multicultural couples and, 177–178
    negative cycle deescalation and, 16
    working with LGBTQIA+ relationships, 200, 212
    working with multicultural couples, 184–186, 185*f*
    working with older adult couples, 220–221
Illness, couples experiencing
    beginning phase of therapy, 310–313
    current phase of therapy, 319–320
    initial assessment and case formulation, 307–310
    intermediate phase of therapy, 314–319
    overview, 305–307, 320–321
Improvement, 120
In vitro fertilization (IVF) issues, 141, 142, 143, 144, 146, 152, 154
Independence, 147
Individual sessions
    common factors approach and, 104
    discernment counseling and, 125–132, 133–135
    integrative behavioral couple therapy (IBCT) and, 256
    integrative psychodynamic couple therapy with personality dysfunction, 51–53
    working with Black couples, 141, 143–145, 151–152

working with couples experiencing spirituality issues, 290–291
working with military and veteran couples, 256
Inequality, 82–83
Infidelity. *See also* Betrayal
common factors approach and, 104
working with couples experiencing issues of sexuality, 275, 283–284
Initial assessment and case formulation
common factors approach, 103–105
discernment counseling, 122
emotion-focused therapy for couples, 11–14
Gottman method, 64–65
integrative behavioral couple therapy (IBCT), 254–257
integrative couple therapy, 28–31
integrative psychodynamic couple therapy with personality dysfunction, 46–53
integrative relational–neurobiological approach, 82–84
transition to parenthood (TTP), 236–240
working with Black couples, 141–146
working with couples experiencing illness, 307–310
working with couples experiencing issues of sexuality, 273–275
working with couples experiencing spirituality issues, 289–292
working with Latinx couples, 160–164
working with LGBTQIA+ relationships, 199–202
working with military and veteran couples, 254–257
working with multicultural couples, 178–181, 182*f*
working with older adult couples, 218–221
working with young adult couples, 236–240
Insecurity, 40
Insight
personality dysfunctions and, 45
working with couples experiencing illness, 312
Integrating common factors. *See* Common factors approach
Integration, 23–25
Integrative approaches. *See* Integrative behavioral couple therapy (IBCT); Integrative couple therapy; Integrative psychodynamic couple therapy; Integrative relational–neurobiological approach; Integrative systemic therapy

Integrative behavioral couple therapy (IBCT)
concluding phase of therapy, 266–268
initial assessment and case formulation, 254–257
intermediate phase of therapy, 260–266
overview, 252–254, 268–269
Integrative couple therapy
beginning phase of therapy, 31–33
concluding phase of therapy, 40–41
initial assessment and case formulation, 28–31
intermediate phase of therapy, 33–39
overview, 26, 41–42
Integrative psychodynamic couple therapy
beginning phase of therapy, 53–54
concluding phase of therapy, 58–59
initial assessment and case formulation, 46–53
intermediate phase of therapy, 54–58
overview, 44, 59–60
Integrative relational–neurobiological approach
beginning phase of therapy, 84–88, 85*f*, 257–260
concluding phase of therapy, 96–97
initial assessment and case formulation, 82–84
intermediate phase of therapy, 88–96
overview, 79–82, 97
Integrative systemic therapy, 139–140, 141. *See also* Systemic approaches
Intensive therapy, 273
Interactional cycles. *See also* Circular coercive cycle; Demand–withdrawal cycle; Vulnerability cycle
common factors approach and, 102, 105
discernment counseling and, 120–121
emotion-focused therapy for couples and, 14–19, 23–25
Gottman method and, 69–70
integrative psychodynamic couple therapy with personality dysfunction, 46, 60
integrative relational–neurobiological approach and, 83, 97
LGBTQIA+ relationships and, 204–205
overview, 306
working with couples experiencing illness, 318–319
working with couples experiencing issues of sexuality, 276
working with couples experiencing spirituality issues, 292–293, 296, 300–301

Interactional cycles (*continued*)
  working with military and veteran couples, 260–263
  working with young adult couples, 234, 238–239, 245, 250
Intercultural couples. *See* Multicultural couples
Intercultural Exeter model, 178
Intercultural therapy. *See also* Multicultural couples
  beginning phase of therapy, 181–187, 182*f*, 185*f*
  concluding phase of therapy, 190–191
  intermediate phase of therapy, 187–190
  overview, 176–177, 191–194
Interdependence, 147
Interfaith couples, 178–181, 193. *See also* Intercultural therapy; Multicultural couples; Religion; Spirituality issues
Intergenerational wounds, 79, 80, 93–96
Interlocking vulnerability cycles, 79–80. *See also* Vulnerabilities
Intermediate phase of therapy
  common factors approach, 108–114
  discernment counseling, 129–135
  emotion-focused therapy for couples, 19–23
  Gottman method, 68–75
  integrative behavioral couple therapy (IBCT), 260–265
  integrative couple therapy, 33–39
  integrative psychodynamic couple therapy with personality dysfunction, 54–58
  integrative relational–neurobiological approach, 88–96
  transition to parenthood (TTP), 244–248
  working with Black couples, 148–152
  working with couples experiencing illness, 314–319
  working with couples experiencing issues of sexuality, 277–284
  working with couples experiencing spirituality issues, 296–301
  working with Latinx couples, 168–170
  working with LGBTQIA+ relationships, 206–210
  working with military and veteran couples, 260–266
  working with multicultural couples, 187–190
  working with older adult couples, 226–230
  working with young adult couples, 244–248
Interpersonal block, 10

Interpersonal neurobiology, 81. *See also* Integrative relational–neurobiological approach; Neurobiology
Interracial couples. *See also* Multicultural couples; Race
  beginning phase of therapy, 14–19, 203–206, 275–277
  concluding phase of therapy, 23–25, 210–212, 284–285
  initial assessment and case formulation, 11–14, 199–202, 273–275
  intermediate phase of therapy, 19–23, 206–210, 277–284
Intersectional contexts
  overview, 12, 16–17, 18
  working with couples experiencing spirituality issues, 303
  working with LGBTQIA+ relationships, 197–198, 199, 212–214
Interventions
  common factors approach and, 102–103
  emotion-focused therapy for couples and, 10–11
  integrative behavioral couple therapy (IBCT) and, 254
  working with couples experiencing issues of sexuality, 271, 277–279
  working with couples experiencing spirituality issues, 293–294
  working with multicultural couples, 194
Interviews, 64. *See also* Assessment
Intimacy. *See also* Connection; Emotional intimacy; Physical intimacy; Sex; Sexuality issues
  common factors approach and, 104
  LGBTQIA+ relationships and, 198
Intimate partner violence, 303
Intrapersonal block, 10
Invalidation, 12–13
Islamaphobia, 193–194

J

Jealousy
  beginning phase of therapy, 164–168
  concluding phase of therapy, 170–172
  intermediate phase of therapy, 168–170
  working with Latinx couples, 157–158, 159, 164–168, 172–174
Joining mind-set, 37
Judgment, 84–85
Justice, 198

L

Language
- LGBTQIA+ relationships and, 196n, 200
- working with couples experiencing issues of sexuality, 273–274, 276
- working with Latinx couples, 160–161, 172
- working with multicultural couples, 181

Latinx couples. *See also* Minority populations; Multidimensional ecological comparative approach (MECA); Race
- beginning phase of therapy, 164–168
- concluding phase of therapy, 170–172
- initial assessment and case formulation, 160–164
- intermediate phase of therapy, 168–170
- overview, 157–159, 172–174

LGBTQIA+ relationships. *See also* Affirmative care
- beginning phase of therapy, 203–206
- concluding phase of therapy, 210–212
- initial assessment and case formulation, 199–202
- intermediate phase of therapy, 206–210
- overview, 196–199, 212–214

Listening. *See also* Communication
- common factors approach and, 106
- personality dysfunctions and, 45
- working with multicultural couples, 180

Logic, 311–313
London Intercultural Couples Centre, 177–178
Loneliness
- Gottman method and, 72
- integrative couple therapy and, 39

Losing relational strategies, 205–206
Loss
- Gottman method and, 72–73
- working with couples experiencing spirituality issues, 300–301
- working with older adult couples, 231

M

Machismo, 172. *See also* Gender; Masculinity
Magic Question, 88–89
Maladaptive patterns of personality, 44. *See also* Personality dysfunctions
Marathon therapy, 64, 77–78
Masculinity, 157, 163, 165, 172–173. *See also* Gender
Mastery, 9. *See also* Identity
Masturbation, 281
Maturity of ego defenses, 44
Meaning in life, 217

Medical issues. *See* Illness, couples experiencing
Mentalization, 44
Mexican transnational couples. *See* Latinx couples
Middle phase of therapy. *See* Intermediate phase of therapy
Middle-class Black couples. *See* Black couples; Class
Military and veteran couples
- beginning phase of therapy, 257–260
- concluding phase of therapy, 266–268
- initial assessment and case formulation, 254–257
- intermediate phase of therapy, 260–266
- overview, 252–254, 268–269
- transition to parenthood (TTP) and, 236–237, 239

Mindfulness
- common factors approach and, 102
- working with couples experiencing issues of sexuality, 278
- working with Latinx couples, 173

Mind-sets, 146–147
Minority populations, 12. *See also* Black couples; Latinx couples; LGBTQIA+ relationships; Race
Minority stress, 197
Mixed-agenda couples, 119, 120, 153–154. *See also* Discernment counseling
Modern emotion theory, 9
Money issues
- integrative psychodynamic couple therapy with personality dysfunction, 48
- integrative relational–neurobiological approach and, 83, 89–90
- working with Black couples, 142–144, 146, 148–153, 154
- working with older adult couples, 218
- working with young adult couples, 245–247

Motivation for change, 27, 33, 41. *See also* Change
Motivational systems, 9. *See also* Attachment; Attraction; Identity
Multicultural couples. *See also* Cultural factors; Intercultural therapy; Interracial couples
- beginning phase of therapy, 181–187, 182f, 185f
- concluding phase of therapy, 190–191
- initial assessment and case formulation, 178–181, 182f
- intermediate phase of therapy, 187–190
- LGBTQIA+ relationships and, 198
- overview, 176–178, 191–194

Multidimensional approach to relational spirituality, 288. *See also* Spirituality issues
Multidimensional ecological comparative approach (MECA), 157, 158–159, 161–162, 163–164, 173–174. *See also* Latinx couples
Multidirected partiality, 82, 83, 94

N

Narrative approach, 218
Negative cycle deescalation, 14–19. *See also* Interactional cycles
Neurobiology, 79, 80–81, 87–88, 97. *See also* Integrative relational–neurobiological approach
New normal concept, 317–319
Nonjudgmental stance, 5

O

Observation, 46
Older adult couples
　beginning phase of therapy, 221–226
　concluding phase of therapy, 230–232
　initial assessment and case formulation, 218–221
　intermediate phase of therapy, 226–230
　overview, 216–218, 232–233
Omissions, 37–38
Oppression, 198, 212, 213–214
Others, including in therapy, 103

P

Pain, 25
Parent–child role reversals
　common factors approach and, 109
　integrative psychodynamic couple therapy with personality dysfunction, 50–51
　integrative relational–neurobiological approach and, 88, 94, 95–96
Parenting. *See also* Transition to parenthood (TTP); Young adult couples
　common factors approach and, 103, 104, 106–108, 109–111
　Gottman method and, 65
　working with Latinx couples, 162–163
　working with LGBTQIA+ relationships, 212
　working with military and veteran couples, 255, 262
　working with multicultural couples, 186
Patterns of interaction. *See* Interactional cycles

Pelvic floor therapy, 284
Perfectionism, 49–50
Personality dysfunctions
　beginning phase of therapy, 53–54
　concluding phase of therapy, 58–59
　initial assessment and case formulation, 46–53
　intermediate phase of therapy, 54–58
　overview, 44–46, 59–60
Photos, 38–39
Physical intimacy. *See also* Intimacy; Sex; Sexuality issues
　common factors approach and, 104, 112–114
　working with military and veteran couples, 263–265
Physiological arousal
　Gottman method and, 64, 69, 77
　integrative couple therapy and, 32–33, 38
Pleasure, 280–284
Pleasure disorders, 282–283, 284, 285
PLISSIT model (Permission, Limited Information, Specific Suggestions, and Intensive Therapy), 272–273, 285
Pluralistic integrative practice, 216, 218
Positive behaviors, 18
Positive emotional experiences, 24–25
Positives, 30–31, 33
Positivity, 75–76
Postpartum depression (PPD), 235
Posttraumatic growth, 315
Posttraumatic-stress disorder (PTSD), 252–253, 254–255, 265–266
Power. *See also* Powerlessness
　empowerment, 260
　integrative relational–neurobiological approach and, 90–91
　working with Latinx couples, 165, 173
　working with LGBTQIA+ relationships, 199, 211, 213, 214
　working with multicultural couples, 185–186, 193–194
Powerlessness. *See also* Power
　Gottman method and, 72–73
　working with multicultural couples, 193–194
Problem solving
　discernment counseling and, 120
　integrative couple therapy and, 28
　working with Black couples, 149
　working with military and veteran couples, 260
Processing arguments, 71–72
Protective buffering, 308
Protective walls, 11

Psychodynamic exploration, 50–51
Psychodynamic perspective. *See also* Integrative psychodynamic couple therapy
 personality dysfunctions and, 45
 working with couples experiencing issues of sexuality, 273
Psychoeducation
 behavioral psychoeducation, 50–51
 emotion-focused therapy for couples and, 12
 working with couples experiencing illness, 311
 working with military and veteran couples, 260
 working with older adult couples, 223
 working with young adult couples, 234, 241
Psychological mindedness, 44
Psychological problems, 137
Pursue–withdraw cycle
 emotion-focused therapy for couples and, 15–16
 working with military and veteran couples, 260–263
 working with young adult couples, 238–239, 241, 243–244, 245–247

Q

Queer relationships. *See* Affirmative care; LGBTQIA+ relationships
Queer theory, 198
Questionnaires. *See also* Assessment
 Gottman method and, 64
 integrative behavioral couple therapy (IBCT) and, 257–258, 259–260, 266
 integrative psychodynamic couple therapy with personality dysfunction, 51
 working with Latinx couples, 161

R

Race. *See also* Black couples; Interracial couples; Latinx couples; Minority populations; Racism
 emotion-focused therapy for couples and, 12
 overview, 155, 157
 working with multicultural couples, 179–181
Racism. *See also* Race
 multicultural couples and, 177–178
 working with Latinx couples, 174
 working with LGBTQIA+ relationships, 197–198, 213
 working with multicultural couples, 179–181, 193–194

Reactivity, 28, 87–88
Reappraisal, 92
Reassurance, 295, 296, 299
Recommitment, 263, 267
Reengagement, 297–299
Referrals, 136–137
Reframing, 21–23
Rejection, 280
Relapse prevention
 emotion-focused therapy for couples and, 24–25
 integrative couple therapy and, 40–41
Relational claims, 92–93
Relational ethics, 92
Relationship, therapeutic. *See* Therapeutic alliance; Therapeutic relationship
Relationship skills, 60
Religion. *See also* Interfaith couples; Religiosity; Spirituality issues
 overview, 289
 working with Latinx couples, 162, 163
 working with multicultural couples, 177, 179, 180–181, 193
Religiosity, 197–198, 288. *See also* Interfaith couples; Religion; Spirituality issues
Repair attempts, 64
Repair of arguments, 71–72
Resentment, 67
Resilience. *See also* Strengths
 working with military and veteran couples, 256, 268
 working with older adult couples, 219–220
Resistance
 integrative relational–neurobiological approach and, 81
 working with couples experiencing issues of sexuality, 280–281
 working with young adult couples, 240, 241
Respect, 168–169
Responding, 106. *See also* Communication
Responsibilities, household
 integrative relational–neurobiological approach and, 82–83, 89
 working with couples experiencing spirituality issues, 291
 working with older adult couples, 221
 working with young adult couples, 243–244, 251
Retirement transition, 219–221. *See also* Older adult couples

Role reversals, parent–child
  common factors approach and, 109
  integrative psychodynamic couple therapy with personality dysfunction, 50–51
  integrative relational–neurobiological approach and, 88, 94, 95–96

S

Safety
  integrative relational–neurobiological approach and, 81
  working with couples experiencing spirituality issues, 291–292, 297–299
  working with Latinx couples, 164
  working with military and veteran couples, 257
Scaffolding, 154
Screening, 121, 122. *See also* Assessment
Second-order change, 210. *See also* Change
Secrets
  integrative couple therapy and, 35–39
  working with Black couples, 141–142
Selective attention, 28
Self-awareness, 193
Self-coherence, 9. *See also* Identity
Self-criticism, 48
Self-disclosure
  common factors approach and, 117
  integrative couple therapy and, 42
  working with couples experiencing illness, 316
  working with multicultural couples, 192–193
  working with young adult couples, 251
Self-esteem. *See also* Identity
  emotion-focused therapy for couples and, 9
  integrative psychodynamic couple therapy with personality dysfunction, 55
  personality dysfunctions and, 44
  working with Latinx couples, 164, 171
Self-pleasure, 281
Self-protective habits. *See also* Habits
  integrative relational–neurobiological approach and, 81–82, 87, 91–92, 93
  vulnerability cycle diagram and, 85–86, 85*f*
Self-reflection, 27
Self-reflexivity, 193
Self-talk, 28
Semantic polarities, 178

Session format. *See also* Beginning phase of therapy; Concluding phase of therapy; Initial assessment and case formulation; Intermediate phase of therapy
  discernment counseling and, 120–121
  Gottman method and, 62, 77–78
Sessions with individual members of couples. *See* Individual sessions
Sex. *See also* Intimacy; Sex therapy; Sexual difficulties; Sexuality issues
  common factors approach and, 112–114
  discernment counseling and, 125–126, 127–128
  Gottman method and, 65
  integrative psychodynamic couple therapy with personality dysfunction, 50, 53–54, 58, 60
  integrative relational–neurobiological approach and, 83
  working with military and veteran couples, 263–265
  working with young adult couples, 236
Sex date, 277–279, 284
Sex therapy. *See also* Sexual difficulties
  beginning phase of therapy, 275–277
  concluding phase of therapy, 284–285
  initial assessment and case formulation, 273–275
  intermediate phase of therapy, 277–284
  overview, 271–273, 285
Sexism, 197–198, 213
Sexual difficulties. *See also* Sex therapy
  beginning phase of therapy, 275–277
  concluding phase of therapy, 284–285
  initial assessment and case formulation, 273–275
  intermediate phase of therapy, 277–284
  overview, 285
Sexual orientation, 12. *See also* LGBTQIA+ relationships
Sexuality issues, 271–273. *See also* Physical intimacy; Sex; Sexual difficulties
Shame
  emotion-focused therapy for couples and, 20–23
  integrative relational–neurobiological approach and, 82
  working with couples experiencing issues of sexuality, 276–277, 280–281, 285
  working with couples experiencing spirituality issues, 297
  working with LGBTQIA+ relationships, 211–212, 213–214

Sickness. *See* Illness, couples experiencing
Skills training, 260, 269
Sociocultural attunement, 117. *See also* Attunement
Sociocultural factors. *See also* Cultural factors; Systemic approaches
   LGBTQIA+ relationships and, 198
   working with Latinx couples, 158–159
Sociopolitical systemic context
   LGBTQIA+ relationships and, 197
   working with Black couples, 139–140
   working with Latinx couples, 158–159
Softening process, 299–301
Solution-focused approach, 223, 232
Somatic therapy, 278–279
Soothing self-talk, 28
Sound relationship house theory, 63
Spirituality, 289. *See also* Religion; Spirituality issues
Spirituality issues. *See also* Interfaith couples; Religion
   beginning phase of therapy, 292–296
   concluding phase of therapy, 301–302
   initial assessment and case formulation, 289–292
   intermediate phase of therapy, 296–301
   LGBTQIA+ relationships and, 197–198
   overview, 287–289, 302–303
Stage-of-treatment compass, 10, 11
Stages of change, 119. *See also* Change
Stonewalling, 64
Strengths
   discernment counseling and, 124
   emotion-focused therapy for couples and, 18
   Gottman method and, 64, 75–76
   integrative couple therapy and, 30–31, 41
   integrative psychodynamic couple therapy with personality dysfunction, 48
   integrative relational–neurobiological approach and, 82, 84
   working with couples experiencing illness, 315
   working with Latinx couples, 162
   working with LGBTQIA+ relationships, 202, 213–214
   working with military and veteran couples, 255–256
   working with older adult couples, 219–220, 221, 223
   working with young adult couples, 249
Stress
   Gottman method and, 75
   initial assessment and case formulation, 308
   transition to parenthood (TTP) and, 235
   working with couples experiencing spirituality issues, 292
   working with military and veteran couples, 257
   working with young adult couples, 245–247
Stuckness, 105
Substance use, 285. *See also* Addiction
Summary. *See also* Communication
   common factors approach and, 106
   Gottman method and, 70
   integrative couple therapy and, 30–31
   integrative psychodynamic couple therapy with personality dysfunction, 47, 49
   working with LGBTQIA+ relationships, 203–204
Survival strategies
   integrative relational–neurobiological approach and, 87, 90
   LGBTQIA+ relationships and, 198
Systemic approaches
   integrative relational–neurobiological approach and, 79
   multicultural couples and, 178
   working with Black couples, 139–140
   working with Latinx couples, 158–159
   working with LGBTQIA+ relationships, 198, 213–214
Systemic interactional theory, 9

T

Talk-to-Each-Other Model, 44
Task compass, 10
Termination, 254. *See also* Concluding phase of therapy
Theoretical approaches, 2
Therapeutic alliance. *See also* Common factors approach; Therapeutic relationship
   overview, 100, 101, 117
   working with couples experiencing spirituality issues, 290–291, 292, 302–303
   working with multicultural couples, 187–188
   working with older adult couples, 232
   working with young adult couples, 240, 244, 250
Therapeutic approaches, 2, 6
Therapeutic relationship. *See also* Alliance formation; Therapeutic alliance
   common factors approach and, 108
   emotion-focused therapy for couples and, 10
   integrative couple therapy and, 34–35, 41

Therapeutic relationship (*continued*)
  integrative psychodynamic couple therapy with personality dysfunction, 46, 51
  integrative relational–neurobiological approach and, 82, 84
  working with couples experiencing illness, 315–317, 320–321
  working with Latinx couples, 157, 165
  working with multicultural couples, 191–192
Therapist factors, 102
Thought, 9
Three C's (calm, curiosity, and caring), 56
Time-outs
  common factors approach and, 107–108, 115
  Gottman method and, 69, 77
  integrative relational–neurobiological approach and, 81, 90
  working with LGBTQIA+ relationships, 206
Top-down approach, 269
Touch, 278–279, 282
Toxic masculinity. *See* Gender; Masculinity
Transference allergy, 50–51, 55
Transgenerational trauma, 183–184. *See also* Trauma
Transition to parenthood (TTP). *See also* Parenting; Young adult couples
  beginning phase of therapy, 240–244
  concluding phase of therapy, 249–250
  initial assessment and case formulation, 236–240
  intermediate phase of therapy, 244–248
  overview, 234–236, 250–251
Transitions. *See* Retirement transition; Transition to parenthood (TTP)
Transparency
  integrative couple therapy and, 40
  working with Black couples, 149–150
  working with multicultural couples, 193
Trauma
  Gottman method and, 64–65
  integrative behavioral couple therapy (IBCT) and, 256, 265–266
  integrative relational–neurobiological approach and, 79
  working with couples experiencing issues of sexuality, 282–283
  working with military and veteran couples, 256, 265–266
  working with multicultural couples, 183–184
  working with older adult couples, 219–220

Trust
  common factors approach and, 104, 108, 112
  contextual therapy and, 80
  Gottman method and, 66, 76
  integrative couple therapy and, 35–39, 40
  working with Black couples, 147–148, 152
  working with couples experiencing illness, 318
  working with couples experiencing issues of sexuality, 275, 284
  working with couples experiencing spirituality issues, 294–296, 299, 300–301
  working with Latinx couples, 168–169
  working with military and veteran couples, 260
Trustworthiness, 84, 97. *See also* Trust
Tune-up sessions, 41

U

Underlying feelings, 19–23
Unified detachment
  integrative behavioral couple therapy (IBCT) and, 254
  working with military and veteran couples, 260–262, 268
Usable countertransferences, 49. *See also* Countertransference

V

Validation
  common factors approach and, 108
  emotion-focused therapy for couples and, 12–13, 14, 15, 18–19, 20–23, 25
  Gottman method and, 70
  integrative relational–neurobiological approach and, 83, 91
  working with couples experiencing spirituality issues, 293, 294, 295–296, 297
  working with LGBTQIA+ relationships, 202
  working with military and veteran couples, 261
  working with young adult couples, 239–240
Values
  integrative relational–neurobiological approach and, 92
  working with couples experiencing spirituality issues, 293
Veteran couples. *See* Military and veteran couples
Video recordings of sessions, 64
Viewing, 102

Violence
  working with couples experiencing spirituality issues, 303
  working with Latinx couples, 164
Virtual sessions, 28
Voice, 13–14
Vulnerabilities
  common factors approach and, 109–114
  emotion-focused therapy for couples and, 11, 19–23, 25
  integrative behavioral couple therapy (IBCT) and, 254
  integrative relational–neurobiological approach and, 79–80, 87, 89–90
  LGBTQIA+ relationships and, 198
  overview. See Vulnerability cycle
  working with couples experiencing spirituality issues, 296, 301, 303
  working with military and veteran couples, 260
  working with older adult couples, 222
Vulnerability cycle. *See also* Integrative relational–neurobiological approach; Interactional cycles; Vulnerabilities
  beginning phase of therapy, 84–88, 85*f*
  concluding phase of therapy, 96–97
  diagram illustrating, 85–86, 85*f*
  initial assessment and case formulation, 82–84
  intermediate phase of therapy, 88–96
  neurobiology of, 87–88
  overview, 81, 97
Vulvovaginitis, 281

W

White heteropatriarchy, 197–198, 203, 207, 212–213, 214
Wise mind, 312
Withdrawal. *See also* Avoidance; Demand–withdrawal cycle
  integrative couple therapy and, 33, 38–39
  integrative psychodynamic couple therapy with personality dysfunction, 48
  integrative relational–neurobiological approach and, 91–92, 93
  working with couples experiencing spirituality issues, 297–299
  working with LGBTQIA+ relationships, 204–205, 207, 209–210
  working with young adult couples, 238–239
Working alliance. *See* Therapeutic alliance

Y

Young adult couples. *See also* Parenting; Transition to parenthood (TTP)
  beginning phase of therapy, 240–244
  concluding phase of therapy, 249–250
  initial assessment and case formulation, 236–240
  intermediate phase of therapy, 244–248
  overview, 234–236, 250–251